"Venomous" Bites from Non-Venomous Snakes

"Venomous" Bites from Non-Venomous Snakes
A Critical Analysis of Risk and Management of "Colubrid" Snake Bites

Scott A. Weinstein
Department of Toxinology, Women's and Children's Hospital,
North Adelaide, South Australia, Australia

David A. Warrell
Nuffeld Department of Clinical Medicine,
University of Oxford, United Kingdom

Julian White
Department of Toxinology, Women's and Children's Hospital,
North Adelaide, South Australia, Australia

Daniel E. Keyler
Hennepin County Medical Center
Department of Medicine
Division of Clinical Pharmacology
Minneapolis, Minnesota, USA
and
Department of Experimental & Clinical Pharmacology
University of Minnesota, Minneapolis, Minnesota USA

ELSEVIER

AMSTERDAM • BOSTON • HEIDELBERG • LONDON • NEW YORK • OXFORD
PARIS • SAN DIEGO • SAN FRANCISCO • SINGAPORE • SYDNEY • TOKYO

Elsevier
32 Jamestown Road London NW1 7BY
225 Wyman Street. Waltham, MA 02451, USA

First edition 2011

British Library Cataloguing-in-Publication Data
A catalogue record for this book is available from the British Library

Library of Congress Cataloging-in-Publication Data
A catalog record for this book is available from the Library of Congress

ISBN: 978-0-12-387732-1

For information on all Elsevier publications
visit our website at elsevierdirect.com

This book has been manufactured using Print On Demand technology. Each copy is produced to order and is limited to black ink. The online version of this book will show color figures where appropriate.

Working together to grow
libraries in developing countries

www.elsevier.com | www.bookaid.org | www.sabre.org

ELSEVIER   BOOK AID
International   Sabre Foundation

Contents

Dedication

This contribution is respectfully dedicated to the fond memory of Professor Sherman A. Minton, Madge R. Minton, and Professor Alan W. Bernheimer. All were innate naturalists, humble, talented scientists, brilliant teachers and mentors and, most importantly, generous, treasured friends.

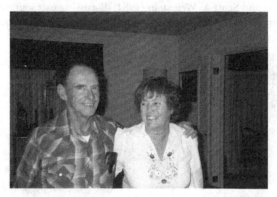

Sherman A. and Madge R. Minton, 1985. An outstanding herpetologist of historical importance, Sherman (1919–1999) was a pioneer in twentieth-century research of venomous snakes and snake venoms. He had a special interest in the medical importance of colubrid snakes and pioneered the modern investigation of their secretions/venoms. A highly respected faculty member in the Department of Microbiology and Immunology at the Indiana University School of Medicine, he was a compassionate physician and accomplished microbiologist/parasitologist. Madge (1920–2004) was a keen herpetologist, pilot, ethnologist, and lapidary-gemologist. She served in the Women Airforce Service Pilots (WASP) program during World War II, while Sherman was a naval medical officer on the USS *Brooks* deployed on the Coral Sea. Their shared intense passion for herpetology and toxinology formed one of the deep links of their greater than 50-year loving partnership. Their professional collaborations produced two popular books and multiple scientific contributions, and also contributed significantly to the conservation of the herpetological fauna of Indiana. Sherman published over 130 papers, including a major comprehensive monograph on the herpetology of Pakistan, and coauthored and edited several books on snakebite as well as regional herpetology guides. To date, his book, *Amphibians and Reptiles of Indiana*, is the most comprehensive study of the herpetology of that state. His engaging autobiography was published posthumously (For detailed information on Sherman A. Minton's life and career, see: Bechtel, 1999; Stewart, 2000; Karns, 2001; Weinstein, 2003, and Minton, 2001; photo copyright to Brian Marian and Scott A. Weinstein).

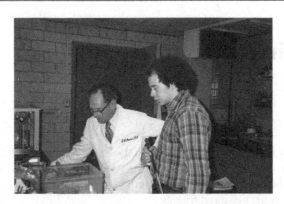

Sherman A. Minton and Scott A. Weinstein (1984) discussing extraction of venom samples from a pair of midget faded rattlesnakes, *Crotalus oreganus concolor* (photo copyright to Brian Marian).

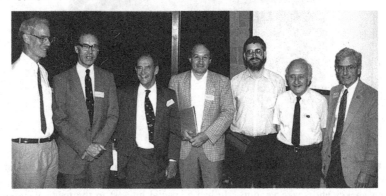

Group photo at the First World Congress of Herpetology, Canterbury, UK (1989), after the symposium on venomous snakes. Pictured from left: Herbert Rosenberg, David A. Warrell, Sherman A. Minton, Dietrich Mebs, Julian White, Elazar Kochva, and David L. Hardy, Sr. (photo copyright to David A. Warrell).

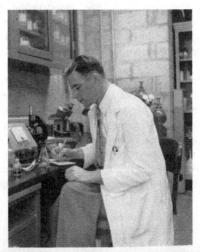

◄ **Alan W. Bernheimer (date unknown).** One of the great microbiologists of the twentieth century, Alan (1914–2006) was one of the pioneers of modern bacterial toxinology. Strongly interested in hemolytic toxins, his research had no boundaries and encompassed the study of toxins from numerous micro-organisms as well as cnidarians (jellyfish, anemones), hymenopterans (especially ants), and snake venoms. He was recipient of a National Institutes of Health career award, and a two-time recipient of the Eli Lilly Award, given to outstanding microbiologists for their noteworthy accomplishments. He contributed over 125 scientific papers and edited several books (see Linder [2006] for further information about Alan W. Bernheimer's life and career; photo copyright to Alan W. Bernheimer, Jr.).

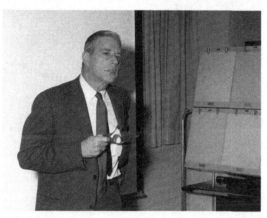

Alan W. Bernheimer (1967). Alan was appointed Professor of Microbiology at New York University School of Medicine in 1941, and remained Professor Emeritus until his passing in 2006. In addition to his insightful approach to research, he was a talented, patient teacher and was popular among the medical and graduate students who attended his information-packed microbiology lectures. He was also an erudite lepidopterist (with a particular interest in South American butterflies) and a talented creative/experimental ("reflectographs") photographer. His wife, Harriet (1919–2009), was an accomplished microbiologist specializing in characterization of the biological roles of the capsular antigens of *Streptococcus pneumoniae* (photo copyright to Alan W. Bernheimer, Jr.).

Preface

Fear of and fascination with venomous snakes has influenced human perceptions of religion, spirituality, and medicine. One of the most common hazards spanning the dynasties of ancient Egypt was injury by snake or scorpion. The Brooklyn Papyrus, written during the thirtieth dynasty (380–343 BCE), constitutes what may be considered one of the earliest known treatises dedicated to the treatment of snakebites. Treatments consisted of emetics, incantations, and spells, with a focus on relieving the victim of spiritual and physical "poison." Unlike the relatively brief comments regarding treatment of snakebites in the earlier Smith surgical papyrus of the eighteenth dynasty (*circa* 1550 BCE), the Brooklyn papyrus included a section on the identification of medically important venomous snakes intended as a guide to direct treatment. During the early Renaissance, the enigmatic alchemist/botanist/astrologer/ medical practitioner, Philippus Aureolus Theophrastus Bombastus von Hohenheim[1] (1493–1541; popularly known by his mercifully contracted Roman appellation, Paracelsus), contemplated the use of venoms during his search for the Azoth, the spiritual medicine of man. The common thread between the earliest clinical perceptions of envenomation and latter views during the Middle Ages was the prevailing belief that snakebites poisoned both the spiritual and physical being. The toxic effects of viper bites were believed to be due to "enraged spirits."

The first systematic investigation of snake venoms was performed by the seventeenth-century Italian physician, Francisco Redi (1626–1698). Redi's experiments revealed the toxic nature of snake venoms, established a relationship between dose, body weight, and toxicity, and demonstrated the enhanced lethal effect of venom introduced near a blood vessel. Interest in the pathophysiology and improved management of snakebites focused attention on the further characterization of venoms, but it was not until 1938 that Karl Slotta (1895–1987) and Heinz Fraenkel-Conrat (1910–1999) succeeded in isolating a toxin, crotoxin, from venom of the medically important tropical rattlesnake or cascabel (*Crotalus durissus terrificus*).

Improvements in protein biochemical separation and characterization methods rapidly advanced the knowledge of venoms, and often provided a pharmacological basis for the clinical effects observed in victims of medically significant snakebites. An

---

[1] Paracelsus is often credited with being the founder of toxicology; although he embraced nonscientific theories, and his greatest interest was probably astrology, he advanced the first systematic study of poisons. His famous quotation: "Alle Ding' sind Gift, und nichts ohn' Gift; allein die Dosis macht, daß ein Ding kein Giftist" ("All things are poison and nothing is without poison, only the dose permits something not to be poisonous"), revealed his understanding of the thin border between the beneficial effects of therapeutics and their potential toxicity.

understandably disproportionate emphasis on biomedically relevant venom properties narrowed the focus of venom research, for the most part excluding snakes with oral secretions of unknown or little-known medical importance. The very limited funding afforded to snake venom research further restricted the scope of investigation. Snakes that possess enlarged posterior maxillary teeth ("rear fangs") and rarely cause human mortality or morbidity were largely ignored. However, although this limited interest in the "mild venom" or "toxic saliva" of "rear-fanged" snakes resulted in sparse research of their oral secretions, these snakes did make their importance known. In the late nineteenth to early twentieth centuries, several inquisitive herpetologists and physicians began to question whether some snakes perceived as "harmless," such as hognose snakes (*Heterodon* spp.) and South American racers (*Philodryas* spp.), were "mildly venomous." South African investigators began to report life-threatening cases of boomslang (*Dispholidus typus*) envenomation. At the time, this poorly known species was viewed only as an arboreal species included in the amorphous, taxonomically incorrect family, the Colubridae. This family, consisting of 65–70% of the worlds' living snake species, was a convenient "dumping ground" for many snakes of allied as well as unrelated taxonomic affinities. Thus, the superfamily of snakes, Colubroidea, and the artificial family beneath, Colubridae, comprise the majority of the world's snake species and are a significant contributor to snakebites in humans, in terms of absolute numbers.

The descriptions of *D. typus* envenomation were disconcerting indeed. These detailed a terrible hemorrhagic disease with suffering extending over days. In 1957 and 1975, the deaths of two prominent herpetologists after bites by *D. typus* and Kirtlands' twig, bird, tree, or African vine snake (*Thelotornis kirtlandii*) gradually increased interest and concomitant research attention on these snakes. This also expanded the awareness of highly toxic species among those "colubrids" termed "rear-fanged," "opisthoglyphous," or "aglyphous" that were perceived as "mildly venomous." Some authorities have resisted recognition of any significant potential hazard of most snakes that lack canaliculated front fangs (e.g., hollow fangs with an internal lumen, or canal, for delivery of venom under high pressure). The Duvernoy's glands that produce toxic oral secretions in "rear-fanged" snakes are without significant muscle attachment, and thus function as low-pressure systems. Therefore, the delivery of these secretions has sometimes, unfortunately and subjectively, been viewed as "inefficient," rather than being considered as distinctive systems whose adaptive performance is reflected by their functional morphology.

Some tantalizing information emerges intermittently about occasional medically significant bites by species previously thought to be "nonvenomous." A slowly growing body of basic biomedical and clinical information is revealing the prospective wealth of knowledge that may be derived from studies of non-front-fanged colubroid snakes. Some species produce neurotoxins with marked specificity for prey such as lizards or birds. Others have potent procoagulant toxins that cause life-threatening effects in humans. Most of these snake species are still considered "harmless," with only a few species with "fangs," and others as noted above, having the capacity to cause lethal envenomation in humans. Yet for most species, there is little or nothing in the academic or medical literature documenting the risk they may pose.

This book is the first study exclusively dedicated to critical analysis of the medical risks of non-front-fanged colubroid snakes. By providing a comprehensive review of this entire assemblage of snakes, with particular attention given to their capacity, real or rumored, to cause harm to humans, the book seeks to fill a palpable gap in the toxinological, medical, and herpetological literature. The oral glands and their secretions/venoms, as well as associated delivery apparatuses, are considered in relation to available clinical, toxinological, and herpetological information. A patient-centered, evidence-based approach is applied to analyzing documented case reports of bites inflicted by approximately 100 species. This analysis identifies some of these species whose medical importance has been incorrectly exaggerated or underestimated, and assigns evidence levels to the quality of published case reports. Clinical management of medically significant bites from non-front-fanged colubroids is methodically reviewed, and specific recommendations are provided. Special attention is given to the assessment of controversial treatments (e.g., provision of blood and blood products) and contraindicated treatments (e.g., heparin) as well as the approach to the patient with venom-induced acute kidney injury.

The authors are authoritative clinical toxinologists, as well as being enthusiastic herpetologists. Three are practicing physicians, and one is a clinical pharmacologist. They contribute to this volume well over a century of combined experience in venom research, management of envenomations, general medical practice, and biomedical investigation. The authors' experience is broad and interdisciplinary: all have had personal contact and/or field experience with many of the snakes studied in this book; with their Duvernoy's secretions/venoms, isolation of some of the constituent components, and with their pharmacology, as well as with hands-on management of envenomation both in First World "centers of excellence" and in remote community "clinics" lacking any modern clinical instrumentation. They have endeavored to tease out fact from fiction or supposition, in order to present a comprehensive dissertation on the impact of non-front-fanged colubroid snake bite on humans.

This book is relevant to a wide range of readers and health professionals; from medical doctors managing cases (emergency medicine, primary care, intensive care, toxicology, rural medicine, tropical medicine), through life scientists (toxinologists, biologists, natural historians), to the increasing numbers of amateur and professional herpetologists as well as casual snake-collecting enthusiasts who keep these snakes in captivity. This book fills a sizable gap in the literature, yet we hope that it also offers something of a visual feast, illustrating many species of snakes, as well as providing both practically useful information, and instilling a joy of discovery for the interested reader. It is our intention that this volume in the Elsevier Insight Series should serve to inform as well as offer a guide to the compassionate and evidence-based treatment of the patient affected by colubroid snake bite, whether it be in an urban or rural setting.

Scott A. Weinstein
David A. Warrell
Julian White
Daniel E. Keyler

Acknowledgments

Several scarce references were obtained with the persistent help of Alan Staples, MEc. The invaluable help of the library personnel of the Women's and Children's Hospital, North Adelaide, South Australia, and that of the Medical Research Library of the State University of New York, Downstate Medical Center, Brooklyn, New York, especially Ms. Juannetta LaGree, is gratefully acknowledged. Prof. Ken Kardong provided essential information, critique, and inspiration. The early inspiration and encouragement of the late Carl Kauffeld, Prof. Edmund D. Brodie, Jr., the late Dr. George Ruggieri, S.J., Prof. Hobart Smith, and Prof. Herndon Dowling is gratefully acknowledged by SAW. Special thanks to Dr. Sam Alfred, Don Becker, Tomer Beker, Prof. Jonathan Campbell, Prof. Richard C. Dart, Dr. Robert Haddock, Dr. Robert W. Henderson, Dr. Khal Ismail, Dr. David Kaufman, FACP, Prof. William Lamar, Kevel Lindsay, Dr. Gad Perry, Louis Porras, Dr. Robert Powell, Dr. Naftali Primor, Dr. Gordon Rodda, and Shane Shiers. We are especially grateful for the invaluable help of Dr. David Kizirian, Robert Pascocello and the Department of Herpetology, American Museum of Natural History, New York, New York. We are grateful for the respective generous photographic and artistic contributions of Arie Lev and Kevin M. McAllister. We thank Alexander Westerström for directing us to and translating several references in Russian and for providing an image. For the courtesy of their generous photo contributions, we thank Maik Dobiey, Dr. Kraig Adler, Dr. Wolfgang Wüster, the late Dr. Yoshio Sawai, Dr. Gordon Rodda, Dr. Ahmed Khalil Ismail, Mark O'Shea, Daniel Jablonski, Dr. Javier José Carrasco Araújo, Dave Nixon, Matt Wilson, Dr. Robert Powell, Dr. Gad Perry, Alec Earnshaw, Jackson Shedd, Brent W. Bumgardner, Alan W. Bernheimer, Jr., Dr. Marcelo Duarte, Gary Sargent, Dave Ball, Christopher E. Smith, Shukla Chaitanya, John White, Dr. Barney Oldfield, Peter Ellen, Robert and Ann Simpson, Prof. Jimmy Thomas, Dr. S. Mishima, Laura Hermann, Dr. Zoltan Takács, Richard Maude, Jeffrey B. LeClere, Jake Scott, Trevor D. Keyler, Kim McWhorter, and Tomer Beker. Helpful comments and/or moral support were offered by: Herbert and Lenore Weinstein (especially for their unwavering encouragement, and for tolerating innumerable legless and multilegged creatures in their home for many years), Brian Marian, Jack Streitman, Virginia Elder, Brenda Gross, Prof. Ken Kardong, Prof. David Chiszar, Dr. Brad G. Stiles, Dr. Paul Moglia, Dr. Elizabeth Reynolds, Dr. Regina Linder, Dr. Annandita Nandi, Dr. Adele Cavalli, Dr. Galina Venikova, Dalia Zwick, PhD, PT; Norman and Ruth Pachtman, Dr. Joseph McArdle, Dennis Brown, Parashos Kalaitzis, JD; Michael Boyll, Sylvia Johns, Tracy D., Gerie Z. Shearrow, Dr. Edward RL Chu, Dr. David Kaufman, Dr. Richard Mayer, Dr. Charles Cartwright, Dr. Peter Dellabella, Dr. Diane Liu, Dr. Nicola Chynoweth,

Dr. Russell Waddell, Joy Rosen, Beverly A. Wright, Veronika Bandera, Peter Mirtschin, Peter Papps, Dr. Vaughan Williams, Dr. Sam Sandowski, Dr. Zev Zelenko, Andrew Wilson, and Meryann Lane. Essential translation was graciously provided by Christian D. Murillo and Maria R. Murillo (Portuguese) and Dr. Marco Pravetoni (French). The ancillary support of Dr. Adam Henner and Dr. Rajesh Kakani is grate- fully acknowledged. The online archives of the Museum of Comparative Zoology, Harvard University and the American Museum of Natural History were invaluable resources. Preparation of the manuscript was enhanced by the encouragement and comestible support of SAW's friends in Bay Terrace and Fresh Meadows, Queens, New York: Harrys Leroy, Ashley Venezia, Chris D. Murillo, Mike, Tina, Alex Morales, Eric, Karyn, Adiib Debbarh, Lauren, Lawrence, Diana, Matthew Bode, Harrison, Angela Chung, Victoria James, Jamie Hillgardner, Richard Kugblenu, Richard Eggers, Raquel Noriega, Megan, and Yovadys Perez.

About the Authors

Scott A. Weinstein, BA, MSc, PhD, MBBS, MD, Dip, ABFM

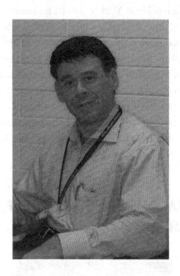

Scott Weinstein was consumed from earliest childhood by an interest in reptiles and amphibians. A member of the New York Herpetological Society by age 11, he was one of a lucky cadre of young members who were gently mentored by the well-known curator of the Staten Island Zoo, the late Carl Kauffeld. His studies of "rear-fanged colubrids" started in Junior High School where he started to compare the sparse information in the available herpetology literature with collected living specimens. These interests rapidly focused on the biology of venomous snakes and herpetological toxinology. This led to his studies in herpetology with Prof. Edmund D. Brodie, Jr. at Adelphi University (Garden City, NY), where he earned his BA in biological sciences and comparative religion. Shortly thereafter, he became the late Prof. Sherman A. Minton's last student at the Indiana University School of Medicine where he earned an MSc in Medical Microbiology and Immunology. His PhD in Medical Microbiology and Immunology was earned with the late Prof. Alan W. Bernheimer at the Sackler Institute of Graduate Biomedical Sciences of New York University School of Medicine (New York, NY), his MBBS was earned at Flinders University School of Medicine, Adelaide, Australia, and the Board of Regents of the University of the State of New York conferred his MD. He completed family medicine residency at South Nassau Communities Hospital, Oceanside, NY, and served as chief resident.

He also completed two postdoctoral research fellowships; one at NYU Medical Center and another at the US Army Medical Research Institute of Infectious Diseases (Fort Detrick, Frederick, MD). His research has included: purification and characterization of novel snake venom neurotoxins; elucidation of components and the biomedical properties of Duvernoy's secretions from non-front-fanged colubroids; venom immunity in ophiophagous nonvenomous snakes; and field studies of reptiles and amphibians. He currently is clinical toxinologist at the Women's and Children's Hospital in Adelaide, South Australia, where he is a consultant in the management of envenomations, and intermittently practices traditional family medicine, urgent care, and occupational medicine in his native New York City. In addition to his lifelong interests in toxinology and herpetology, Dr. Weinstein has a strong interest in the medical management of special-needs populations (e.g., those with disabilities), infectious diseases (especially academic and clinical venereology), and substance dependency medicine. He still participates in field herpetology whenever possible, and has always remained active in captive propagation of a wide variety of living specimens. As is common with many herpetologists and toxinologists, he also has traveled extensively. He has contributed more than 50 peer-reviewed publications in toxinology, herpetology, and medicine, and is board certified in family medicine by the American Board of Family Medicine (ABFM).

David A. Warrell, MA, DM, DSc, FRCP, FRCPE, FRGS, HonFZS, FMedSci, HonFCeylonCP

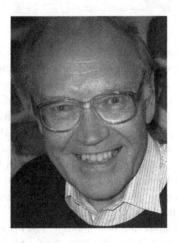

Professor David Alan Warrell is professor emeritus of Tropical Medicine and Honorary Fellow of St Cross College, University of Oxford, UK. After training at Oxford, St Thomas' Hospital and the Royal Postgraduate Medical School in London, he lived, worked, researched, and traveled in Ethiopia, Nigeria, Kenya, South Africa,

Thailand, Burma, Sri Lanka, Bangladesh, Papua New Guinea, Brazil, Ecuador, Peru and other tropical countries, founding the Oxford University-based Tropical Medicine Research Program whose units in Thailand (since 1979) and elsewhere to study malaria and other major tropical diseases. He became director of the Oxford Tropical Network in 1986, and later head of The Nuffield Department of Clinical Medicine, University of Oxford. He has been the Delegate for Medicine and Music at Oxford University Press, and is senior editor of the *Oxford Textbook of Medicine* (fifth edition, 2010) as well as the *Oxford Handbook of Expedition and Wilderness Medicine* (first edition, 2008). He has published more than 400 research papers, articles, reviews, and textbook chapters on malaria, rabies, relapsing fevers, meningococcal meningitis, cryptococcal meningitis, HIV, other tropical and infectious diseases, comparative respiratory physiology, respiratory diseases, herpetology, venomous animals, envenoming, and plant and chemical poisoning. He is a consultant to the World Health Organization (WHO) on snakebite, rabies, and malaria; the British Army, UK Medical Research Council, Foreign and Commonwealth Office, Earth Watch International (conservation), Zoological Society of London, Royal Geographical Society, and ToxBase UK. He also served as the past president of the Royal Society of Tropical Medicine and Hygiene, and International Federation for Tropical Medicine. His principal research interest remains the pathophysiology and treatment of envenoming. In November 2010, David Warrell was awarded the William Osler Memorial Medal by the University of Oxford.

Julian White, MBBS, MD, FATM

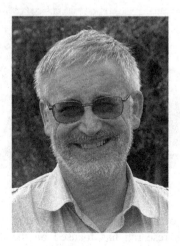

Professor White is director of the Toxinology Department of the Women's and Children's Hospital in Adelaide, South Australia, a position he has held since 1990. He has been involved with managing cases of envenoming, notably snakebite, since

1976 and currently is consulted about several hundred cases per year, including over 100 snakebites. However, prior to completing his medical degrees at the University of Adelaide, he was heavily involved in herpetology and, to a lesser extent, arachnology. He founded the South Australian Herpetology Group in 1974, and has collected and kept a wide variety of animals, especially reptiles, including numerous species of venomous snakes. His involvement with clinical toxinology remained a passionate sideline until he was invited to found the Toxinology Department, Women's and Children's Hospital, Adelaide, in 1990, though throughout these earlier years he was involved in both basic (venom) and clinical toxinology research. Amongst his many publications, he ranks the 1995 CRC *Handbook of Clinical Toxicology of Animal Venoms and Poisons*, which he edited with Prof. Jurg Meier, as his most important contribution. In 1997, together with Dr. John Williams, he founded the international clinical toxinology short course, which has run regularly ever since. In 2002, the Clinical Toxinology Resources website (www.toxinology.com) was launched through his efforts. An occasional consultant to the WHO since 1988, and a frequent invited speaker at international meetings, Prof. White remains active in providing clinical advice in envenoming cases, teaching clinical toxinology, producing publications in the field, and supporting research. He is currently the secretary treasurer of the International Society on Toxinology.

Daniel E. Keyler, BS, PharmD

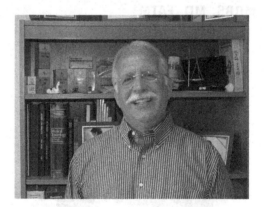

Dr. Keyler is codirector of Toxicology Research with the Minneapolis Medical Research Foundation. His research has focused on the development of antibodies and vaccines as immunological and therapeutic approaches to reducing drug-, and toxicant-induced toxicity as well as for the treatment of substance dependency. He holds a BS degree from Purdue University in Science, and BS Pharmacy and Doctor of Pharmacy degrees from the University of Minnesota. He is a professor in the Department of Experimental and Clinical Pharmacology with the University of Minnesota, College of Pharmacy, and has authored numerous publications in peer-reviewed journals. He has also authored multiple book chapters involving immunotherapeutics, animal toxins, venomous snakebite, and the medical management of snakebite victims. He has been actively involved with venomous snakes for over 30 years. His interest in the science of herpetology was spurred early on by the late Prof. Sherman A. Minton, with whom he kept in touch with via consultations until Prof. Minton's passing in 1999. Dr. Keyler has a lifelong passion for timber rattlesnakes (*Crotalus horridus*), and has had multiple research grants to study timber rattlesnakes in the Upper Mississippi River Valley. He serves on a national committee (Timber Rattlesnake Conservation Action Plan) for their conservation. The medical treatment of venomous snakebites has been a significant component of his professional career, and he has been involved in the medical treatment of over 250 venomous snakebites, including exotic species. He served as chair of the Envenomations SIG with the American Academy of Clinical Toxicology 2002–2007, and is a founding member with the Medical Advisory Committee to the Online Antivenom Index. He is also an author concerning medical management reviews of snakebites for the Antivenom Index. Currently, he is working with Animal Venom Research International and the country of Sri Lanka with respect to developing an efficacious polyvalent antivenom developed from venomous species within the country.

Introduction

Most extant snakes belong to the superfamily, Colubroidea, that contains the approximately 3,000 species of advanced snakes [i.e., those with identifiably derived traits (e.g., a duplex retina, left lung reduction, modification of cranial osteology, etc.)] including all of the medically important venomous snakes, such as elapoids (including atractaspidids) and viperoids. Living families of advanced snakes all appear in the fossil record in the Cenozoic (well after the disappearance of the great sauropod dinosaurs), beginning with those previously grouped together as colubrids[1] [during the Oligocene, approximately 34 million years ago (mya)], followed by elapids (cobras, mambas, seasnakes, coral snakes, kraits, and allies) and viperids (vipers and pit vipers), both at about the start of the Miocene (approximately 23 mya). Although still a subject of controversy, viperids currently are thought to derive early within the radiation of advanced snakes, and elapids more directly from colubrids (Cadle, 1987; Heise et al., 1995; Kardong, 1979; Kraus and Brown, 1998; Weinstein et al., 2010; Zahradnicek et al., 2008). Clinically important cases of envenomation by snakes are most often caused by bites from elapid and viperid species (see Minton, 1974; Russell, 1980; White, 1995; Chippaux, 1998; Mebs, 2002; and Warrell, 2004 for reviews). Recent speculations suggest that at least 1.2 million persons are bitten by snakes annually, with hundreds of thousands affected with long-term morbidity and between 20,000 and 100,000 fatalities (Kasturiratne et al., 2008).

The medical importance of the largest discrete and polyphyletic group of snakes, referred to previously as the family Colubridae for convenience, is verified only for a handful of the approximately 2,000–2,500 taxa in this diversified and taxonomically artificial assemblage (Warrell, 2004; Weinstein and Kardong, 1994; Weinstein et al., 2010). The broad range of estimated snakebite fatalities reflects a general lack of consistently reported data from specific geographic regions (e.g., Third World countries) significantly affected by envenoming. The inconsistent availability of this information is commonplace when considering medically significant bites from species (non-front-fanged colubroids) previously, or currently, assigned to the Colubridae.

---

[1] Studies of snake systematics have provided firm evidence of the long-held perception of polyphyly among the inaccurately assembled family, the Colubridae, as this generally referred to all Colubroidea that were not included in the families Acrochordidae, Elapidae, or Viperidae. See ahead for a brief discussion of the instability of colubroid taxonomy.

Complicating the interpretation of many reported cases of bites from these snakes are the often lacking confirmation of species identifications and the continuous changes in colubroid taxonomy based on molecular systematics (Lawson et al., 2005; Pyron et al., 2011; see ahead). An undetermined percentage of colubrid snakes secrete toxins from an apparatus capable of generating only low pressure because of little or no direct muscle attachment to the gland secretory system or compression by surrounding muscles. This gland, Duvernoy's gland, may or may not be associated with grooved posterior enlarged maxillary teeth (Mackessy, 2002; McKinstry, 1978, 1983; Weinstein and Kardong, 1994). Fatal envenomings or serious morbidity inflicted by the African Dispholidini, the boomslang, *Dispholidus typus*; twig, bird, or vine snakes, *Thelotornis kirtlandii* and *T. capensis*; and the Asian natricids, the red-necked, and tiger keelbacks, *Rhabdophis subminiatus* and *R. tigrinus* have been extensively documented (see ahead and Minton, 1986, 1990; Weinstein and Kardong, 1994; and Mackessy, 2002 for reviews). Accumulating data suggest that *Philodryas*.spp. (the South American racers— a useless but frequently used common name for members of this genus and other genera as well; see later)[2] probably are medically important in South America (Salomão et al., 2003; Warrell, 2004). The clinical relevance of other colubrid taxa [e.g., *Malpolon monspessulanus* (Montpellier snake; Gonzáles, 1979; Pommier and De Haro, 2007), *Boiga irregularis* (brown tree snake; Fritts and McCoid, 1999; Fritts et al., 1990, 1994)] is supported by relatively limited evidence. Aside from this small sampling of non-front-fanged colubroids with proven capacities to produce human mortality and morbidity, few documented, evidence-based cases support the medical importance of other "colubrid" species (Warrell, 2004; Weinstein and Kardong, 1994; Weinstein et al., 2010).

In this book, in order to assess potential medical risk posed by various non-front-fanged colubroid taxa, we critically evaluate selected cases in which documented bites were inflicted by some of these snakes. It is important to note that this study does not strive to review all reported cases of "colubrid" bites published in the literature. Rather, we have chosen published cases that contain sufficient detail about the bite, identification of the species involved, and the outcome. We have included some cases that lack information about symptoms or signs, and/or that were anecdotally reported, because of the scarcity of information about bites by some taxa and in order to demonstrate important points about the evaluation of such cases (e.g., lack of correlation of reported symptoms with clinical findings). We have also included some previously unpublished cases that we have either personally managed or on which we were consulted.

Methods

The literature concerning colubrid bites published between 1870 and 2010 was searched using the terms "colubrid" and "bites"; "rear-fanged snakes"; "colubrid" and "envenomation" or "envenoming"; "Duvernoy's secretions"; "opisthoglyphous" and

---

[2]A variety of genera are commonly called racers or whipsnakes. Table 2.1 contains a selection of common and locally used names for all non-front-fanged colubroid species considered in this book. "Common names are common only when used" (Sherman A. Minton).

"snakes"; "nonvenomous" and "nonpoisonous" "snakes" and "bites" and "envenomation." A further search for specific species of colubrid snakes used scientific nomenclature and common names (e.g., boomslang, mangrove snake, twig snake) combined in a boolean with "bite," "envenoming," or "envenomation." Search engines included Scirus, Scopus, PubMed, and Google. Additional searches were performed with the assistance of the authors' personal and institutional libraries. Selected books were reviewed, and descriptions of bites with significant detail were occasionally included. Anecdotal reports were rejected unless they included interesting or important information that was not available elsewhere. We have generally excluded cases posted on the Internet and those without verifiable provenance. However, several representative cases from Internet fora are included as an informative exercise (Appendix A).

Reviewed cases were assessed using a modified interpretation of the Strength of Recommendation Taxonomy (SORT) system criteria (Ebell et al., 2004). Evidence rankings were assigned as follows:

- Level A—Multiple well-documented cases that contain thorough clinical detail and evaluation by a medical professional. This level usually includes qualified review and/or treatment in a medical facility and carefully reported clinical accounts in the medical literature.
- Level B—Limited number of well-documented cases that contain thorough clinical details and evaluation by medical professionals.
- Level C—Case report prepared/interpreted by a nonmedically qualified/credentialed author or/and limited clinical information and/or lack of demonstrated linkage between the described symptoms/signs and the inflicted bite.
- Level D—Published report without appropriate clinical or medical evaluation; report based on anecdotal information.
- IE—Insufficient evidence for basic evaluation; purely anecdotal information.

Mixed-level rankings (e.g., C/D) reflect features of both evidence levels. For example, a single report regarding a given species that has unconfirmed identification of the snake responsible for the reported bite; an isolated case reviewed by a medically qualified individual, but lacking in any significant medical effects or detail facilitating evaluation of the case; or a report that contains detailed serious symptoms but without any significant medical assessment, thereby without linkage between the subjectively reported symptoms and the reported bite. Inclusion of a lower level of evidence implies the need for further information in order to fully evaluate the medical risk potential of any given species.

Hazard Index is based on modification of criteria of Weinstein et al. (2009):

- Level 1—Serious and potentially fatal envenoming is possible.
- Level 2—Systemic envenoming is possible, but uncommon.
- Level 3—Mild-to moderate localized effects, and frequently associated with a protracted bite.
- Level 4—Typically only mild lacerations, reactive erythema and edema, and occasional (very infrequent) bites with slightly more significant effects, such as mild ecchymoses.

1 An Overview of the Artificial Assemblage, the Colubridae: A Brief Summary of Taxonomic Considerations

The taxonomy of this former assemblage is in dynamic transition and subject to frequent and often conflicting recommended rearrangement. This very large artificial grouping often functioned as a sort of "disposal depot" (colloquially known as a "taxonomic garbage can" or "rag bag") for taxa of unestablished affinities. This resulted in the incorrect assignment of many diverse and phylogenetically unrelated ophidian species. For over 30 years, numerous taxonomists have devoted increasing attention to resolving this complex issue by using methods involving morphological (based on osteology, dentition, hemipenal morphology, lepidosis/meristics, etc.) or molecular (analysis of nuclear or mitochondrial DNA sequences—sometimes inferred from ribosomal RNA sequences—allozyme electrophoresis, immunodiffusion, etc.) methods or, less commonly, combined morphological and molecular systematics (Cadle, 1988; Dessauer et al., 1987; Dowling et al., 1983, 1996; Heise et al., 1995; Jenner and Dowling, 1985; Kraus and Brown, 1998; Lawson et al., 2005; Pinou et al., 2004; Vidal et al., 2000, 2007, 2010; Zaher, 1999; Zaher et al., 2009).

Discussion of the current status of these ongoing reassignments is far too voluminous to detail here. However, some recommended changes are summarized in Table 1.1. Analyses of previous taxonomic assignments have increasingly been subject to more of a "splitting" (e.g., division of a given species, genus, subfamily, or family into separate entities) approach, rather than "lumping" these together. For instance, the crayfish-eating snakes (*Regina* spp.) of the tribe Thamnophiini are polyphyletic, and the Thamnophiini itself has at least three major clades (Alfaro and Arnold, 2001). Ongoing phylogenetic investigations will probably modify numerous subfamilies, genera, and re-define existing lineages (Hedges et al., 2009; Pyron et al., 2011). It should be noted that several medically important species have been recently reassigned. For example, Vidal et al. (2007) and Zaher et al. (2009) recommended raising the previous subfamily, Natricinae, to a full family, Natricidae (see Table 1.1). This family contains *Rhabdophis tigrinus* and *R. subminiatus*, two species that have inflicted fatal or life-threatening bites (Section 4.2). Such reassignments reinforce the call for the use of precise and current taxonomy in clinical toxinology (Wüster et al., 1998). Some species can be reassigned; this can lead to controversy and confusion in the literature. For example, historically, the front-fanged mole vipers, burrowing asps, or stiletto snakes (*Atractaspis* spp., approximately 18 species; Plate 1.1A), were first considered viperids or elapids, then reassigned to the colubrid subfamily, Aparallactinae (the centipede-eating snakes), then placed in

"Venomous" Bites from Non-Venomous Snakes. DOI: 10.1016/B978-0-12-387732-1.00001-4

Table 1.1 Summary of Proposed Taxonomic Reassignments for the Superfamily Colubroidea and Other Medically Relevant Taxa[a,b]

Superfamily Colubroidea

Colubridae

  Colubrinae (including *Boiga, Dispholidus, Hierophis, Platyceps, Thelotornis*)*

  Grayiinae

  Calamarinae

Dipsadidae

  Dipsadinae (including *Leptodeira, Sibynomorphus*)*

  Heterodontinae (*Heterodon*)*

  Xenodontinae (including *Alsophis, Boiruna, Clelia, Hydrodynastes, Phalotris, Philodryas, Tachymenis*)*

Natricidae (including *Natrix, Rhabdophis, Thamnophis*)*

Pseudoxenodontidae

Superfamily Elapoidea

Elapidae

  Elapinae

  Hydrophiinae

Lamprophiidae

  Atractaspidinae*

  Lamprophiinae

  Psammophiinae* (including *Malpolon*)

  Pseudoxyrhophiinae

Superfamily Homalopsoidea

Homalopsidae (including *Cerberus, Homalopsis, Enhydris*)*

Superfamily Viperoidea

Viperidae

  Azemiopinae

  Causinae

  Crotalinae

  Viperinae

[a] Taxa discussed in the text are marked with an asterisk.
[b] Further revision of the Colubroidea is underway and may modify the relationships shown here. For instance, Pyron et al. (2011) supported the earlier definition of the Colubroidea, and thus recognized the subfamily status of a number of clades. This includes the Natricinae, rather than the full family, Natricidae as assigned by Vidal et al. (2007), and Zaher et al. (2009).

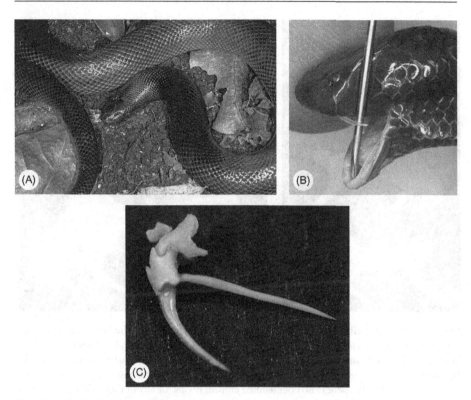

Plate 1.1 (A–C) Mole viper, burrowing asp, or stiletto snake (*Atractaspis* spp.). These unusual fossorial snakes have long been subject to taxonomic revision. They possess notably enlarged, canaliculated fangs that are freely rotatable on the maxilla. This makes manual handling impossible as gripping these snakes behind the head in the conventional manner allows a penetrating jab from the laterally highly mobile fang(s) (Plate 1.1A, *A. fallax*, **Kenya**; Plate 1.1B, West African mole viper; slender burrowing asp, *A. aterrima*, **Nigeria**; Plate 1.1C, **fangs from** Reinhardt's burrowing asp; variable burrowing adder; itiuiu, *A. irregularis*, **Niangara, Congo**). Their venoms contain a wide array of components, including multiple isoforms of cytotoxins and novel vasoconstrictor peptides (e.g., sarafotoxins). Envenomations may be severe; life-threatening cases are well-documented. Current taxonomic reassignments have recommended placement of these snakes from their own family Atractaspididae into a subfamily, Atractaspidinae, of the Lamprophiidae, thereby including one other taxonomically problematic front-fanged genus, *Homoroselaps*. However, some investigators consider *Homoroselaps* spp. as members of the Elapidae. Many little-known colubroids remain of uncertain taxonomic affinity (see text). Photos copyright to David A. Warrell (Plate 1.1A and B) and Arie Lev (Plate 1.1C; AMNH specimen #12355).

their own family, Atractaspididae (Underwood and Kochva, 1993). These distinctive snakes are now assigned by some investigators to the superfamily Elapoidea, as a sub-family (Atractaspidinae) of the Lamprophiidae (www.reptile-database.org/; see Table 1.1). The lamprophiids include a number of species that are commonly kept in captivity.

Among the approximately 8-12 genera (depending on the author [s]) grouped within the atractaspidids are taxa with mid-maxillary enlarged, grooved, and noncanaliculate

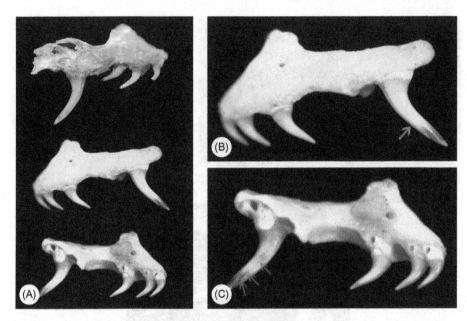

Plate 1.2 (A–C) Maxilla and enlarged posterior maxillary teeth of the Natal black snake
(*Macrelaps microlepidotus*)**.** The natural history of this rare semifossorial species is poorly
known. A non-front-fanged colubroid, it has traditionally been grouped with the unusual front-
fanged genus, *Atractaspis* (see text). There are a number of anecdotal cases of bites by this
species. Unfortunately, there is no documented clinical review of any of these victims. Effects
have allegedly included loss of consciousness and possible cranial nerve involvement, but
further information is required in order to critically evaluate the potential hazard associated
with bites from this uncommon species. As illustrated in the comparison of two specimens
in Plate 1.2A, the most posterior maxillary teeth are markedly enlarged and gently recurved.
They contain a shallow groove that extends along almost the entire medial-posterior surface
of the tooth (the position of the groove from an antero-lateral view is indicated by the arrow
in Plate 1.2B). The groove is visible (arrows) in Plate 1.2C. The uppermost specimen in Plate
1.2A is AMNH #5897; the other specimen in Plate 1.2A and Plate 1.2B and C is AMNH
#18227. See Appendix E for locality data; photos copyright to Scott A. Weinstein.

dentition (e.g., the Natal black snake, or Natal swartslang, *Macrelaps microlepidotus*,
Plate 1.2A–C), and front-fanged ("proteroglyphous") canaliculated morphology (e.g.,
the dwarf garter snakes, *Homoroselaps* spp.), with *Atractaspis* spp. exhibiting markedly
enlarged distensible canaliculated fangs (Plate 1.1B and C) and notably elongated venom
glands. Deufel and Cundall (2003) noted the similarities between unilateral fang use in
Atractaspis and unilateral "slashing envenomation by some rear-fanged snakes." However,
the loss of pterygoid teeth and associated maxillary movement resulted in the inability of
Atractaspis spp. to perform "pterygoid walk" prey transport.[1] These authors remarked

---

[1] "Pterygoid walk" prey transport refers to the alternating pterygoidal movements employed during active
deglutition of a seized prey item. This generally advances the maxillae, thereby drawing the grasped prey
into the snake's esophagus, and facilitates swallowing.

that "*Atractaspis* spp. appear to represent the evolutionary endpoint of a functional conflict between envenomation and transport in which a rear-fanged envenomating system has been optimized at the expense of most, if not all, palatomaxillary transport function" (Deufel and Cundall, 2003). Therefore, although all of the fossorial and/or nocturnal genera included in this group share many traits: slender body form with short tails, and lacking a loreal scale; possessing smooth, shiny scales; relatively small heads and eyes (Shine et al., 2006; see Plate 1.1A), and their monophyly is supported by morphological and molecular data (McDowell, 1986; Underwood and Kochva, 1993; Vidal et al., 2008; Zaher, 1999; Zaher et al., 2009), some genera possess markedly different dentitional morphology that notably influences their potential medical importance. Bites from *Atractaspis* spp. have caused serious envenomings (Kochva, 1998; Kurnick et al., 1999; Wagner et al., 2009; Warrell et al., 1976a), while the medical importance of uncommonly encountered genera such as *Homoroselaps* and *Macrelaps* is unclear. Bites from *M. microlepidotus* have been reported to cause loss of consciousness, and the species is considered "potentially lethal" by some authors (Vitt and Caldwell, 2008), although all of these cases are anecdotal, without any formal medical evaluation or verification (Branch, 1982; Chapman, 1968; FitzSimons, 1919, 1962; FitzSimons and Smith, 1958; Visser and Chapman, 1978). FitzSimons (1919) stated that *M. microlepidotus* bites were insignificant, and Chapman (1968) described a bite with minimal local effects. Similarly, the single well-documented bite from a dwarf-spotted garter snake (*Homoroselaps lacteus*) consisted of only local pain and edema (Branch, 1982). Thus, the atractaspidids are a distinctive series of snakes assigned to a shared taxonomic status on the basis of strong morphological and molecular systematic evidence. However, this taxonomy has placed together several species previously considered either "colubrids," elapids, or viperids. Therefore, the revised biological classifications of many species previously considered part of the "Colubridae" may result in reassignments that can impact their perceived clinical importance by altering previous taxonomic relationships, or by formulating new perceptions on the basis of relationships to newly reassigned taxa.

It must be noted that to date, some of these reassignments (such as those involving *Atractaspis* spp.) are not universally adopted or recommended by consensus and may be subject to further changes or returned to their previous classification(s). Therefore, the clinician must be proactive in seeking a thorough biological history (through consultation with a knowledgeable toxinologist or professional herpetologist and/or via current literature) for any colubroid of unknown clinical importance involved in a medically significant bite. This may provide clues about the potential medical importance of the species involved as derived from observations of bites by related taxa. It emphasizes the need for careful verification of recommended taxonomic reassignments prior to their publication and general adoption. Such a standard may frustrate taxonomists eager to achieve recognition of their findings, but this caution may also temper incorrect, premature assertions that can affect categorization of an "envenomed" patient.

2 Differences Between Buccal Gland Secretion and Associated Delivery Systems of "True" Venomous Snakes and "Colubrid" Snakes: Low- Versus High-Pressure Gland Function and Canaliculated Versus Solid Dentition

A half-truth, like half a brick, is always more forcible as an argument than a whole one. It carries better.

Stephen Leacock

2.1 Basic Considerations Regarding Gland Structure and Function

The functional morphology of venom glands in "front-fanged" or "true" venomous snakes (viperids, elapids, and atractaspidids) differs notably from the gland apparatus and associated dentition of other colubroids. An unknown number of these species lack their homologous counterpart, the Duvernoy's gland (Kardong, 1996; Taub, 1966; Weinstein and Kardong, 1994; Weinstein et al., 2010; Zalisko and Kardong, 1992). Taub (1967) reported that about 17% (approximately 30 species) of colubrid snakes studied (120 genera, 180 species) lacked evidence of Duvernoy's glands and, in some discrete groups, as many as 90% examined lacked these glands.

Most Duvernoy's glands lack any significant storage capacity, exhibit a duct system distinguishable from that of venom glands of front-fanged snakes, and usually have no direct striated muscle insertion to pressurize the fundus of the gland. The consequence is a low-pressure secretion-injecting system (Kardong, 1996; Kardong and Lavin-Murcio, 1993; Taub, 1967; Weinstein and Kardong, 1994; Weinstein et al., 2010). Figure 2.1 (Panels A–C) illustrates the basic functional morphology of a typical Duvernoy's gland with its limited muscle attachment and associated dentition. Some members of the tribe, Dispholidini (Section 4.3), are exceptions to this, as they do have some limited striated muscle attachment on the gland fundus and thereby have

"Venomous" Bites from Non-Venomous Snakes. DOI: 10.1016/B978-0-12-387732-1.00002-6

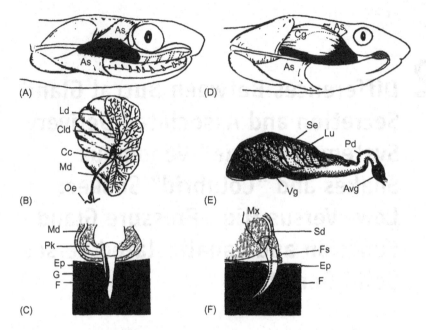

Figure 2.1 Comparison of a Duvernoy's gland system in an "opisthoglyphous" ("rear-fanged" = non-front-fanged) snake (left) and a venom gland system in a model "proteroglyphous" or "solenoglyphous" snake (right). Panel A. In the non-front-fanged ("opisthoglyphous") snake, Duvernoy's gland (shaded) is located in the temporal region. Adjacent striated muscles (e.g., *adductor superficialis*) run medially past the gland, but usually are not directly attached. *Dispholidus typus* is an exception to this, as it does have limited muscle attachment to the gland. Panel B. A cross-sectioned view of the Duvernoy's gland that reveals the arrangement of the internal duct system draining the extensive parenchyma. A single duct departs from a small, central cistern within the gland, and runs to a cuff of oral epithelium surrounding the posterior maxillary tooth (F). Panel C. When the posterior maxillary tooth penetrates the integument of the prey or human victim, the cuff of the oral epithelium remains on the surface, thereby receiving Duvernoy's secretion, which flows around the tooth that may (as depicted here) or may not be grooved (an "open system" with inherently low pressure). Panel D. The venom gland (shaded) of this model proteroglyphous or solenoglyphous snake includes a main venom gland, main duct accessory venom gland, and secondary duct that empty into the base of the canaliculated (hollow) fang. Striated jaw muscles (e.g., *adductor externus superficialis* in "proteroglyphous" elapids or *compressor glandulae* in "solenoglyphous" viperids) act directly upon the venom gland to raise the intraglandular pressure and send a pulse of venom from the gland through the duct to the fang. Panel E. A sagittal view of the venom gland reveals the secretory epithelium, and extensive storage reservoir of venom. Panel F. When the fang penetrates the integument of the prey, the attachment of the venom duct to the fang tightens in order to maintain the relatively high-pressure head, and venom passes down the hollow core of the fang to be delivered deeply into the tissues (a "closed system" with inherently high pressure). Abbreviations: jaw muscles, *adductor mandibulae externus superficialis* (As), *compressor glandulae* (Cg), accessory venom gland (Avg), central cistern (Cc), common lobular duct (Cld), epithelium of prey integument (Ep), fang or enlarged maxillary tooth (F), fang sheath (Fs), groove on surface of maxillary tooth (G), lobular duct (Ld), lumen holding secretory product (Lu), main duct (Md), maxilla (Mx), oral epithelium (Oe), pocket of oral epithelium around tooth (Pk), primary venom duct (Pd), secondary venom duct (Sd), secretory epithelium (Se), main venom gland (Vg). After Weinstein and Kardong (1994) used with permission.

some pressurization of the system (Fry et al., 2008; Taub, 1966; Weinstein et al., 2010). The muscle insertion into the venom glands typical of front-fanged snakes exerts a high-pressure head (often in excess of 30 psi; Kardong, 2009) facilitating rapid delivery of a significant volume of pre-stored venom bolus through the associated venom ducts and canaliculate fangs (Figure 2.1, Panels D–F) that may be fixed (essentially, permanently erect, "proteroglyphous," Plate 2.1A–E) or erectile with varying mobility (or, distensibility) according to size or species ("solenoglyphous," Plate 2.2A; Kardong,

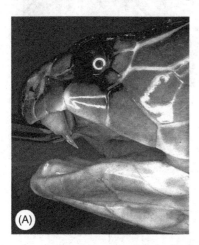 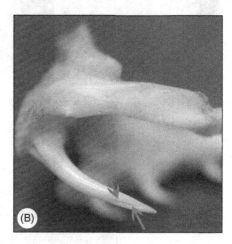

Plate 2.1 (A and B) Fangs of the common Asian cobra (*Naja naja*). The fixed, erected, canaliculated fangs are representative of the "proteroglyphous" dentition present in the Elapidae. Many elapid species have short fangs, but some such as the coastal taipan (*Oxyuranus scutellatus*) have long, slightly recurved fangs. Many elapid venoms contain multiple isoforms of postsynaptic or presynaptic neurotoxins. These venoms may be delivered less deeply than those administered by the often larger fangs of viperids, but this does not decrease their *in vivo* lethality.
(A) Profile of fangs of *Naja naja*, Sri Lanka.
(B) Close-up of fang of *Naja naja*, North India. Note the elongated oval-shaped bevel (arrows) that closely resembles that of a hypodermic needle. The canaliculated (hollow or containing a lumen) morphology facilitates deep injection of venom into the integument of prey or human victim (see text).
(C) Fangs of the yellow-lipped sea krait (*Laticauda colubrina*), Madang, Papua New Guinea. Hydrophiine sea snakes and laticaudiines (sea kraits) exhibit the "proteroglyphous" dentition associated with high-pressure venom glands. Bites from laticaudiines are rare, but may be life threatening when they occur (see text).
(D) Yellow-lipped sea krait (*Laticauda colubrina*), Madang, Papua New Guinea. While hydrophiine sea snakes are ovoviviparous, the laticaudiines are oviparous, and come ashore to lay their eggs in rock crevices. Their venoms contain postsynaptic neurotoxins (e.g., erabutoxins), and phospholipases A_2 myotoxins.
(E) Close-up view of fangs of the olive sea snake (*Aipysurus laevis*), Roebuck Bay, Western Australia. The fixed canaliculated fangs of this hydrophiine sea snake are closely set (arrows), probably to establish a firm grip on struggling prey and possibly increase the likelihood of effective venom delivery to the fishes of multiple niches belonging to at least 17 families and six different morphological types that comprise a major part of the diet of this species (Heatwole and Cogger, 1993). *Aipysurus laevis* also preys on crustaceans, cephalopods, and fish eggs. Plate 2.1A, C, and D, photos copyright to David A. Warrell; Plate 2.1B, AMNH specimen #64418; and Plate 2.1E, AMNH specimen #86176, photos copyright to Arie Lev.

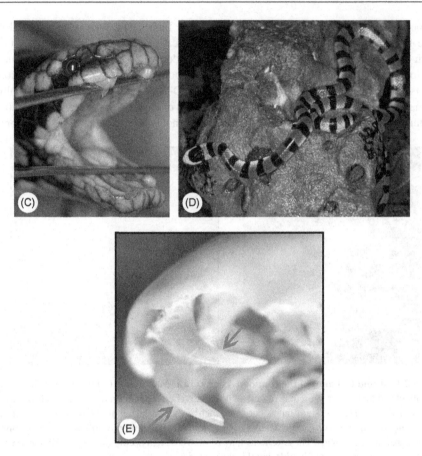

Plate 2.1 C–E (*Continued*)

1979; Weinstein and Kardong, 1994). Some elapids exhibit incomplete fang cannula without complete fusion of the venom duct groove (Bogert, 1943). None of the
known colubroids of the former colubrid assemblage possess such dentition. The teeth
associated with Duvernoy's glands are never canaliculate (i.e., never with a lumen),
but instead are solid, often enlarged, and sometimes deeply grooved (Fry et al., 2008;
Weinstein and Kardong, 1994; Weinstein et al., 2010; Young and Kardong, 1996).

Duvernoy's gland morphology may vary considerably among non-front-fanged
colubroid species, and enlarged teeth associated with glands may be present mid- [e.g.,
Pampas snake, boipemi, cobra espada comum (other names as well), *Tomodon dorsatus*, Plate 2.3A–D], or notably posterior (e.g., *Malpolon monspessulanus*, Plate 2.4A–C),
in the maxilla (Broadley and Wallach, 2002; Fry et al., 2008; McKinstry, 1978; Taub,
1967; Weinstein et al., 2010). Several medically important species (i.e., some members
of the tribe, Dispholidini, see Section 4.3) have multiple enlarged, deeply grooved posterior maxillary teeth with modifications probably adapted for enhanced conduction of
secretions into inflicted bite wounds (Broadley and Wallach, 2002; Meier, 1981; Section
4.3). It is important to note that other medically important species (e.g., *R. tigrinus* and

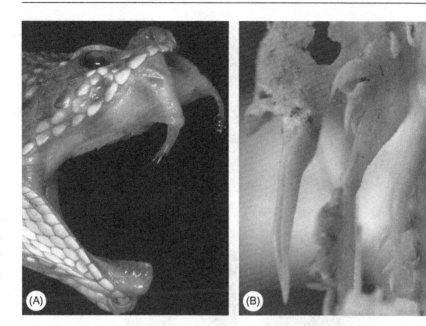

Plate 2.2 (A) **Tropical rattlesnake; Neotropical rattlesnake; cascabel; cascavel; maraca-boia; numerous other names (*Crotalus durissus collilineatus*) (Brazil) with fangs erected.** Central and South American rattlesnakes have markedly variable venoms among different populations. Some secrete venoms that contain the potent heterodimeric presynaptic neurotoxin, crotoxin, historically, the first toxin isolated from any snake venom. Other populations lack this toxin, and secrete venoms that only contain toxins common to many *Crotalus* spp. (procoagulants, hemorrhagins, hypotensive peptides, and numerous other components). Bites from these snakes can cause severe systemic envenoming. Given their sizable fang structure, venom reservoir, and potent venom, fatalities are common. Note the distensible, strongly recurved, canaliculated front-fangs typical of "solenoglyphous" dentition. The fang on the right side of the photo is expressing a drop of venom at the fang aperture. (B) **Close-up view of Western diamondback rattlesnake (*Crotalus atrox*) anterior maxilla and fangs.** This specimen has fangs that contain a visible groove that corresponds with the venom canal or lumen. Viperid and elapid fangs have significant morphological variability. Several hypotheses have attempted to establish evolutionary models for the development of dentition adapted for venom delivery. One of these suggests that selective apoptosis (programmed cell death) contributes to the formation of a fang lumen, or an external groove (see text). Plate 2.2A, photo copyright to David A. Warrell; Plate 2.2B, AMNH specimen #137173, photo copyright to Arie Lev.

R. subminiatus) lack grooves in their enlarged posterior maxillary teeth (Section 4.3). This supports the accuracy of Stejneger's contention that the presence of a grooved "rear fang" is not strictly necessary for the introduction of Duvernoy's secretion into a bite-inflicted wound (Stejneger, 1893).

Although their morphology is variable (Fry et al., 2008; Weinstein et al., 2010), the typical storage capacity of venom glands also emphasizes the functional difference between these and Duvernoy's glands (Figure 2.1). One notable aspect of this difference is in the much broader range of potential venom yields from front-fanged

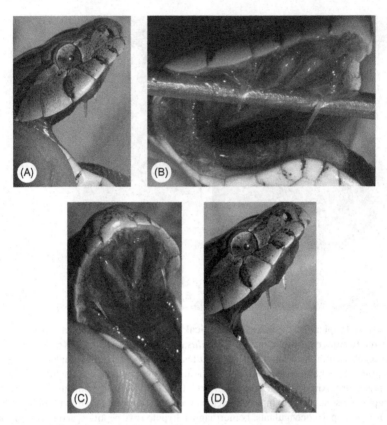

Plate 2.3 (A–D) Pampas snake, false viper or mock viper (*Tomodon dorsatus*), Ibiuna, Brazil. The enlarged teeth positioned midway on the maxillae (see Plate 2.3A–D) demonstrate the variability of adaptive dentition among colubroid snakes. The terms, "rear-fanged," or "opisthoglyphous," do not accurately describe the dentition present in many species of non-front-fanged colubroid snakes. *Tomodon* spp. are members of the tribe, Tachymeninii, and to date the documented cases of bites from these snakes have caused only mild effects (see Table 4.1).
Photos copyright to David A. Warrell.

snakes compared to those of Duvernoy's secretions of other colubroids. For example, although occasional large yields are obtained, manual extraction of venom from the eastern brown snake (*Pseudonaja textilis*, Plate 2.5) typically yields only about 2 mg of lyophilized venom solids (Peter Mirtschen, personal verbal communication with SAW and JW; SAW, personal observations), while extraction of some large viperids or elapids [e.g., an adult eastern diamondback rattlesnake, *Crotalus adamanteus* (Plate 2.6A and B), West African Gaboon viper, *Bitis rhinoceros* (Plate 2.7A–C), and hamadryad or king cobra, *Ophiophagus hannah* (Plate 2.8), respectively], will often yield large volumes, sometimes in excess of 1 g of venom dry weight (Minton, 1974; Minton and Minton, 1980; Russell, 1980; Minton and Weinstein, unpublished observations). Members of the former colubrid assemblage usually produce far lower

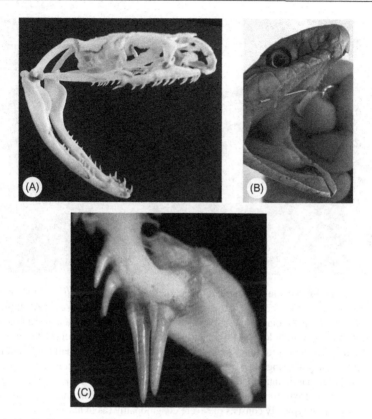

Plate 2.4 (A–C) Skull of *Malpolon monspessulanus* and close-up of enlarged posterior maxillary teeth. The teeth are notably enlarged and posterior on the maxillae (Plate 2.4A and B, Spain). Note the deep groove that is present for almost the entire length of the teeth (Plate 2.4C, Bulgaria). Plate 2.4A and B, copyright to Javier José Carrasco Araújo; Plate 2.4C, photo copyright to Zoltan Takács.

volumes of Duvernoy's secretions, and thus potential ranges of yields are far narrower (see Appendix B for Duvernoy's secretion yields of some representative species). The largest yields are usually produced by large adult specimens of the brown tree snake (*Boiga irregularis*, Section 4.4), and to date these are usually less than 20 mg dry weight even with parasympathomimetic stimulation of the Duvernoy's glands (Chiszar et al., 1992; Mackessy et al., 2006; Weinstein et al., 1991; see later). This also emphasizes the lack of any significant storage capacity in the majority of colubrid species studied to date. Unlike the case with many viperids and elapids, attempts to increase yields by manual pressure on the Duvernoy's glands do not usually succeed. Thus, it is unlikely that manual pressure exerted on the head of a snake during attempts to remove it while inflicting a protracted or sustained bite would substantially increase the volume of secretion. Such concerns (e.g., per bites inflicted by the green palm snake, *Philodryas viridissimus*; Means, 2010; see later) should probably focus on avoiding increased maxillary mobilization (e.g., "walking" of the jaws on the bitten site)

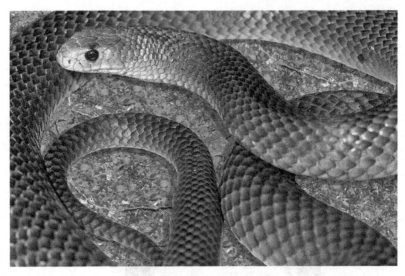

Plate 2.5 Eastern brown snake (*Pseudonaja textilis*). *Pseudonaja textilis* and its congener, *P. nuchalis* (western brown snake), are the most medically important snakes in Australia. *Pseudonaja textilis* is also found in West Papua and Papua New Guinea, and has a notorious reputation. The color morphology of this elapid is widely variable from all shades of brown to black with multiple tinted color tones (ochre, rust, yellow). They have small fangs, but possess highly toxic venom containing the most potent snake venom toxin characterized to date (textilotoxin, a presynaptic multimeric neurotoxin, the murine i.p. LD50 is 0.001 mg/kg) as well as other neurotoxins (e.g., pseudonajatoxin A, a postsynaptic neurotoxin). However, human envenomation typically consists of severe coagulopathy (as in hazard level 1 colubrids), and very rarely includes neurotoxic effects. Envenomation may result in rapid systemic complications (seizures, cardiac effects, collapse, and arrest). However, some 80% of bites result in no envenomation ("dry bites").
Photo copyright to David A. Warrell.

as this may stimulate increased secretion via secondary anatomical influences (see later). Duvernoy's secretion yields from a variety of non-front-fanged colubroid taxa were reviewed by Weinstein and Kardong (1994) and are selectively reviewed later (also see Appendix B).

In view of the lack of muscular compression, release of Duvernoy's secretion appears to result primarily from autonomic stimulation (Rosenberg, 1992). However, as the gland tightly adheres to the overlying skin and the quadratomaxillary ligament runs from the posterior aspect of the gland and inserts on the distal end of the quadrate, contraction of jaw adductors may contribute to gland pressurization (Weinstein et al., 2010). Some observations suggest that in other species there may be additional (secondary) sources of pressurization due to anatomical relationships between "venom ducts" and surrounding structures (Fry et al., 2008). Fry et al. (2008) suggested that in cross-sectional analyses, the "venom duct" of some taxa was more crenated and was surrounded by concentric layers of connective tissue suggestive of pressure regulation.

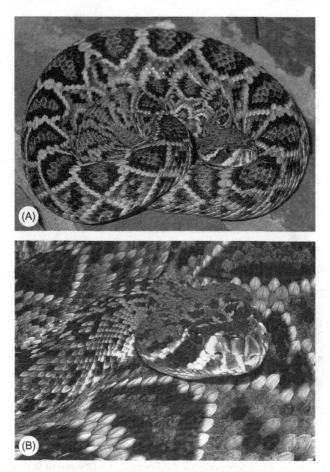

Plate 2.6 (A and B) Eastern diamondback rattlesnake (*Crotalus adamanteus*), Florida, USA. The largest venomous snake of North America, this impressive crotaline viperid can produce large volumes of venom. Manual extraction can yield over 1 g of venom solids. Bites from this species commonly produce significant morbidity, and may be fatal. Photos copyright to David A. Warrell.

This seemed to be particularly developed in *D. typus, Stenorrhina freminvillei* (Central American blood snake or alacranera), and *T. capensis*.

The released secretion is conveyed by a duct into a loose cuff of buccal mucosa near or around the adjacent teeth (Figure 2.1, Panel C). Some taxa have multiple ducts that transmit secretion to the vicinity of the adjacent maxillary teeth (Fry et al., 2008). The secretion is thereby conducted by capillary action along the surface of the tooth, a process sometimes facilitated by dental grooves. Thus, in contrast to venom delivery in front-fanged venomous snakes, Duvernoy's secretion is not injected, but rather inoculated into the bite wound inflicted in the integument of the bitten prey or human victim (Kardong, 2009).

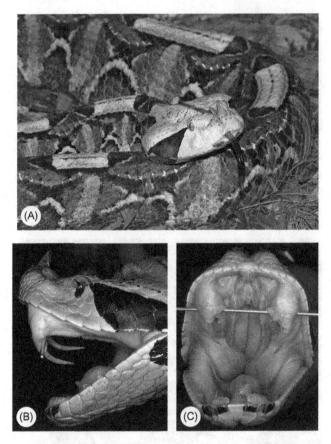

Plate 2.7 (A–C) **West African Gaboon viper** (***Bitis rhinocerous***). Probably the most heavy-bodied viper, this viperine viperid has the longest fangs (≥6 cm) of any venomous snake, and can produce large volumes of toxic venom. The almost hook-like, mobile fangs ("solenoglyphous" dentition; see Plate 2.7B and C) are often used in the manipulation of prey during deglutition. Popular in private collections in the USA and Europe, bites from this species are life threatening, with well-documented fatalities. This taxon is also medically important in its range, as is the East African form, *B. gabonica*.
Photos copyright to David A. Warrell.

2.2   Overview of Hypotheses for the Evolution of Venom-Delivery Systems

Changes in ophidian morphology (e.g., increasing appearance of slender body forms) during the Miocene, concomitant with decreasing reliance on constriction for prey subjugation, have been presented as contributing selection pressures for the development of venom-delivery systems (Savitzky, 1980). The evolution of venom and an apparatus for its delivery has been the subject of speculation, hypothesis, and scholarly research for several hundred years and has been reviewed by a number of authors. Recent contributions continue to expand knowledge of the molecular biology, morphology, function,

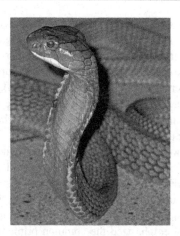

Plate 2.8 King cobra, or hamadryad; taw-gyi mwe haut, yanjing wang she, ular tedong selar; others (*Ophiophagus hannah*), Trang, Thailand. Native to Southeast Asia (India, Burma/Myanmar, Nepal, Bangladesh, Malaysia, Indo-China, Thailand, Indonesia, and the Philippines), *O. hannah* is the largest of venomous snakes, and has been documented to reach a length of 5.7 m long. The venom contains long-chain postsynaptic neurotoxins, a multitude of enzymes, is known for a species-specific hemorrhagin, hannahtoxin, but is moderately toxic (murine i.p. LD_{50} is approximately 1.5–1.7 mg/kg). However, clinically a bite may result in severe envenomation due to the potentially large venom yield (average ≈420 mg dry wt., but may well exceed 1 g). The natural diet of this impressive serpent is typically restricted to other snakes (thus the genus name), especially Indian rat snakes, or dhaman (*Ptyas mucosus*), and, opportunistically, varanid lizards. Although currently considered monotypic, ongoing research suggests that there may be several species or clades of these elapids.
Photo copyright to David A. Warrell.

and biochemistry of the evolution of venom and venom-delivery systems (Bogert, 1943; Fry et al., 2003, 2006, 2008, 2009a; Jackson, 2002, 2003; Jackson and Fritts, 1995; Kardong, 1979, 1980a; Kardong and Luchtel, 1986; Kochva, 1965, 1978, 1987; Kochva et al., 1980; Kuch et al., 2006; Mackessy and Baxter, 2006; Mebs, 1978, 2002; Minton and Minton, 1980; Vonk et al., 2008; Weinstein et al., 2010). Current theories advance a single evolutionary appearance of the primordial venom-delivery system with subsequent radiation and taxon-specific modification of the venom-delivery system [Fry et al., 2006, 2008; also advocated in the mid-twentieth century by Bogert (1943) and others through dentitional/osteological studies]. Other researchers have used phylogenetic and/or functional morphological studies or analyses in order to support appearance of Duvernoy's glands early in colubroid evolution, and independent evolution of high-pressure venom glands multiple times in viperids, elapids, and atractaspidids (Cadle, 1988; Jackson, 2002, 2003; Kardong, 1982; Kraus and Brown, 1998; Weinstein et al., 2010, and others). The reader is referred to the cited studies for details regarding these interesting but still unresolved hypotheses.

Anatomical studies of venom glands from viperids, elapids, and atractaspidids, as well as Duvernoy's glands from other colubroids, have demonstrated a likely common origin from dental glands (Kochva, 1978). Some authors have considered a venom gland origin from the rictal gland, rather than a precursor Duvernoy's gland (McDowell, 1986). However, embryological evidence (as well as the co-occurrence of rictal glands and venom glands among many representative venomous colubroids) argues against this (Jackson, 2003). Also, Duvernoy's glands and venom glands of viperids, elapids, and atractaspidids all are innervated by the same cranial nerve [maxillary branch (V_2) of the trigeminal nerve] (Kochva, 1965; Taub, 1966), and supplied with blood by vessels branching from the internal carotid artery (Kochva, 1965). In *Natrix tessellata* (dice water snake, tessellated water snake), the anterior teeth arise from the anterior portion of the maxillary dental laminae, and the posterior "fang" (which is associated with the Duvernoy's gland) from the posterior section (Jackson, 2003).

In *N. tessellata*, Duvernoy's gland is not homologous with the mammalian parotid gland because it has a different embryonic origin (Gygax, 1971). This argues for recognition of the gland [named after the French morphologist/anatomist, George Louis Duvernoy (1777–1855); Taub, 1966] as a separate entity, rather than perpetuating the term "parotid gland" commonly used for Duvernoy's gland up until the mid-twentieth century. Some authors have emphasized the common primordium of the venom gland and associated fangs. This is the case even in species in which the adult fang ends up at the anterior end of the mouth, with the gland posterior to the eye (Jackson, 2003). Although Duvernoy's gland has been long-recognized as a structure distinctive to some colubroids other than those with front fangs (viperids, elapids, and atractaspidids), Duvernoy's glands have been described in some atractaspidids, based on their macroscopic coarsely lobulated appearance and dorsolateral position, at the corner of the mouth (Greene, 1997; Haas, 1931; McDowell, 1986). The high-pressure venom glands of atractaspidids are very different from those of viperids and elapids in lacking a discrete accessory gland, possessing a distinct histochemical profile (Kochva, 1978), and having a gland compressor muscle that is derived from the *adductor externus medialis* (Jackson, 2003), while the *compressor glandulae*, *adductor externus profundus*, and *pterygoideus* functions as the venom gland compressor in viperids, and the *adductor externus superficialis* (*levator anguli oris*) in elapids. However, the interpretation of co-existence of these glands is problematic (Underwood, 2002; Weinstein et al., 2010), and may be a misinterpretation of a rictal gland. Confirmation and further careful morphological analysis of the buccal glands of various *Atractaspis* spp. is desirable, as possible concomitant presence of both glands may serve different or complimentary functions.

2.3   Theories Considering the Evolution of Canaliculated Fangs and Enlarged Grooved Teeth

Studies of the development, formation, and specialized adaptation of snake teeth have facilitated improved understanding of the evolution of the "business end" of venom-delivery systems. Buchtová et al. (2008) found that ophidian tooth formation differed from that of rodents. The majority of snake teeth were found to bud off a deep, ribbon-like dental lamina rather than as separate tooth germs. Asymmetries in cell proliferation and extracellular matrix distribution before and after ingrowth of the dental lamina suggested that localized signaling by a secreted protein was involved (Buchtová et al., 2008). Using two pythonids [African rock python, *Python sebae* (Plate 2.9A), and ball or regal python, *P. regius* (Plate 2.9B)] and a colubrine colubrid (corn snake,

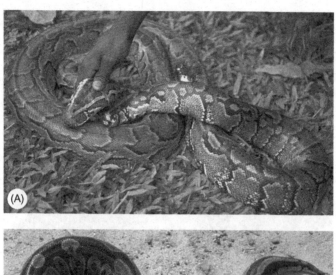

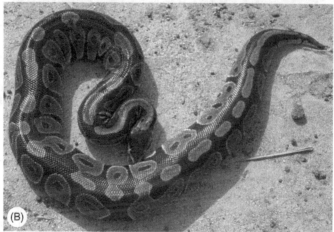

Plate 2.9 (A and B) Representative pythonid snakes. The Pythonidae are members of the superfamily, Henophidia. These snakes lack Duvernoy's glands or venom glands, as well as any dentition adapted for delivery of oral secretions (this does not obviate the presence of enlarged teeth; see Plate 2.11A and B). Studies of tooth replacement in pythons have enhanced the understanding of the evolution of ophidian dentition including the fangs or modified maxillary teeth of colubroids.

(A) African rock python (*Python sebae*), Nigeria. Native to portions of central-sub-Saharan and South Africa, this is an impressive constrictor that can attain a body length of just over 6 m. Revered in many West African countries and kept peridomestically as totems, they are known to take large prey such as small antelope, monkeys, and wart hogs. There are rare reports (most are anecdotal) of this species having eaten children and killed adults.

(B) Ball, royal or regal python (*Python regius*), Nigeria. *Python regius* is a small docile species that is among the most popular snakes in amateur private collections. The species has been subjected to selective captive breeding in order to propagate some of the most colorful and unusual pattern morphologies [thus the term "designer snakes" (also see Plate 4.79A–F)]. Plate 2.9A and B, photos copyright to David A. Warrell.

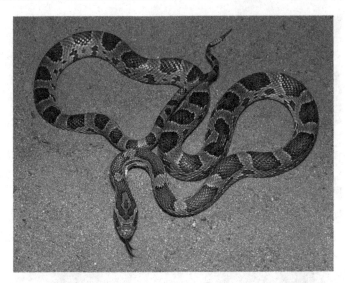

Plate 2.10 Corn, or red rat snake (*Pantherophis guttata*). One of the most common colubrine snakes maintained in private collections, it has been genetically selected for numerous color and pattern morphs. Although its bite is of no medical significance as it lacks Duvernoy's glands and venom glands, as well as any modified dentition, it has also been employed as a model in order to study the molecular development of ophidian teeth. Photo copyright to Julian White.

Pantherophis guttata, Plate 2.10), the authors cloned Sonic hedgehog genes (SHG)[1] and traced their expression in these species. The expression of SHG was found to define the position of the future dental laminae. Expression was noted in the inner enamel epithelium and the stellate reticulum of the tooth anlagen, but was absent from the outer enamel epithelium and its derivative, the successional lamina (Buchtová et al., 2008). This suggested that signals other than SHG are responsible for replacement tooth formation (Buchtová et al., 2008). Although these data were derived from study of two henophidians (pythonids) and one colubrine without specialized dentition or a discrete Duvernoy's gland, it is likely that the molecular mechanisms of tooth formation are very similar in other extant ophidians.

It is also important to note that enlarged teeth can evolve for other likely functions such as grasping, or stabilizing the grip on seized prey. Such adapted dentition, as seen in the aptly named boiid, *Corallus caninus* (Emerald tree boa, Plate 2.11A and B), certainly can inflict a painful, edematous wound accompanied by transient bleeding and erythema, as has been proven to some collectors (including one of the authors, SAW)

---

[1] "Sonic hedgehog" is named after a character from a popular video game. The original hedgehog gene was found in the fruit fly, *Drosophila*, and named for the appearance of the mutant phenotype that caused an affected embryo to be covered with pointy, spine-like projections or denticles (e.g., resembling those of a hedgehog). This gene is one of three homologues, all of which encode proteins integral to development and of the vertebrate notochord and other embryonic determinants of morphology. These, and other homeobox genes, directly influence the commitment of a given cell population to a defined cell lineage.

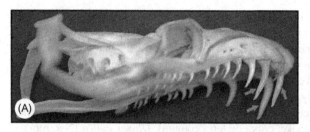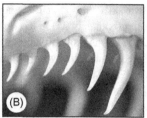

Plate 2.11 (A and B) The enlarged anterior maxillary dentition of the emerald tree boa (*Corallus caninus*). Although the teeth are enlarged and recurved (arrows), there are no grooves or other modifications. These teeth are probably used in order to aid grasping or stabilizing prey. These arboreal snakes can inflict a painful wound including edema and erythema. Therefore, a bite by a snake with large teeth and lacking oral secretions of any appreciable toxicity can still produce mild local effects as a result of purely physical trauma. AMNH specimen #R57788, photo copyright to Arie Lev.

who have maintained captive specimens of this attractive species. However, there may be no apparatus for producing or administering any specialized oral secretion. Henophidians, such as *C. caninus*, lack Duvernoy's glands as well as "true" venom glands; thus, they are truly nonvenomous and do not produce "mildly toxic saliva."[2] Therefore, it is important to remain aware that physical trauma inflicted from bites by snakes with large teeth, and without toxic secretion, can be incorrectly assigned with a "toxic" potential due to misinterpretation of localized trauma (see later).

In some species, evidence suggests that prey preference may influence the specific nature of specialized dentition, and these adaptive modifications may facilitate prey handling. Lizards with tightly overlapping scales [e.g., those with cycloid scales, such as scincid lizards (skinks)] may present as hard-bodied prey items that are difficult to grasp. Modified teeth may serve to maintain a firm grip, prevent escape, and aid deglutition. In some species, such as the common wolf snake (*Lycodon aulicus capucinus*), the combination of several dentitional modifications [e.g., enlarged anterior maxillary teeth, an arched maxilla, and enlarged (ungrooved) posterior maxillary teeth] may increase the likelihood of successful prey capture, control, and ingestion (Jackson and Fritts, 2004). In other species (e.g., the Asian mock viper or leopard snake, *Psammodynastes pulverulentus*), dentitional adaptations are probably used in concert with Duvernoy's secretions in order to subjugate prey (Savitzky, 1983; see later). The Asian slug-eating snakes (family Pareatidae) comprise a group of gastropod specialists (or "malacophagous" snakes) with a distinct lineage (Vidal et al., 2007). Some of these snakes (e.g., *Pareas iwasakii*;

---

[2] Antiserums against venoms from elapids such as *Dendroapsis* spp. (mambas), *Naja* spp., and *Haemachatus haemachatus* (ringhals, ringhals spitting cobra) have shown some limited immunoelectrophoretic cross-reactivity with oral secretions from the Bahaman boa, *Epicrates striatus strigilatus* (Eleuthera Island boa; see Minton and Weinstein, 1987). Although it has no medical or apparent biological significance, the phenomenon may reflect "exaptation" or "preadaptation." This is discussed later in relation to consideration of toxins present in the oral secretions of nonvenomous lizards.

Iwasaki's slug or snail-eating snake; Iwasaki-sedaka-hebi) have a larger number of teeth (approximately 25) in the right maxilla than in the left (approximately 17.5) (Hoso et al., 2007). This probably allows the species to extract snails from shells that possess a right-sided whirl (clockwise). Some snail species (e.g., the air-breathing or pulmonate snails, *Satsuma* spp.) that have evolved left-sided (or sinistral) whirls exhibit some functional protection against predation by these snakes due to the reliance on right-dominant prey seizure and extraction (Hoso et al., 2007). Some gastropod specialists, such as *Atractus reticulatus* (reticulate ground snake; cobra de terra comum), *Dipsas indica* [Neotropical snail-eater; cobra-cipo (this name is commonly used for *P. olfersii*, and other species; see Table 4.1 for examples of commonly used regional names)], and *Sibynomorphus mikanii* (Mikan's tree snake, or dormideira preta) also exhibit wide morphological/histochemical variability in their infralabial glands that may reflect secretion constituent diversity and dietary specialization (de Oliveira et al., 2007). In the event of biting a human victim, such dentitional modifications, adaptations, and concomitant glandular variability, which probably facilitate specific prey capture certainly may influence the extent of any possible local effects, with or without the introduction of Duvernoy's secretions (see later).

A recent hypothesis suggested that an alteration of the timing of developmental events (specifically, a heterochronic mechanism; Jackson, 2007) might provide a basis for the appearance of specialized dentition in colubroids. This concept advanced the development of ungrooved and grooved teeth of colubroid snakes from an ancestral tubular fang via attachment of replacement tubular fangs to the maxilla at an earlier developmental stage than previously considered (termed "precocial ankylosis") (Jackson, 2007). The evolution of the canaliculated fang provided a means of penetrating the prey's (or foe's) integument and deeply injecting venom, containing a wide array of biologically active components, including highly potent toxins. Therefore, the evolution of the high-pressure venom system combined with the formation of an enclosed venom canal, or lumen (resembling the action of a hypodermic syringe needle), provided an adaptation allowing the subjugation, and in some species, predigestion, of large, strong prey with a probable reduced risk of defensive or retaliatory injury inflicted on the snake. Some studies support enclosed venom canal formation by invagination of a groove along the surface of the tooth or epithelial wall of the developing tooth with eventual fusion, thereby forming the enclosed canal, while others suggest that direct, successive deposition of materials (e.g., dentin) form the tubular fang from tip to base—therefore the canal develops directly, without any folding ("brick chimney hypothesis," Jackson, 2002; Zahradnicek et al., 2008). Using the expression of SHG, early development of the fangs was followed in *Cryptelytrops* (Malhotra and Thorpe, 2004; *Trimeresurus*) *albolabris* (white-lipped pit viper, Plate 2.12) (Zahradnicek et al., 2008). These authors found that the fang lumen was formed by an early invagination of epithelial cells into the dental mesenchyme. The epithelial cells proliferated in order to enlarge the canal, with subsequent apoptosis (programmed cell death) forming the functional lumen (Zahradnicek et al., 2008). The two sides of the invaginating epithelium never come into contact, thus leaving the orifice open. These researchers compared the mechanism by which the fang orifices form with that of the open groove on the posterior maxillary teeth of *D. typus* (Plate 2.13). Zahradnicek et al. (2008) speculated that the process of orifice formation in viperids represents the ancestral

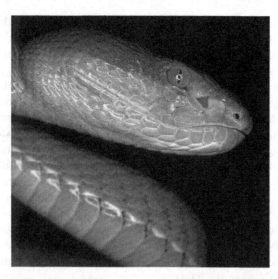

Plate 2.12 White-lipped green pit viper; bai chun zhu ye qing; ngu khiaw hang mai; others (*Cryptelytrops albolabris*), Thailand. A small, wide-ranging, Southeast Asian crotaline viperid that is common and responsible for many bites primarily associated with local morbidity. An arboreal species, it has a prehensile tail, and will frequently use it as an anchor to tree branches, recoiling into a flexed sigmoid body position. It is commonly maintained in private collections.
Photo copyright to David A. Warrell.

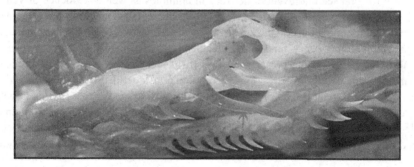

Plate 2.13 Close-up of the enlarged posterior maxillary teeth of the boomslang (*Dispholidus typus*). Note the deep groove (arrow) that traverses the majority of the length of the tooth, and the blade-like modification of the edges. Several theories considering the development of specialized ophidian teeth include programmed cell death (apoptosis) of epithelial cells, and the resulting formation of a functional lumen/canal that facilitates the delivery of venom. AMNH specimen #75722, photo copyright to Arie Lev.

plesiomorphic state. In this view, enclosed fang lumens developed by a change in the shape and size of the initial invagination.

Recent data have shed additional light on the shared developmental mechanisms for specialized dentition among colubroids with either posterior enlarged grooved or ungrooved maxillary teeth ("rear fangs") associated with low-pressure Duvernoy's glands, or anterior-positioned canaliculated fangs associated with high-pressure venom glands. A study of SHG expression showed that front fangs develop from the posterior end of the upper jaw and are strikingly similar in morphogenesis to rear fangs, consistent with their proposed homology (Vonk et al., 2008). These researchers found that the anterior part of the upper jaw of front-fanged snakes lacked SHG expression. Ontogenetic allometry displaces the fang from its posterior developmental origin to its adult front position, consistent with an ancestral posterior position of the front fang (Vonk et al., 2008). The authors reported that the posterior maxillary teeth of "rear-fanged" snakes develop from an independent posterior dental lamina and retain their posterior position. Based on their data, they hypothesized a model for the evolution of snake fangs in which a posterior subregion of the tooth-forming epithelium became developmentally uncoupled from the remaining dentition. This allowed the posterior teeth to evolve independently and in close association with the venom gland (Vonk et al., 2008). As this could lead to notable modification in different lineages, the authors proposed that their model partly accounted for radiation of advanced snakes in the Cenozoic era, with the resulting marked diversification in extant colubroids (Vonk et al., 2008).

Some investigators have noted the presence of paired grooves and compound serrations on the posterior teeth of *Uatchitodon schneideri*, an archosauriform[3] species from the Late Epoch of the Triassic Period (also known as the Upper Triassic and previously as the Keuper Period, approximately 230–200 mya) that is known only from dental specimens (Mitchell et al., 2010). These authors advanced the hypothesis that the described dentitional modifications were markers of the evolutionary pathway/ trajectory for oral secretion/venom delivery in amniotes as well as evidence of venom conduction in early diapsid[4] reptiles (Mitchell et al., 2010). Therefore, the aforementioned dental modifications on the fossilized teeth of *U. schneideri* were hypothetically assigned a venom-delivery function (Mitchell et al., 2010). In this, another relevant hypothesis is based on the presence of toxins (of shared classes) in oral secretions/ venoms of some lizards (e.g., the known venomous helodermatids, but also including some varanoids, iguanids, and others; see later) as well as snakes that (in this hypothesis) constitute a venom-secreting lineage of squamate reptiles belonging to a single clade (Fry et al., 2006). Thus, as mentioned previously, some researchers have suggested early evolution and subsequent derivation of venom-delivery systems (Fry et al.,

---

[3] The archosaurs, or "ruling reptiles", probably originated in the late Permian Period (approximately 250 mya), and their sauropod descendants (e.g., dinosaurs) thoroughly dominated the Mesozoic Era [approximately 250–65 mya; it was composed of the Cretaceous (about 146–65 mya), Jurassic (about 208–146 mya), and Triassic (about 245–208 mya) Periods]. The only surviving archosaurian descendants are birds and crocodilians. Relevant to the hypotheses about the evolution of venom-delivery systems is the thecodontal (teeth implanted into dentitional compartments or sockets in the jaws) condition as well as other cranial properties present in archosaurians (see Romer, 1956).

[4] Aside from the order Testudinata [turtles, terrapins, and tortoises, with only extant species recognized in the synonymous order Chelonia, are anapsids (named as most lack temporal openings in their skulls)] and a few extinct lineages, all reptiles are or were diapsids (including all of the dinosaurs), meaning that they possess(ed) two temporal openings (fenestrae) in their skulls.

2006; Mitchell et al., 2010). However, due to the limited information about the biological function(s) of some of these dental modifications and oral secretion properties in extant as well as in extinct species with very limited fossil remains, these interesting data and related hypotheses should be very cautiously considered and subjected to careful scrutiny in order to verify the proposed functions/roles (see later).

2.4 Duvernoy's Glands and Venom Glands: A Question of Semantics?

In emphasizing phylogenetic considerations, some authors have suggested abandoning terms (opisthoglyphous, rear-fanged, etc.) accentuating the enlarged maxillary teeth present in some of these colubroid taxa (Vidal et al., 2000). Others have proposed rejection of specific recognition of Duvernoy's glands, preferring to group these with venom glands as defined for venomous front-fanged species such as elapids and viperids (Fry et al., 2003, 2008). Kardong (1996), Weinstein and Kardong (1994), and Weinstein et al. (2010) have conversely suggested that Duvernoy's glands are distinctive structures associated with various types of delivery apparatus. These authors emphasized the aforementioned functional morphological differences between the Duvernoy's gland low-pressure systems in comparison with that of the high-pressure "true" venom glands (Figure 2.1). Delivery of venom or secretion volumes sufficient to cause human morbidity or mortality are certainly influenced by the nature of the delivery system as outlined above. It is noteworthy that non-front-fanged colubroid taxa widely recognized as venomous in a clinical and biological sense (e.g., *D. typus, T. kirtlandii,* and several others; see later) exhibit notably serous Duvernoy's glands with some limited muscle attachment, some venom storage capacity, a highly toxic secretion (venom), and enlarged, often grooved, posterior maxillary teeth (see Section 4.3). Therefore, the distinctive morphology of the oral glands and related delivery apparatus of these diverse snakes clearly influence their potential medical importance.

3 A Summary of the Toxinology of Duvernoy's Secretions: A Brief Overview of the History of Colubrid Oral Secretion Research

The formal scientific study of snake venoms has been a quiet but reasonably steady endeavor since the mid-nineteenth century. Since the isolation of the presynaptic neurotoxin, crotoxin, from venom of the tropical rattlesnake (*Crotalus durissus terrificus*) by Slotta and Fraenkel-Conrat in 1938, much has been learned about the composition of snake venoms. Venoms from advanced snakes such as viperids, elapids, and atractaspidids have received consistent attention from toxinologists, separation scientists (e.g., protein biochemists), pharmacologists, and other investigators. Oral secretions from other colubroids have received far less comprehensive investigation. As noted previously, many of these other species were artificially grouped together and likely have a wide array of biologically active oral secretion components. An unknown number of these snakes produce secretions or venoms/toxins of varying potency and unknown potential medical importance. Some early authors considered the possibility of "poisonings" inflicted by "harmless" snakes (Quelch, 1893). Scientific and medical interest in the potential toxicity of colubrid secretions and venoms dates from the late nineteenth century (Mackessy, 2002; Weinstein and Kardong, 1994). When considering the effects of a "jubo" [a species of West Indian racer, probably the Cuban racer, *Alsophis* (*Cubophis* Hedges et al., 2009) *cantherigerus*] perceived as nonvenomous, the Cuban physician Don Felipe Poey commented on the ability of seemingly harmless snakes suddenly to transform their "salivary glands" into "hazardous glands" when sufficiently provoked (Poey, 1873). Some mid-nineteenth century naturalists partitioned snakes into three classes: *Innocua* (considered "harmless"), *Suspecta* (not known to be venomous, but with "poisonous saliva" or with "slight" venomous quality), and *Venenosa* (known to be venomous) (Nicholson, 1874). However, others held the view that colubrid snakes collectively posed no threat. For example, Schlegel (1828) concluded that as the structures of the "parotid gland" (Duvernoy's gland) of colubrid snakes were similar to the structure of other salivary glands, and the bites of any colubrid snake were not known at the time to be fatal to man, these snakes were not truly venomous. This view persisted into the early twentieth century. Abercromby (1910) stated "With the Opisthoglypha the removal of the fangs is unnecessary, as their poison is so slight, and the grooved fangs, being at the back of the mouth, seldom enter you when they bite." This assertion did not prevent Martins (1916) from investigating the effects in animal models of Duvernoy's secretions from the Patagonian racer (*Philodryas patagoniensis*). Beginning in the early twentieth century, several

"Venomous" Bites from Non-Venomous Snakes. DOI: 10.1016/B978-0-12-387732-1.00003-8

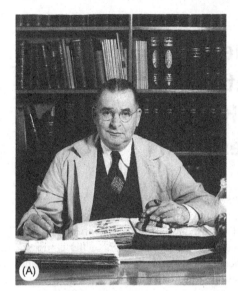
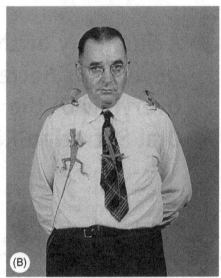

Plate 3.1 (A and B) Karl Patterson Schmidt (1890–1957). One of the influential American herpetologists of the twentieth century, Karl P. Schmidt was introduced to museum-based systematics as a scientific assistant at the American Museum of Natural History in New York City. He later became the Assistant Curator of Reptiles at the Chicago Field Museum, where he ultimately assumed the role of Chief Curator of Zoology. A graduate of Cornell University, he received Doctor of Science from Earlham College in 1952, and was elected to the National Academy of Sciences in 1956. His contributions to herpetology amounted to greater than 200 journal publications and several books, including the broadly popular *Living Reptiles of the World*, a book coauthored with Robert F. Inger, written for a general audience. His tragic fatal envenomation by a boomslang (*D. typus*), well known in herpetological history due to his own detailed, handwritten notes documenting the symptomatic time course of venom-induced coagulopathic effects, increased interest in the potentially lethal consequences of bites from non-front-fanged colubroid snakes. Date of photos unknown; copyright to Kraig Adler.

investigators noted the unexpected fatal consequences of human envenomings inflicted by colubrid snakes of certain genera (*Dispholidus* and *Thelotornis*; FitzSimons, 1909, 1912; FitzSimons and Smith, 1958; Pope, 1958). The tragic deaths in 1957 and 1975, respectively, of the prominent herpetologists, Karl Patterson Schmidt (1890–1957; Plate 3.1A and B) and Robert Friedrich Wilhelm Mertens (1894–1975; Plate 3.2) focused increased attention on the toxic potential of some colubrid species previously viewed as "mildly venomous" or having "mildly toxic saliva" (Weinstein and Kardong, 1994).

Researchers in the 1960s and early 1970s initiated closer examination of the potential toxicity of secretions produced by various colubrid species. Minton and Minton (1969) and Mebs (1978) considered the occurrence of toxic secretions among the Colubridae and began investigating their properties. Important contributions were made by a small cadre of researchers, including Taub (1966), Minton (1974), and Mebs et al. (1978), who examined the toxicity of colubrid oral gland secretions and

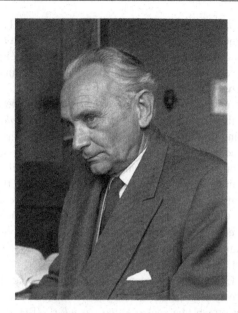

Plate 3.2 Robert Friedrich Wilhelm Mertens (1894–1975). One of the most important and prolifically published herpetologists of the twentieth century, Robert Mertens began his career as a research assistant at the Senckenberg Museum, Frankfurt am Main, Germany. In less than 10 years, his intense intellect and energy led to his rapid progression to Curator of Herpetology at the museum. He eventually became Director of the Senckenberg Research Institute and Nature Museum as a full professor. Among some of the specimens maintained in his home vivarium was a Kirtlands' twig snake (*T. kirtlandii*). While feeding a lizard to this specimen, he received a brief bite on a finger. This led to a protracted course of consumptive coagulopathy including disseminated intravascular coagulation, and a hemorrhagic cerebral infarct that ultimately resulted in his death. During his final days, he wrote a diary entry, "Für Herpetologen Einzig Angemessene ende" ("A fitting end for a herpetologist"). He had received an inconsequential bite from the same snake just weeks before the fatal envenomation. Date of photo unknown; copyright to Kraig Adler.

the possible role of various species in human envenoming. McKinstry (1978, 1983) reviewed colubrid species that possessed toxic secretions and glands that may be associated with enlarged grooved or ungrooved, posterior maxillary teeth. Vest (1988) reported lethal potency and bioactivity of secretions from *Hypsiglena torquata* (night snake). Boquet and Saint Girons (1972) and Minton and Weinstein (1987) found that many of these secretions exhibited complex immuno-identity with medically important elapid venoms. However, little immunological relationship was found between colubrid secretions and those of viperids. Although bites by many of these non-front-fanged colubroids cause only minor local edema and lacerations, the species of the genera currently known to be most toxic to humans (*Dispholidus*, *Thelotornis*, and *Rhabdophis*) produce consumptive coagulopathy due to Factor X and prothrombin activators and, in some, due to probable disintegrins and rhexic hemorrhagins present in these venoms (Bradlow et al., 1980; Ferlan et al., 1983; Kamiguti et al., 2000;

Kornalik and Táborská, 1978; Sawai et al., 1985; Zotz et al., 1991). Thus, the majority of well-documented medically important effects are due to procoagulant toxins functioning as those often observed in some viperid and Australian elapid venoms. These venoms have been previously reviewed (Mackessy, 2002; Weinstein and Kardong, 1994) and are considered further in Section 4.3.

Knowledge of the nature of constituent toxins present in these secretions began to accumulate with the fractionation of venoms from *Malpolon monspessulanus* (Montpellier snake) and *Spalerosophis* spp. (diadem or camel snakes; approximately five species) (Rosenberg et al., 1985). Much of the work on secretions and venoms from these colubroids has been hampered by limited availability of secretions and very low yields obtained by extraction. Rosenberg et al. (1985) addressed this problem by recommending the use of parasympathomimetic agents, such as pilocarpine, while collecting the secretion using a capillary pipette. This technique has been modified and used effectively in order to procure samples for more extensive pharmacological and biochemical/structural analyses (Fry et al., 2003; Hill and Mackessy, 1997, 2000; Pawlak et al., 2006, 2009).

Use of FPLC, HPLC, online mass spectroscopy, and other separation modalities facilitated the continuing analysis of several colubrid secretions/venoms, including that of the ecologically important brown tree snake, *Boiga irregularis* (Broaders et al., 1999; Fry et al., 2003; Hill and Mackessy, 2000; Mackessy et al., 2006; Pawlak et al., 2006, 2009; Weinstein and Smith, 1993; Weinstein et al., 1991). Renewed attention to this understudied area resulted in studies of other colubrid species of regional medical importance [e.g., *Philodryas olfersii* (Lichtenstein's or green racer) in Brazil (Ribeiro et al., 1999) and Argentina (Acosta de Pérez et al., 2003); *P. patagoniensis* (Patagonian racer) in Argentina (Peichoto et al., 2005); and *Thamnodynastes stigilis* (northern coastal house snake) in Venezuela (Lemoine et al., 2004a)]. Comprehensive reviews of colubrid secretions and venoms and reported colubrid envenomations (Mackessy, 2002; Minton, 1990; Warrell, 2004; Weinstein and Kardong, 1994) stimulated further investigations.

With the advent of proteomics and genomic arrays, the study of these secretions and venoms has accelerated and advanced. Properties and/or partial primary sequences of several saliva and venom/secretion components were reported by Hill and Mackessy (2000). A complete sequence for a "three-finger-fold" postsynaptically active neurotoxin[1] ("colubritoxin") isolated from secretion of the radiated rat snake [*Coelognathus* (*Elaphe* Fitzinger, 1833) *radiatus*; Utiger et al., 2005] was elucidated by Fry et al. (2003). Lumsden et al. (2005) reported weak postsynaptic and prejunctional neurotoxicity induced by a three-finger toxin ("boigatoxin A" isolated from Duvernoy's secretion of the mangrove snake, *Boiga dendrophila*) in rat skeletal muscle and smooth muscle (vas deferens), respectively. Avian and/or saurian-specific three-finger neurotoxins, "denmotoxin" and "irditoxin," were structurally and functionally characterized from *B. dendrophila* and *B. irregularis* secretions, respectively (Pawlak et al., 2006, 2009), confirming previous observations suggesting the presence of neurotoxins in their secretions

---

[1] "Three-finger-fold" neurotoxins were previously classified as various types of short-chain or long-chain postsynaptic neurotoxins. These were structurally grouped according to the numbers of amino acids and disulfide bonds comprising a given characterized toxin.

(Broaders et al., 1999; Weinstein et al., 1993). Previous investigations had suggested the presence of postsynaptically active neurotoxins in other colubrid secretions, such as those from *Boiga blandingi* (Blanding's tree snake—Broaders et al., 1999; Levinson et al., 1976; Weinstein and Smith, 1993), *P. olfersii* (Prado-Franceschi et al., 1996), *Heterodon platirhinos* (eastern hognose snake; Young, 1992), *Thamnodynastes stigilis* (Lemoine et al., 2004a), and others. Recent electrophysiological investigations have demonstrated the presence of neurotoxins in secretions from *Trimorphodon biscutatus* (lyre snake), *Telescopus dhara* (large-eyed or Israeli cat snake), *Psammophis mossambicus* (olive whip snake) and several additional *Boiga* spp. (Lumsden et al., 2004) as well as the African beaked snake, *Rhamphiophis oxyrhynchus* (Lumsden et al., 2005). In addition, the Duvernoy's secretion ("venom") of some species, such as the Puerto Rican racer, *Alsophis* (*Borikenophis*; Hedges et al., 2009) *portoricensis*, contains components such as cysteine-rich secretory proteins (CRISPs) that probably function as ion channel regulating proteins. One of these had sequence homology with tigrin, a CRISP isolated from venom of *R. tigrinus* (Weldon and Mackessy, 2010). Another CRISP isolated from secretion of *P. patagoniensis* was myotoxic (Peichoto et al., 2009). "Helicopsin," a CRISP characterized from Duvernoy's secretion of *Helicops angulatus* (South American or broad-banded water snake; water mapepire) caused rapid death of mice following i.p. injection (minimal lethal dose was 0.4 mg/kg, tested in a small group of mice; Estrella et al., 2010).

Some Duvernoy's secretions exhibit prey-specific immobilization functions. Neill (1954) described the quiescent effect on prey of *Rhadinea flavilata* (pinewoods or yellow-lipped snake) oral secretions. As a specific example, fish are a favored prey of *Helicops* spp. (South American water snakes). When fish are injected with oral secretions from *Helicops* spp., they show decreased opercular activity and a 30-min period of immobilization followed by death (Albolea et al., 2000). Reports of immobility and/or death induced as a result of bites inflicted on squamate prey species by *Diadophis punctatus* ssp. (ringneck snakes) suggest the use of Duvernoy's secretions in prey subjugation (Anton, 1994; Gehlbach, 1974; Mackessy, 2002). O'Donnell et al. (2007) reported lethal effects of *D. p. occidentalis* (northwestern ringneck snake) oral secretions injected intra-abdominally into the natricine colubrid, *Thamnophis ordinoides* (northwestern gartersnake), a natural prey species. It is noteworthy that all doses used by these investigators resulted in 100% mortality of the injected snakes within 3 h. Several observers have reported active engagement of the enlarged posterior maxillary teeth of *A. portoricensis* during prey capture with seized anoline lizards exhibiting concomitantly decreased struggling movements (Rodriguez-Robles, 1992; Rodriguez-Robles and Thomas, 1992; Weldon and Mackessy, 2010; see later). However, it can be observed that often there is a wide variation in observations that are interpreted as use of Duvernoy's secretions in prey handling. For example, oral secretions of *S. mikani* immobilized slugs (Salamão and Laporta-Ferreira, 1994), and a black-fronted nunbird (*Monasa nigrifrons*) grasped by a green vine snake (*Oxybelis fulgidus*), appeared immobilized (without constriction) and was swallowed by the snake without significant struggle (Endo et al., 2007). On the other hand, an *O. fulgidus* seized the head of a large Central American whiptail lizard (*Ameiva festiva*), and held its "frantically" moving prey for an estimated 15 min. The lizard succumbed shortly thereafter, and was swallowed by the snake in approximately 10 min (Pineda Lizano, 2010). A Central American cat-eyed snake (*Leptodeira septentrionalis polysticta*) immobilized a Mexican blue-spotted treefrog (*Smilisca cyanosticta*) by "chewing" the frog's hind-leg "until the rear fangs were engaged" (Hernández-Ríos et al., 2011). Three minutes after being seized by the snake, the frog's movements ceased, and it was swallowed (Hernández-Ríos et al., 2011). Differences in observations of natural prey handling may be related to the prey specificity of toxins present in Duvernoy's secretions or venoms, and/or the individual prey-specific capture strategy, as well as the successful introduction of Duvernoy's secretions into the seized prey. In comparison with their lethal potency for mice, Duvernoy's secretions from *B. irregularis* had markedly higher toxicity for scincid and gekkonid lizards as well as domestic chickens, suggesting prey specificity of these secretions (Mackessy et al., 2006). As noted above, the presence of prey-specific toxins in oral secretions of these snakes has been established by the characterization of saurian and avian-specific neurotoxins from Duvernoy's secretions of *B. dendrophila* and *B. irregularis* (Pawlak et al., 2006, 2009). Thus, as evidence of active biological use of Duvernoy's secretions in prey subjugation is accumulated, combined with verified toxicity in various natural prey species, some of these secretions will accommodate the current defining criteria for "venom" and will likely be so classified.[2]

The similarity of chromatographic and antigenic complexity of venoms from viperids, elapids, and the Duvernoy's secretions from other colubroids has been noted by investigators (Fry et al., 2003; Mackessy, 2002; Weinstein and Smith, 1993). Characterization of a Duvernoy's gland transcriptome from *P. olfersii* revealed venom constituents and complexity similar to that of viperids (Ching et al., 2006). An earlier genomic analysis reported toxin classes common to many venomous front-fanged colubroid taxa present among the non-front-fanged colubroids examined (Fry et al., 2003). Transcriptomic and proteomic analysis of Duvernoy's secretion ("venom") of the dog-faced water snake (*Cerberus rhynchops*) characterized a new group of proteins, the "ryncolins" (the proposed protein family was named "veficolins," for "venom ficolins"; OmPraba et al., 2010). These proteins showed sequence homology with ficolin, a mammalian protein with collagen-like and fibrinogen-like domains, prompting speculation that ryncolins might induce platelet aggregation and/or initiate complement activation (OmPraba et al., 2010). A recent comparative evaluation of Duvernoy's gland ("venom gland") morphology and transcriptomes of representative colubroid genera supported the concept of shared toxin classes among many genera of advanced snakes, including former colubrid genera, viperids, and elapids (Fry et al., 2008).

Continuing analysis of Duvernoy's secretions and venoms from these diverse snake species may identify a pool of biomedically useful components. The characterization of these may provide tools useful in laboratory medicine (especially in blood coagulation studies), and possibly, pharmacotherapeutics. Such investigations may also clarify some of the medical effects observed after bites inflicted by some of these non-front-fanged colubroid species.

---

[2] To date, expert consensus defines venom as a toxic substance produced in a highly developed secretory organ or group of cells that is delivered by the act of biting or stinging, typically via a specialized apparatus. These substances are deleterious to other organisms at a certain dosage and are actively used in prey acquisition and/or defense (Mebs, 1978, 2002; Minton, 1974; Minton and Minton, 1980; Russell, 1980).

4 Medically Significant Bites by "Colubrid" Snakes

4.1 Typical Features of Documented Cases and Evidence-Based Risk

Some circumstantial evidence is very strong, as when you find a trout in the milk.

Thoreau (1850)

Review of several hundred published case reports or accounts of bites by "colubrid" snakes indicated that these reported incidents involved at least 100 taxa (Table 4.1). When critically reviewed, the vast majority of these (approximately 71.5%) featured only minor pain, puncture wounds/lacerations, and very mild local effects (e.g., slight reactive edema, brief bleeding), without any lasting sequelae. Most reported symptoms/signs resolved within 24h after the bite. Approximately 24 taxa (28.5% of the cases reviewed) inflicted bites that resulted in medically significant effects. Although this is notably subjective, a medically significant bite is defined as one with clinically detectable pathology sufficient to cause the patient distress along with some observed progression of the symptoms/signs. In a relatively small number of these cases, the symptoms/signs did not fully resolve for several days, weeks, or even months.

"Venomous" Bites from Non-Venomous Snakes. DOI: 10.1016/B978-0-12-387732-1.00004-X

Table 4.1 Summary of Published Cases of Medically Significant Colubrid Bites

Taxa Frequent, Common Name(s)	Reports (Cases)	Reported Effects {Comments}	Reference	Evidence Rating[a]
Ahaetulla nasuta (Plate 4.1A and B) Green whip snake, Green vine snake, Asian vine snake; ahaetulla, kan kuthi pambu; pachchai pambu; as gulla (regional names for this species are influenced by local beliefs and often refer to it as "eye plucker"; see text)	2 (7)	BL, E, P ("slight"), Pr {3/6 persons bitten reportedly had no symptoms. Subaraj (2008) and Campden-Main (1970) reported no effects from bites inflicted by *A. prasina*. Available information indicates mild, transient local effects}	Abercromby (1910); Deraniyagala (1955); Whitaker (1970); De Silva and Aloysius (1983); Daniel (1983)	C/D
Alsophis (Cubophis, Hedges et al., 2009) ***cantherigerus*** (Reinhardt and Lütken, 1862) Cuban racer; jubo	1 (2)	E, P {Bite wounds described as "troublesome lesions." This species may be the *A. angulifer* of Minton (1990). Neill (1954) described "streaks" (possibly minor ecchymoses) and erythema from a bite by *Alsophis* spp.}	Poey (1873); Neill (1954); Jaume and Garrido (1980); Jaume (1983)	C/D
Alsophis (Borikenophis, Hedges et al., 2009) ***portoricensis*** (Reinhardt and Lütken, 1862) (Plate 4.2A–F) Puerto Rican racer; culebra corredora; culebra corredora puertorriqueña (Plate 4.3A–C illustrate *A. sibonius*; Plate 4.3D–E show *A. rufiventris*)	3 (8) Note: One of the victims in the case series reported by García-Gubern et al. (2010) was bitten by an unverified species, likely an *A. portoricensis*	Bs, E, Ecc, HM, P, PA, Pr {In the case reported by Heatwole and Banuchi (1966), the victim's wound was incised and drained. There was reportedly rapid progression of edema from arm to axilla, and involving the upper pectoralis. Patient was given "gas gangrene polyvalent antitoxin" that likely caused delayed Type III immune complex disease. The patient was treated with steroids and antibiotics. García-Gubern et al. (2010) reported six *A. portoricensis* bites (five verified and one presumed) that occurred from 1998 to 2007. All of the bites were protracted (the snake remained attached for 1–4 min) and	Heatwole and Banuchi (1966); Rodríguez-Robles and Thomas (1992); García-Gubern et al. (2010); Weldon and Mackessy (2010); this report	B/C

were inflicted on the victims' fingers. Four of six victims had edema that progressed from the affected hand to the elbow, and the edema reportedly reached the shoulder in 2/6. All of the victims reported symptom resolution within 10 days, although one patient described persistent episodic "cold sensitivity" at the wound site. Local blistering occurred in one patient, and all laboratory investigations in the series were unremarkable. None of the victims had neurovascular compromise. Three of the victims were below age 21 years, and one (13 years) reported two episodes of vomiting after being bitten (see Sections 4.4—4.6 regarding autonomic responses to snake bite). Another pediatric patient (age 15 years) was a Type 1 diabetic, but fortunately had an uncomplicated course. It is noteworthy that one of the pediatric victims was transferred for surgical evaluation (e.g., fasciotomy) in order to rule out compartmental syndrome (see the reviewed case of *Philodryas viridissimus* bite for relevant discussion about the need for careful evaluation of snake bite local effects). Fortunately, the edema and ecchymoses resolved, and he was discharged. Treatment of these patients included: antihistamines, nonsteroidal anti-inflammatory drugs, steroids, antibiotics, and tetanus prophylaxis. Rodriguez-Robles and Thomas (1992) briefly described their respective bites from *A. portoricensis*

(Continued)

Table 4.1 (*Continued*)

Taxa Frequent, Common Name(s)	Reports (Cases)	Reported Effects {Comments}	Reference	Evidence Rating[a]
		(neither was medically reviewed). They reported minor local effects (e.g., "burning sensation, itching, swelling"), and mentioned "impaired coagulation" without any supporting laboratory investigations that are required for a diagnosis of coagulopathy. These cases are not included in those tallied here. Weldon and Mackessy (2010) also communicated an anecdotal case that described many of the aforementioned signs/symptoms as well as "arthralgia." An *A. portoricensis* bite is further detailed in Section 4.2, and the effects of this bite are illustrated in Plate 4.4}		
Amplorhinus multimaculatus Multi-spotted snake, Cape reed snake	1	Er, E, P ("burning") {The limited available information suggests mild local effects}	Blake (1959); Marais (1992)	C/D
Apostolepis spp. South American burrowing snakes (approximately 26 species; this common name is applied to many diverse genera)	1 (14)	E, Er, L, P, "local hemorrhage" {Reported as part of a retrospective review (see text), original case documentation unavailable and species identification/verification are unknown. "Local hemorrhage," P, Er were respectively the most commonly recorded signs/symptoms (33.3%, 28.6%, and 28.5%)}	Salomao et al. (2003)	C/D

Atractus spp. Central and South American ground snakes (approximately 112 species; shares this general common name with other genera, e.g., *Liophis* spp.)	1 (29)	L, P {Reported as part of a retrospective review (see text), original case documentation unavailable and species identification/verification are unknown. Recorded symptoms/signs suggest very mild effects}	Salomao et al. (2003)	C/D
Balanophis ceylonensis (*Rhabdophis*, Wall, 1921, *Amphiesma*, Wall, 1921) Sri Lankan keel-back, flower or blossom krait; nihaluwa; others	1	E, Er, HA, P {Limited information suggests mild local effects and minor autonomic (possibly anxiety-driven) response}	De Silva and Aloysius (1983)	C/D
Boiga (*Toxicodryas*, Trape and Mané, 2006) *blandingi* (Plate 4.5A and B) Blanding's tree snake, Blanding's cat snake, Temankeema, others	3 (3)	BL, L, P {Goodman (1985) experienced a mild, insignificant bite but cautioned regarding the potential hazard posed by this species. A similar subjective caution was articulated by Spawls (1979). See Section 4.2}	Pitman (1974); Spawls (1979); Goodman (1985); Weinstein and Smith (1993)	C
Boiga ceylonensis Sri Lankan cat snake, Ceylon cat snake; nidi mapila	1	BL, E, Pr {De Silva (1976b) reported insignificant effects from bites by this species)	Whitaker (1970)	C/D
Boiga cyanea (Plate 4.6) Green cat-eyed snake, green cat snake	1	BL, Er, L {Bite experienced by one of the authors (SAW) was inflicted by a 90-cm female specimen. Minor bleeding, mild pain, and erythema resulted from the bite. There were no sequelae and the symptoms/signs resolved in <24h. Similarly, the few anecdotally reported bites (not included in the tally here) included only mild local effects. Interestingly, De Lisle (1984) described the bite inflicted by a captive *B. cyanea* on another specimen. The bitten *B. cyanea* gradually succumbed, and this was ascribed to the effects of the bite}	This report	C

(Continued)

Table 4.1 *(Continued)*

Taxa Frequent, Common Name(s)	Reports (Cases)	Reported Effects {Comments}	Reference	Evidence Rating[a]
Boiga dendrophila (Plate 4.7A–D) (including approximately nine subspecies) Mangrove snake, Mangrove cat snake, Gold-ringed catsnake, ular tetak mas; ular katam tebu; oraj taliwangsa; oraj santja manuk; tetak emas; bangkit (many others depending on locale and subspecies)	2 (2)	P, E {The case reported by Monk (1991) included "metallic taste, joint pain, and slight fever." Trestrail (1982) mentioned an admission of an individual bitten by a captive *B. dendrophila* without further detail. Minton and Dunson (1978) noted two cases of *B. d. multicinctus* bites with minor local effects. Several cases posted on the internet describe and illustrate significant local effects such as blistering. These cases are not included in the tally here. See Section 4.2 and Appendix A}	Burger (1975); Monk (1991)	C/D
Boiga forsteni (Plate 4.8) Forstens' tree snake, Forstens' cat snake; naga mapila; le mapila; poonai pambu; others	1	"Giddiness" {Limited information; case must be classified as anecdotal. These snakes have a sensationalized reputation on Sri Lanka, and in some regions are greatly feared. There is no available information that supports any medical significance of their bites}	De Silva and Aloysius (1983)	D

Boiga irregularis (Plate 4.9A–F) Brown tree snake, Brown cat snake	4 + series ($n = 11$) from unpublished survey (450) Note: There are additional recorded bites, some with limited documentation. Only representative cases with detailed information are included here	E, Ecc, L, N, P, Pt, V {All purported cases (from Guam) that reported exhibiting "neurotoxicity," "lethargy," or "respiratory difficulty" involved infants. An Australian case involving a protracted bite inflicted by a captive specimen featured "persistent vomiting" and "severe" edema. See Section 4.4 for discussion of these cases}	Fritts et al. (1990, 1994); Sutherland and Tibballs (2001); Morocco et al. (2006); this report	B/C
Boiga nigriceps Dark (black)-headed cat snake, Red-eyed catsnake; ular banjang	1	E, Ecc, Er, P {Some symptoms described as "severe." Further information and clinical evaluation of any additional cases are needed. Available information suggests only mild local effects}	Cox (1991)	C/D
Boiruna maculata[b] Mussurana; culebra de sangra; vibora luta, others Note: Both *Clelia* spp. and *Boiruna* sp. are commonly called "mussurana"	1	E, Ecc, Er, H, Ly {Report includes description of "discrete cyanosis" in the area surrounding the bite wound on the left ankle. Patient was an approximately 15-month-old infant bitten at night in her crib. See comparison with *B. irregularis* cases in Section 4.4}	Santos-Costa et al. (2000)	C/D

(Continued)

Table 4.1 (*Continued*)

Taxa Frequent, Common Name(s)	Reports (Cases)	Reported Effects {Comments}	Reference	Evidence Rating[a]
Cerberus rynchops (Plate 4.10A–C) Bockadam, Dog-faced watersnake; Kuna diya kaluwa; Birang; others	Precise number unclear due to multiple anecdotal reports	{Ramachandran et al. (1995) mentioned one case without any detail. Subaraj (2008) and Campden-Main (1970) reported insignificant effects of bites. Saha and Hati (1998) surveyed several districts in West Bengal and reported circumstances surrounding 157 nonvenomous bites from *C. rhynchops*, *Lycodon aulicus*, and *Ptyas mucosus*. There were an indeterminate number of bites from each species in the series, all of which were insignificant. None of these are included here due to lack of clinical detail}	De Silva and Aloysius (1983); There are no well-documented, specifically described cases. This taxon is included due to oft repeated concerns and plentiful presence within natural range.	IE
Chironius spp. (species not designated) Sipo; Cipo; Machete Savane; Liana snake; Tree snake (13 species; common names vary/shared per individual species)	1 (81)	E, L, P, "local hemorrhage" {Reported as part of a retrospective review (see text), original case documentation unavailable and species identification/verification are unknown. Review probably included multiple species. L and P were the most common respective symptom/signs (43.8% and 37.5%)}	Salomão et al. (2003)	C/D
Chrysopelea pelias Twin-barred tree snake, Twin-barred flying snake (Plate 4.11A and B; Plate 4.11C and D illustrate two additional taxa of *Chrysopelea* spp.; some local names for these species may include: dibomina; ular petola; ular jelotong; ule alo; timbulus; others as well)	1	E, HT, P, PA {One episode of HT during presentation was reported. This case must be considered presumed or alleged as the snake was found next to the victim immediately after the reported bite, but was not observed biting the victim. Several authors have described medically insignificant bites inflicted by *C. paradisi* (De Silva, 1990a,b; Gopalakrishnakone and Chou, 1990; Subaraj, 2008)}	Ismail et al. (2010)	C/D

Clelia clelia (Plate 4.12A and B illustrate *C. occipitoleutea*; a taxonomically problematic species) Mussurana; Mustarangue; Mussuvana; Moon snake; others	1	Er, H, "necrosis" {In their retrospective review, Salomão et al. (2003) reported three bites from *Clelia* spp. without detail. These cases are not included in the tally here. Additional data and cases are required in order to assess potential incidence of wound complications such as "necrosis" as reported in this single documented case of a bite by this species}	Chippaux (1986)	C/D
Clelia c. plumbea[b] (*C. plumbea*, Zaher, 1996; Pizzatto, 2005) Mussurana	1	E, H, L {Limited available information}	Pinto-Leite et al. (1991)	C/D
Coluber (Platyceps, Schätti and Monsch, 2004) *najadum* (Schmidt, 1939; Szczerbak, 2003) (Plate 4.13A–C) Dahls' whipsnake; Ghamcheh snake; Light green whipsnake; others	2 (2)	E, L, P (mild) "fatal progressive segmental neuropathy[c]" {In the case published by Chroni et al. (2005), the identity of the snake responsible for the reported bite was not verified, and thus it is only a presumed bite by this species. The patient exhibited delayed pyrexia and myalgia, and was treated with i.v. steroids and tetanus prophylaxis. See Section 4.4 for further comments. There is no question about the identity of the snake in the case illustrated by Trapp (2007) as it is shown delivering the described bite! The bite caused only mild local edema, and puncture wounds. There is no conclusive evidence of any serious medical sequelae from bites by this species}	Chroni et al (2005); Trapp (2007)	C/D

(Continued)

Table 4.1 (*Continued*)

Taxa Frequent, Common Name(s)	Reports (Cases)	Reported Effects {Comments}	Reference	Evidence Rating[a]
Coluber* (*Platyceps*,** Nagy et al., 2004a) ***rhodorachis (Szczerbak, 2003) (Plate 4.14) Jans' desert racer, Cliff racer; Braid snake; Jeier; difen; others	4 (8)	Bs, E, Er, L, Ly, P ("tenderness"), PA {Branch (1982) described the effects as "milder" than those from *Hemorrhois* (*Coluber*) *ravergieri*. In the cases reported by Malik (1995), one featured leukocytosis and two had elevated CK, but there were no specific systemic findings. Further information is required in order to fully evaluate any potential risk associated with this species}	Branch (1982); Pery (1988); Malik (1995); this report (Alexander Westerström, personal verbal communication with DAW, September 2010)	C/D
Coluber rubriceps Red-headed whipsnake, Red whipsnake	1	Er, E (mild), L, P {Mild, insignificant and transient local effects (see Plate 4.15)}	This report (Tomer Beker, personal written communication with SAW, April 2009)	C/D
Coluber* (*Hierophis*,** Nagy et al., 2004a) ***viridiflavus (Schätti and Wilson, 1986) (Plate 4.16A–D) Green whipsnake, Western whipsnake; Gelbgrüne zornnatter	1	Pt, V, Ver {Authors reported that patient exhibited "major muscular weakness" and "neck weakness." Patient was managed in the ICU and authors weighed intoxication versus "toxic saliva" as the primary etiology. See Section 4.4 for further commentary}	Bedry et al. (1998)	C/D
Coniophanes imperialis Black-striped snake; Culebra de raya negra; others	2 (3)	DW, E, Er, P, Pr, PA {"Intense, throbbing pain" was reported by Lee (1996)}	Brown (1939); Lee (1996)	C/D

Species	No.	Effects	References	
Conophis lineatus (Plate 4.17A and B) Guardo camino, Lined road guarder; others	3 (3)	BL ("persistent"), E, Er {A specimen responsible for a bite was misidentified as *Stenorrhina freminvillei* in an original case account (Cook, 1984). The identification was corrected in a subsequent paper (Johnson, 1988). Johanbocke (1974) reported E and Er in upper arm after a bite on digits. Two communicated anecdotal cases included immediate (transient) bleeding, discoloration, and swelling that resolved after 2 h. These are not included in the tally here}	Johanbocke (1974); Cook (1984); Johnson (1988); Lee (1996); this report (Roy McDiarmid, personal verbal communication with DAW, September 2010; also see Warrell, 2004 for additional references)	C/D
Conophis vittatus Striped road guarder; Culebra listada; Culebra de cuatro lineas; others	2 (2)	P, E {Mild local effects}	Taylor and Smith (1938); Johnson (1988)	C/D
Crotaphopeltis hotamboeia (Plate 4.18A–C) Herald snake, Red or white-lipped snake; Rooilipslang; Pimpi; others	1	P, E {Mild, transient local effects. Blaylock (1982) reported two insignificant bites. These are not included in the tally here}	Chapman (1968); Branch (1982)	C/D
Crisantophis nevermanni Dunn's road guarder	1	E {Limited information suggests mild local effects. A diurnal and crepuscular monotypic species with relatively little-known natural history. Reportedly favors saurian prey, but is an opportunistic feeder, and may be semiaquatic}	Villa (1969)	C/D

(Continued)

Table 4.1 (*Continued*)

Taxa Frequent, Common Name(s)	Reports (Cases)	Reported Effects {Comments}	Reference	Evidence Rating[a]
Dendrelaphis papuensis (O'Shea, 1995) (*Ahaetulla papuae*, Neill, 1949) Papuan tree snake	1	E, Er, P {"axillary swelling"; limited information. Available information suggests only mild, transient local effects, and additional clinical information is required in order to fully assess the potential effects of bites by any of the approximately 23 species of *Dendrelaphis*}	Neill (1949)	C/D
Diadophis punctatus (Plate 4.19) Ring-neck snake; culebra de collar (others depending on subspecies and locale)	2 (2)	E, Er, P {Bites by this species are uncommon and available information suggests only very mild, transient local effects. Myers (1965) communicated anecdotal reports of transient "burning" effects of bites, and remarked about the lack of reported protracted bites by this species. *Diadophis* spp. likely have what may be best termed "prey-specific venom" as it probably has some specificity for squamate reptiles, particularly other semi-fossorial snakes. See text}	Myers (1965); Shaw and Campbell (1974)	C/D
Dipsadoboa aulica Marbled tree snake, Cross-barred treesnake	1	P, E {Limited information}	Branch (1982)	C/D
Dispholidus typus[b,d] (Plate 4.20A–G) Boomslang; Gewone boomslang; n' dlondlo; Coracundu; others	25 (63) This is a representative tally of cases selected due to their well-documented	AEM, ALFT, An, ARF, CCo (DIC), H, Ep, BG, BL, F, HA, He, HT, HUS, L, LOC, Mel, N, OL, Sh, Thr {Several patients required dialysis and were given repetitive transfusion of PRBC. Reported also was blephedema, ocular hemorrhage, and periorbital ecchymoses. Several patients	FitzSimons (1919, 1962); Christensen (1955); Pope (1958); Lakier and Fritz (1969); Broadley (1960); Spies et al. (1962); MacKay et al. (1969);	A

(Continued)

	clinical detail and/ or historical importance		
	attempted first-aid using cut/extraction of wound. Matell et al. (1973) treated their patient with blood transfusions, heparin, and monovalent antivenom. Bajaj et al. (1980) treated a presumed *D. typus* bite with polyvalent antivenom. Vaughan and Lobetti (1995) reported a veterinary case per hemorrhagic diathesis in a dog with subsequent reversal from monovalent antivenom. Four communicated cases that have occurred since 2006 are described in the Epidemiology section. These cases are not included in the tally here. See Epidemiology and Section 4.3 for further discussion. Plate 4.20L–O illustrate some of the ecchymotic effects that may be caused by serious *D. typus* envenomation}	Wapnick et al. (1972); Matell et al. (1973); Nicolson et al. (1974); Gomperts and Demetriou (1977); Du Toit (1980); Gerber and Adendorff (1980); Geddes and Thomas (1985); Branch and McCartney (1986); McNally and Reitz (1987); Haagner and Smit (1987); Reitz (1989); Aitchison (1990); this report	
Dryophis nasutus (Smith, 1943) (= **Ahaetulla nasuta** Cox et al., 1998)	1	See *Ahaetulla nasuta*	Whitaker (1970)	C/D
Enhydris (Hypsirhina, Duméril et al., 1854) **enhydris** (Cox et al., 1998) Schneider's water snake; Rainbow water snake; ular ajer (Plate 4.21A and B, **E. bocourti; E. plumbea**)	1	P ("throbbing"), Er {36-year-old victim bitten while attempting to catch "irritated" snake (1 ft in length). Insignificant bleeding ("scarcely 2 drops"). Pain lasted <1h with no further effects noted. See Plate 4.21C for a photo of local effects after a bite by *E. plumbea*}	D'Abreu (1931); Daniel (1983)	C/D
Erythrolamprus spp. (species not designated) False coral snakes (six species; this common name is used for several other genera, e.g., see *Pliocercus*)	1 (10)	Er, L, P "local hemorrhage" {Part of a retrospective review (see Section 4.1), original case documentation is unavailable. Available data (including next table entry), support mild, local effects}	Salomão et al. (2003)	C/D

Table 4.1 (*Continued*)

Taxa Frequent, Common Name(s)	Reports (Cases)	Reported Effects {Comments}	Reference	Evidence Rating[a]
Erythrolamprus aesculapii False-coral snake; boi-cora; bacora , cobra coral; falsa coral de aesculapi	2 (2) Note: The actual number of individual cases is unclear due to possibly duplicated reports. Thus, the number here is conservative	E, P {Available information suggests only mild local effects}	Quelch (1893); Martins (1916); Silver-Júnior (1956)	C/D
Erythrolamprus bizona False coral snake; falsa coral	1	E, Ecc, P {Quelch (1893) anecdotally reported persistent edema and pain from several bites from *Erythrolamprus* spp. These were not detailed and are not included in the tally here}	Gutiérrez and Mahmood (2002)	C/D
***Helicops* spp.** (species unidentified) South American water snakes; South American keel-backs; other names depending on species (16 species; see other entries)	1 (427)	E, Er, L, P, "local hemorrhage" {Reported as part of a retrospective review (see text), original case documentation unavailable and species identification/verification are unknown. Cases likely involve multiple species of *Helicops*; it is unclear if confirmed identification was established of snakes involved in all of these cases. Salomão et al. (2003) attributed reported "local hemorrhage" to action of Duvernoy's secretions along with skin perforation from the inflicted bite}	Salomão et al. (2003)	C/D

Species	No.	Notes	References	
Helicops angulatus South American water snake; Water mapepire; Mountain keel-back; others	3 (4)	E, Ecc, L, P {Two cases were communicated (written, April 2010) by Prof. William Lamar to SAW. One produced minor pain and erythema, the second caused more marked local reaction including boggy edema. An additional case was communicated to DAW (written, September 2010) by Zoltan Tacáks). The bite caused only several uncomplicated puncture wounds, Plate 4.22}	Warrell (2004); Quelch (1893); this report	C/D
Helicops tapajonicus Tapajos water snake	1	E, Er, L, P {Mild local effects}	This report (Prof. William Lamar, personal written communication with SAW, March 2009)	C/D
Hemorrhois (Coluber, Szczerbak, 2003) nummifer (Nagy et al., 2004a) (Plate 4.23A–C) Coin snake, Asian racer	1	E (mild), Er, L, P {Mild local effects. See Plate 4.23D–F}	This report (Tomer Beker, personal written communication with SAW, April 2009)	C/D
Hemorrhois (Coluber, Szczerbak, 2003) ravergieri (Nagy et al., 2004a; Schätti and Monsch, 2004) Mountain racer, Leopard snake; others	3 (3)	BL, E, L, P {Mamonov (1977) reported "bluish" coloration in edematous limb}	Mamonov (1977); Ishunin (1950)	C/D
Heterodon nasicus (Plate 4.24A–C) Western hognose snake, Spreading adder; culebra nariz de cerdo occidental; others	7 (7)	BL, Bs, DW, E, L, Ly, P {Most of these uncommon bites occurred while a captive specimen was offered food. The majority were protracted bites that required forcible removal of the snake from the victim. A few patients reported arthropathy and compromised range of motion of affected extremities that persisted for as long as several months. See Plate 4.24D–J}	Bragg (1960); Morris (1985); Phillips et al. (1997); Walley (2002); Averill-Murray (2006); Warrell (2009); Weinstein and Keyler (2009)	B/C

(Continued)

Table 4.1 (*Continued*)

Taxa Frequent, Common Name(s)	Reports (Cases)	Reported Effects {Comments}	Reference	Evidence Rating[a]
Heterodon platirhinos (Plate 4.25A–D) Eastern hognose snake; Spreading adder; others	1	BL, DW, E, L, N, P {This single case resulted from contact with the snake's open mouth while the specimen was feigning death. The resulting tooth punctures were not due to an actively inflicted bite}	Grogan (1974)	C/D
Hydrodynastes (*Cyclagras*, Peters and Orejas-Miranda, 1970) *gigas* (Leynaud and Bucher, 1999) (Plate 4.26A–D) False water cobra; Brazilian false-water cobra; Boipevacu; Surucucu do pantanal; others	4 (4)	BL, DA, E, Er, L, P, PA {See Plate 4.26E. In the case involving a protracted bite reported by Manning et al. (1999), a 9-h period elapsed before the development of reported serious symptoms (including expanding edema, "muscle paralysis," and "unsteady gait"). See Section 4.4 for further comments regarding this case. Salomão et al. (2003) reported a bite without detail. This case is not included in the tally here}	Minton and Mebs (1978); Manning et al. (1999); Hill and Mackessy (2000); Malina et al. (2008)	C/D
Hypsiglena torquata texana (Plate 4.27) Texas night snake; culebra nocturna (many others depending on subspecies and locale)	1	P (limited information) {Available information suggests only minor local effects. There are two species in the genus *Hypsiglena*, and *H. torquata* has approximately 17 subspecies}	Russell (1980)	C/D
Ithycyphus miniatus Madagascan tiny night snake; Nosy Bé tiny night snake; fandrefiala	1 (2)	BL, E, Ecc, P {Bitten finger described as "enormously" swollen. The symptomatic case as reported occurred after a protracted bite. A quick release bite was reportedly unremarkable}	Mori and Mizuta (2006)	C/D
Langaha madagascariensis Madagascar vine snake; leaf-nosed or spear-nosed snake	1	E, P {Protracted bite; mild local effects. This pseudoxyrhophiine lamprophid is reasonably popular in private collections }	D'Cruze (2008)	C/D

Leioheterodon madagascariensis (Plate 4.28A–G; pictured are three of the approximately four species of *Leioheterodon*). Madagascar brown snake, Madagascar hognose; Menarana	2 (2)	BL ("prolonged"), E, P {Larger specimens may be capable of inflicting a painful and edematous local wound. To date, there is no evidence that this pseudooxyrhophiine lamprophid can inflict bites that cause any systemic effects such as Co}	Malina et al. (2008); Domergue and Richaud (1971)	C/D
Leptodeira septentrionalis Northern cat-eyed snake; falsa mapanare; escombrera manchada; others	1	E, P {This single reported case featured mild, transient local effects}	Minton (1986)	C/D
Leptodeira annulata ashmeadii Banded cat-eyed snake; Ashmead's banded cat-eyed snake; falsa mapanare; dormideira; escombrera; culebra ojo de gato, others	2 (2)	BL, E, Er, P {Limited information and observations suggest transient, mild local effects. Lemoine et al. (2004b) described proteolytic and hemorrhagic acitivites present in *L. a. ashmeadii* Duvernoy's secretion. They also reported "neurotoxic disorders" in mice injected with the secretion. *Leptodeira annulata* Duvernoy's secretion had a murine s.c. minimal lethal dose of 1.0 mg (Mebs, 1968). To date, bites have caused only the mild local effects noted above}	Gorzula (1982); Warrell (2004)	C/D
Leptophis ahaetulla Parrot snake, Green horse-whip snake; ranera perico; verdegallo; green machete; others	3 (3)	BL, E, P, PA {Beebe (1946) reported only slight bleeding without any significant effects after a bite from a *L. a. ahaetulla*}	Zwinenberg (1977); Minton and Mebs (1978); Warrell (2004)	C/D
Leptophis diplotropis Pacific coast parrot snake; ranera del litoral del Pacifico; others	2 (2)	P, BL, PA {"Persistent stinging pain" reported}	Zweifel and Norris (1955); Hardy and McDiarmid (1969); Warrell (2004)	C/D

(Continued)

Table 4.1 (*Continued*)

Taxa Frequent, Common Name(s)	Reports (Cases)	Reported Effects {Comments}	Reference	Evidence Rating[a]
Liophis spp. (species unidentified) (Plate 4.29 shows *L. anomalus*) Central and South American ground snakes (approximately 49 species; shares this general common name with several other genera, e.g., *Atractus* spp.)	1 (258)	E, Er, L, P, Pr, "local hemorrhage" {Reported as part of a retrospective review (see text), original case documentation unavailable, and species identification/verification are unknown. Pr was present in 2.2% of reported cases; L and P were most common (32.6% and 39.1%, respectively)}	Salomão et al. (2003)	C/D
Liophis miliaris[b] (Plate 4.29B and C) Military swamp snake, Military ground snake; cobra d' agua; Jararaca do tabuleiro; others	2 (2) Note: One of these cases is probably included in the previously summarized genus-specific review by Salomão et al. (2003)	BL, Co, E, H, P, PA, Pr {One patient given antivenom due to "serious symptoms of hemorrhage" (Salomão et al., 2003). There is no clinical evidence of any serious effects of bites by this species. Larger specimens may be capable of inflicting bites with more significant local effects}	Santos-Costa and Di-Bernadino (2001); Salomão et al. (2003)	C/D
Liophis poecilogyrus Venezuelan swamp snake, Wied's golden belly snake; culebra verdinegra; mboi capitan, others	1	E, Er, P, PA {Salomão et al. (2003) reported an anecdotal case of *L. poecilogyrus* bite that reportedly resulted in local effects consisting of "throbbing intense pain," swelling, "local hemorrhage," as well as "lack of sensitivity," and "local decrease of temperature." This species probably only causes mild-to-moderate local effects. More information is needed for full evaluation of potential risks associated with specific taxa of *Liophis*}	Amorós (2004)	C/D

Liophis p. sublineatus (Plate 4.30A and B) Stripe-bellied water snake, Yellow-bellied snake; culebra verdinegra; others	1	BL (local), E ("moderate"), Er, P ("ardor"), PA {Bite occurred after capture of a female specimen (snout-vent length 317 mm) in an urban area of Rio Grande of Rio Grande do Sul, Brazil. The victim-author described a brief bite ("a few seconds"), and a 3-h progression of pain that referred from the bitten R thumb to the R axilla. The pain reportedly lasted for 3–4 days, and two ecchymotic foci were described in the forearm and biceps that disappeared on the fifth day postbite. The victim was reviewed in the hospital, but received no specific treatment}	Marques Quintela (2010)	C/D
Liotyphlops spp. (Note: these snakes are in the "primitive" superfamily, Scolecophidia (= Typhlopoidea), family, Anomalepidae; thus, these snakes were not part of the previous Colubridae; species in reported series were unidentified) Dawn blind snakes; other common names according to species (many used for other fossorial species including other blind snakes)	1 (28)	E, L, P "local hemorrhage" {Reported as part of a retrospective review (see text), original case documentation unavailable, and species identification/verification are unknown. The majority of cases included in the review featured P (57.1%) and reportedly primarily involved bites inflicted on children digging up soil and bitten on bare lower extremities. Identification of snakes involved in these reports is of particular importance as these snakes have very few teeth. Therefore, confirmation of identity in these reports is essential}	Salomão et al. (2003)	C/D
Macropisthodon rhodomelas Blue-necked keel-back	1	CP, D, DA, HA {See Section 4.5.1.4 for further comments}	Subaraj (2008)	D

(Continued)

Table 4.1 (*Continued*)

Taxa Frequent, Common Name(s)	Reports (Cases)	Reported Effects {Comments}	Reference	Evidence Rating[a]
Macropisthodon plumbicolor (Plate 4.31A and B illustrates the orange-necked keel-back, *M. flaviceps*) Green keel-back; lead keel-back	1	BL, P {In describing the dentition of *Macropisthodon* spp., Smith (1943) commented, "... it would appear almost as if the development of the posterior fangs had passed the stage when they were really serviceable to their owner. They extend backward almost in a straight line with the long axis of the maxillary bone, and it is only by extreme elevation that they can be brought into service." Thus, Smith (1943) insinuated that the size of these enlarged maxillary teeth may affect their efficient engagement. Plate 4.31C shows the markedly enlarged posterior maxillary teeth of *Macropisthodon rudis* (red keel-back, false habu). Aside from the single report of a *M. rhodomelas* bite, there is little information regarding the effects of bites from these snakes. To date, available information suggests that bites from these snakes cause only mild local effects}	Gay (1978)	C/D
Madagascarophis meridonalis (Plate 4.32) Malagasy cat-eyed snake; Malagasy night snake; others	1 (2)	Bs, E {Report included description of bite wound "necrosis." As noted with reported bites by lesser-known non-front-fanged colubroid taxa, careful clinical review of any future cases is desirable in order to thoroughly assess any risks associated with bites by this pseudoxyrhophiine species}	Domergue (1989)	C/D

Malpolon monspessulanus (Plate 2.4D–F, p. 97) Montpellier snake; yaleh snake; egtateh; others	6 (74)	BL, D, Dp, E, Er, L, Ly, N, Pt/additional cranial nerve palsy, P, PA, "paresis of affected limb" {One case reported "slight nausea" and "muscle spasms" (Newman, 1985). Three cases suggest neurotoxicity, and one of these (Pommier and de Haro, 2007) establishes that this species can inflict a bite that may cause cranial nerve palsies. One case reported by Gonzáles (1982) exhibited "severe symptoms of neurotoxicity" with a reported therapeutic response to steroids and anti-histamines. "Drowsiness" was reported in several cases. The identity of the snake was unverified in almost all of the cases reported by Gonzáles (1982). Only 10 of these are included here and most of these lack confirmation of the species responsible. See Section 4.4 for further comments regarding these cases. Pozio (1988) mentioned an additional case of "suspected" *M. monspessulanus* envenoming in Italy, but without any details. Also, Boulenger (1913) described a French zoologist who reported that "swelling extended within thirty hours up to the shoulder, and was accompanied by fever and nervous troubles" after a *Coelopeltis* (*Malpolon*) *monspessulanus* bite. These are not included in the tally here. A confirmed bite with only minor local effects is shown in Plate 2.4G, p. 97}	Gonzáles (1979, 1982); Newman (1985); Pommier and de Haro (2007); Malina et al. (2008); this report B/C
Malpolon (*Scutophis* Padial, 2006) ***moilensis*** (Largen and Spawls, 2010) (Plate 4.33A and B) Moila's snake, hooded malpolon; talheh snake; others	1	E, L, PA {This case resulted from a protracted bite (see text)}	Perry (1988) C/D

(Continued)

Table 4.1 (*Continued*)

Taxa Frequent, Common Name(s)	Reports (Cases)	Reported Effects {Comments}	Reference	Evidence Rating[a]
Mastigodryas spp. Central and South American tropical racers (common names according to individual taxa; approximately nine species)	1 (27)	Er, L, P {Reported as part of a retrospective review (see text), original case documentation unavailable, and species identification/ verification are unknown. These are included due to a paucity of data regarding this genus. Majority of reported signs was L (44.5%)}	Salomão et al. (2003)	C/D
Natrix natrix European grass snake; ringelnatter	2 (2)	L, "Muscle contractions," P ("tenderness"), PA, "dilated pupils," "weakness" {The case reported by Gardner-Thorpe (1967) was noted in a newspaper account (*Daily Express* July 21, 1967). Reid (1967) commented on the account of this bite inflicted by an initially unidentified snake and the related process of assessing a snake bite as well as the potential use of antivenom. One of the clinicians involved in managing the case, Gardner-Thorpe, responded with a published comment and opined that the dilated pupils and weakness reportedly observed in the afflicted patient were "not caused by fear alone," thus suggesting that the symptoms/signs resulted at least partly from the bite. In a brief report, Satora (2004) described a 17-year-old male bitten on the lower L leg by a *N. natrix* in Poland. The identity of the snake was not independently verified, and was only identified by the victim	Gardner-Thorpe (1967); Satora (2004)	D

on the basis of color and pattern. The presenting complaints were "muscle contractions" and "numbness" in the bitten extremity. Three puncture wounds were observed, and local tenderness was noted at the bite site. The patient was given tetanus prophylaxis, and laboratory investigations were negative. The patient was observed for several hours, the reported numbness and muscle contractions subsided, and the patient was discharged. There are no other well-documented cases or patient-based data to support any medical risks from this species. Interestingly, Phisalix (1922) reported the presence of Duvernoy's glands in *N. natrix*, while Smith and Bellairs (1947) reported the absence of the gland in this species}

Oxybelis aeneus auratus (Plate 4.34A, B–D show *Oxybelis fulgidus*) Vine snakes; cobra cipo; bejuquilla parda; bejuca; bicuda; boitaboia; others depending on species (four species)	3 (3) Note: One case may have been a bite by *O. fulgidus*	Bs, E, L, Pr, PA {Victim introduced fluid from Bs into a laceration made on the unbitten (opposite) thumb. This reportedly produced a Bs. Stebbins (1985) reported transient PA after a bite from an *O. aeneus*, while Fowlie (1965) described Bs and PA after a bite from *O. a. auratus*}	Crimmins (1937); Fowlie (1965); Stebbins (1985); Starace (1998); Chippaux (1986)	C/D
***Oxyrhopus* spp.** (species unidentified; Plate 4.35A–C illustrates three species of *Oxyrhopus*) Central and South American false-coral snakes (approximately 12 species; note the common name shared among several genera of Neotropical snakes)	1 (167)	E, Er, L, P ("stinging") {None of the species in this retrospective series were identified, and this decreases the value of the study. L most common (33.3%); other listed symptoms reportedly of near-equal frequency (≈16%). These snakes can be mistaken for micrurine elapids (see Plate 4.36A–C), and this error may contribute to inappropriate management. See Section 4.5}	Salomão et al. (2003)	C/D

(Continued)

Table 4.1 (*Continued*)

Taxa Frequent, Common Name(s)	Reports (Cases)	Reported Effects {Comments}	Reference	Evidence Rating[a]
Phalotris lemniscatus trilineatus[b] (Plate 4.37A–C) Argentine black-headed snakes; cubeca preta; others	2 (2) Note: One of these cases may have been described by Minton (1990) using this species previous classification as *Elapomorphus bilineatus*	BG, E, H, HA, HT, L, P, Pr, "renal insufficiency," "drowsiness" {Also reported was hypersalivation. In case resulting from a protracted bite, reported by de Lema (2007), the patient (the author) was treated with vitamin K, blood transfusions, homeopathic botanicals, and s.c. "global antiophidic serum." See Section 4.5 for further discussion of this case}	De Lema (2007); Valls-Moraes and De Lema (1997)	D
Philodryas spp. (specific taxa unidentified) South American racers; specific names according to species (18 species; see other entries for examples)	1 (397) Note: The cases included in the cited retrospective review may include some of the *P. olfersii* cases considered separately here	BG, E, Ecc, Er, L, PA, "local hemorrhage," "local paleness" {These cases, involving multiple species, are from a retrospective review conducted by Salomão et al. (2003; see Section 4.1). These authors noted "gum hemorrhage" in 1.3% of cases recorded at Hospital Vital Brazil, 1959–1999. See Section 4.1 for further comments}	Salomão et al. (2003)	C/D
Philodryas baroni (Plate 4.38A–E) Baron's green racer; culebra verde; culebra narigona	2 (2)	E, Ecc, Er, P {Bites reported to date caused only mild local effects}	Kuch and Jesberger (1993); C Malina et al. (2008)	C

Philodryas (Dromicus, Donoso-Barros, 1966) **chamissonis** Chilean green racer; Chilean long-tailed snake; culebra verde Chilena	1	BS, E, HA, N {"Drowsiness" reported in referenced case. Further data are required in order to provide evidence-based assessment of insinuated systemic effects}	Schenone and Reyes (1965); Arzola and Schenone (1994); Kuch (1999); Neira et al. (2007)	C/D
Philodryas olfersii[b] (Plate 4.39A and B) Lichtenstein's racer, Green racer; lora; cobra cipa comum; cobra verde, others	8 (50) Note: Other cases are listed by various authors without sufficient documentation for risk assessment	DW, E, Er, Ecc, L, Ly, P {The majority of bites feature mild–mildly moderate local effects. Recovery in some of these cases may involve several weeks and require careful wound management. The retrospective review of 43 cases by Ribeiro et al. (1999) reported that local pain, edema, erythema, and ecchymoses were respectively the most common presenting symptoms (37.2%, 34.9%, 18.6%, and 9.3%). There were no systemic effects documented. De Araújo and dos Santos (1997) described a bite on the fifth digit of the victim's right hand that resulted in reported "loss of tactile sensitivity," an effect ascribed to progressive edema. The local effects persisted for 10 days, with recovery at 15 days. Silveira and Nishioka (1992) described a bitten patient with "severe local pain." Correia et al. (2010) reported a case involving moderate edema, erythema, and mild ecchymoses of the right hand in which the patient received eight ampoules of polyvalent anti-*Bothrops* spp. antivenom with a subsequent antivenom reaction. One case reported here included widespread ecchymoses (Warrell, 2004; Plate 4.40A and B).	Nickerson and Henderson (1976); Silveira and Nishioka (1992); De Araújo and dos Santos (1997); Ribeiro et al. (1999); Malina et al. (2008); Correia et al. (2010); this report	B/C

(Continued)

Table 4.1 (*Continued*)

Taxa Frequent, Common Name(s)	Reports (Cases)	Reported Effects {Comments}	Reference	Evidence Rating[a]
		There is one purported report of a fatality. This report (Centro de Informações Toxicológicas do Rio Grande do Sul, 1996) does not contain sufficient detail establishing linkage of the anecdotally described victim's death directly with the alleged *P. olfersii* bite. See Section 4.2 for critical comments regarding this oft-cited report}		
Philodryas olfersii latirostris (see *P. olfersii*)	1	BL, N, P ("burning"), V, Ver {The initial mild localized symptoms rapidly subsided. Vertigo, nausea, and vomiting occurred several days after the bite and were assigned as effects of "ophitoxemia." See Section 4.4 for analysis of this case}	Kuch (1999); Peichoto et al. (2007a)	C/D
Philodryas patagoniensis[b] (Plate 4.41) Patagonian racer; culebra de alfa; culebra de los pastos; others	4 (300) Note: The cases included in the cited retrospective review may include some of the *P. patagoniensis* cases considered separately here	BL, E, Er, L, P, Pr {Some authors have alluded to mild Co without providing clinical test results supporting this contention. As in many similar cases, verified reports of abnormal laboratory results are required in order to establish whether or not systemic effects, "mild" or otherwise, directly result from bites of this species. De Araújo and dos Santos (1997) described a bite on a victim's right hand that caused almost immediate Pr. This was followed by progressive edema, and limb movement was "hampered and painful." Recovery occurred after 15 days. In a	Martins (1916); Nishioka and Silveira (1994); De Araújo and dos Santos (1997); de Medeiros et al. (2010)	C/D

		retrospective review of 297 Brazilian cases, de Medeiros et al. (2010) found no coagulopathy, and bleeding was "transitory." Seven of these victims reported "mild dizziness"; see Epidemiology section for further discussion of these cases}		
Philodryas viridissimus (Plate 4.42) Common green racer, Green palm snake; boiobu; lora verde; others	1 (2)	BL (brief), E, L, P, Pr {Both cases described bites from the same snake inflicted on the same victim (the author of the report). Effects were very mild and transient. An anecdotal case with some credible support suggests severe edema, and purported compartmental syndrome with a likely unnecessary fasciotomy. Brief discussion of some features of this report is included in the section on *Philodryas* in Section 4.2}	Warrell (2004); Means (2010)	C/D
Pliocercus (*Urotheca*, Liner, 1994) *elapoides*[b] (Wilson and McCranie, 2002) False coral snake; Imitacoral (this common name is used for other genera; e.g., *Erythrolamprus*)	1	L, Ly, P {Patient was inappropriately treated as he was given several i.m. injections of anti-*Crotalus* spp. antivenom. The very limited available information suggests that bites by these dipsadids cause mild local effects}	Seib (1980)	C/D
Psammophis biseriatus (Plate 4.43A) Two-striped sand snake, Two-striped sand racer; mararinga; others	1	BL, E, Ecc, Ly, P {Simbotwe (1982) noted that several *Psammophis* spp. inflicted insignificant bites}	Spawls (1979)	C/D
Psammophis phillipsii (Plate 4.43B) Olive grass snake, Olive grass racer; joppaguri; others	4 (4)	E, Er, N, P {The identity of the culprit species in one report (FitzSimons, 1962) is unclear and may be *P. sibilans*. Senter (1998) accepted a protracted bite (e.g., allowed the snake to "chew" for approximately 60 s). His symptoms reportedly resolved in 48 h. Several cited cases	FitzSimons (1962); Broadley and Cock (1975); Branch (1982, 1998); Senter (1998)	C/D

(Continued)

Table 4.1 (*Continued*)

Taxa Frequent, Common Name(s)	Reports (Cases)	Reported Effects {Comments}	Reference	Evidence Rating[a]
		(see references) were not specifically quantitated, although these were evaluated in a medical facility and identity of species involved was not confirmed. These are not included in the number of cases reviewed here. Bites by several other species of *Psammophis* have been anecdotally reported (e.g., see Plate 4.43C–F)}		
Psammophis punctulatus (Plate 4.43G) Speckled sand snake; ekrace, ndasiangombe; others	1	BL, L, P (mild) {Mild effects that included multiple bleeding punctures; see Plate 4.43H}	This report	C/D
Psammophis sibilans (Plate 4.43I) Olive grass snake, Olive sand snake; olyfkleurige grasslang, olyfkleurige sandslang; others	Number unclear due to multiple anecdotal accounts	E, P, "malaise" {Cases reported to date are anecdotal. Available information suggests only mild local effects}	Isemonger (1955)	D
Psammophylax spp. (probably *P. tritaeniatus* or *P. rhombeatus*) Skaapsteker or grass snake (identifiers associated with common names (e.g., striped, southern) dependent on species and provenance	4 (2)	E, Ecc, HA, P {The species involved in cases reported by Chapman, 1968, is unclear}	FitzSimons (1912); Branch (1982); Chapman (1968)	C/D
Ptychophis flavovirgatus (Plate 4.44A) Fanged water snake; cobra espada d'agua; cobra d'agua	1 (1)	L, P, E {Bite produced notable local edema, see Plate 4.44B and 4.43C}	This report (Marcelo Duarte, personal written communication with DAW, October 2010)	C/D

| *Rhabdophis subminiatus* (Plate 4.45A–C) Red-necked keel-back; ular pitjung; ular lempeh | 9 (10) | AEM, An, BL, CCo (DIC), E, Ecc, Ep, H, HA, He, Hep, HM, HT, F, L, Mel, N, PA, Thp, V {In case reported by Mather et al. (1978), slight jaundice was noted and several concerning symptoms occurred between 48 and 72h postbite. Hoffmann et al. (1992) noted a lack of ARF or Thp in their patient despite a severe DIC. Their patient also exhibited depleted Protein C. Similarly, Li et al. (2001) noted a lack of serious multiple organ damage despite DIC with "severe" hemorrhage. Smeets et al. (1991) reported myoglobinuria with a normal CK, and a transient rise in creatinine. Most cases involved treatment with multiple units of FFP, PRBC, and platelets. Aside from supporting a steady hematocrit, these infusions were ineffective. The cases reported by Mather et al. (1978), Cable et al. (1984), and Seow et al. (2000) featured protracted bites. The case histories reported by Viravan et al. (1992) support the role of protracted bites influencing the severity of bites from this species. These authors described five insignificant bites from *R. subminiatus*. None of these involved intentional handling of the culprit snake (all were accidental, i.e., victim stepped on snake). These cases are not included in the tally here. See Section 4.3 for further discussion, and description of a recent additional case is included in Section 4.6} | Mather et al. (1978); Cable A et al. (1984); Smeets et al. (1991); Zotz et al. (1991); Hoffmann et al. (1992); Kijjirah et al. (1998); Seow et al. (2000); Li et al. (2001); this study |

(*Continued*)

Table 4.1 (*Continued*)

Taxa Frequent, Common Name(s)	Reports (Cases)	Reported Effects {Comments}	Reference	Evidence Rating[a]
Rhabdophis tigrinus[d] (Plate 4.46A–G) Tiger keel-back, Yamakagashi; Japanese garter snake; Red-sided water snake	12 (24)	An, ARF, BG, BL, BV, CCo (DIC), E, Ecc, H, HA, Hep, HT, F, L, LOC, Ly, Mel, N, P, PA, Thp, V {In the case reported by Mandell et al. (1980), "massive" ecchymoses of right thigh occurred after bruising during postenvenoming "collapse" (two episodes). This report also included a case involving an unidentified species. This case is not included in the tally. Similarly, Kono and Sawai (1975) reported "severe" Ecc in their patient who was treated with multiple transfusions. Plate 4.45C shows severe ecchymoses in a patient with serious *R. tigrinus* envenomation. Kikuchi et al. (1987) reported that one patient exhibited "pre-shock." A fatal pediatric case reported by Ogawa and Sawai (1986) featured brain hemorrhage involving the left temporal and occipital lobes with intraventricular perforative involvement (see Plate 4.46D). Multiple transfusions and dialysis did not alter the fatal course in the case reported by Nakayama et al. (1973) (translated by Mittleman and Goris, 1978). Sakai (2007) reviewed *R. tigrinus* envenoming. See Section 4.3 for further discussion}	Sakamoto (1932); Nakayama et al. (1973); Mittleman and Goris (1974); Kono and Sawai (1975); Mittleman and Goris (1978); Mandell et al. (1980); Mori et al. (1983); Wakamatsu et al. (1986); Kikuchi et al. (1987); Nomura et al. (1989); Matsuda et al. (1990); Orlov et al. (1990); Akimoto et al. (1991); Sakai and Hatsuse (1995); Sakai (2007)	A

Sibynomorphus spp. (Plate 4.47A–D; Plate 4.47A and B illustrate *S. williamsii*) South American slug-eating snakes (12 species; other common names according to species; also see Plate 4.48A and B for an example of a different species of slug-eating snake, *Sibon nebulosa*)	1 (74)	L, P, "local hemorrhage" {Reported as part of a retrospective review (see text), original case documentation unavailable and species identification/verification are unknown}	Salomão et al. (2003)	C/D
Sibynomorphus mikanii[b] (Plate 4.47C and D) Slug-eating snake, Mikan's tree snake; dormideira preta	1 Note: The case reported by Silveira and Nishioka (1992) may be included in the retrospective review of Salomão et al. (2003)	Ecc, L, P {Silveira and Nishioka (1992) reported "mild coagulopathy." This isolated report is in contrast with the review of Salomão et al. (2003) who reported >70 purported cases of bites from *Sibynomorphus* spp. that featured only mild local reactions (see previous entry). Confirmation is desirable of any possible systemic effects resulting from bites of this species. Salomão and Laporta-Ferreira (1994) reported that *S. mikanii* oral secretions (including Duvernoy's secretions) were employed in the immobilization of molluscan prey, thus providing some support for the use of the proposed term, "prey-specific venom," for the secretions of this species}	Silveira and Nishioka (1992); Salomão et al. (2003)	C/D
Stenorrhina freminvillei (see *Conophis lineatus*)				
Symphimus spp. (species unidentified) White-lipped snake (additional names dependent on species [two species])	1	E, P {"Extensive swelling, intense pain" reported. The bite was reportedly delivered in a "particularly delicate location" while the snake was being smuggled in the victim's underwear}	Warrell (2004)	C/D

(Continued)

Table 4.1 (*Continued*)

Taxa Frequent, Common Name(s)	Reports (Cases)	Reported Effects {Comments}	Reference	Evidence Rating[a]
Tachymenis peruviana (Plate 4.49A–D) Peruvian slender snake	Unclear number; largely anecdotal accounts	Unclear, possibly Ecc {An oft cited purported fatal case (Vellard, 1955) has no basis in fact. This reference discusses the effects of *Tachymenis* secretion on several experimental animals. There is no verified fatality from a bite inflicted by this species. See Section 4.3 for further discussion}	Warrell (2004)	IE
Telescopus semiannulatus (Plate 4.50) African tiger snake; gewone tierslang; damara tierslang	2 (2)	BL (minor), E, L, P (mild) {This species is occasionally offered in the commercial snake trade. There is little available information about bites from this species. It is unlikely to have any medical significance. A bite from a small (approximately 30 cm) male Kenyan specimen caused only puncture wounds, slight local P, and transient local bleeding (SAW, personal observations)}	Branch (1982); Broadley (1983); this study	C/D
Thamnodynastes pallidus Mock viper; saperas; candelillas; candelitas; others	1	BL, E, Ecc, Er, HA, L, P {Protracted bite with reportedly marked edema. Reported also was strong metallic taste associated with hypersalivation and headache. There was no additional evidence of systemic effects or detail regarding the aforementioned symptoms. Wound was treated with icepack (note: this is positively contraindicated), and patient received i.v. steroids	Diaz et al. (2004)	C/D

as well as p.o. analgesia. The edema notably decreased after 36h postbite. Laboratory studies have suggested neurotoxic and hemorrhagic activities in *T. stigilis* (Northern coastal house snake, Lemoine et al., 2004a). However, aside from the aforementioned limited report, clinical effects of bites by *Thamnodynastes* spp. to date are limited only to mild and uncommonly moderate local effects. As noted with all other non-front-fanged taxa, it is critically important to carefully clinically assess and document all medically significant bites}

Thamnodynastes strigatus (Plate 4.51A–C) Coastal house snake; culebra de casa; ubiracoa; corredeira; others	1	BL, E, P {Plate 4.51D shows the localized edema that occurred after a bite by *T. strigatus*. The only other significant effect was local pain}	This report	C/D
***Thamnodynastes* spp.** (species not indicated) South American house snakes; mock vipers (Tribe Tachymenini, approximately 19 species)	2 (143)	E, Er, L, P, "local hemorrhage" {Case reported by Warrell (2004) described rapidly spreading edema with resulting difficulty in ambulation due to involvement of lower extremity. The retrospective series reviewed by Salomão et al. (2003) likely included multiple species. See previous entry for *T. pallidus* as it suggests somatosensory amplification, or aberrant systemic effects (unlikely)}	Warrell (2004); Salomão et al. (2003)	C/D
Thamnophis elegans terrestris (Plate 4.52A–C illustrate *T. e. elegans*) Coastal garter snake; culebra de agua nomada occidental terrestre	3 (3)	Ecc, E {Accounts and observations suggest mild, transient local effects}	Minton (1976); Gans (1978); De Lisle (1984)	B/C

(Continued)

Table 4.1 (*Continued*)

Taxa Frequent, Common Name(s)	Reports (Cases)	Reported Effects {Comments}	Reference	Evidence Rating[a]
Thamnophis elegans vagrans (Plate 4.52D) Wandering garter snake; culebra de agua nomada	2 (2)	Bs, E, Ecc, L, P {Limited, but well-documented case reports suggest that occasional bites may cause mild-moderate transient local effects. Most bites are insignificant as noted with bites by other *Thamnophis* spp. See later and Section 4.2}	Vest (1981a); Gomez et al. (1994)	C
Thamnophis marcianus Marcy's garter snake; sochuate; others	2 (3)	BL (slight), E, L, P {Two bites by two different specimens caused miniscule puncture wounds, brief, scant BL, and insignificant pain (SAW, personal observations); medically insignificant}	Warrell (2004); this study	C/D
Thamnophis proximus Western ribbon snake; culebra acuatica	1	E, P {Medically insignificant}	Warrell (2004)	C/D
Thamnophis sirtalis similis (Plate 4.53) Blue-striped garter snake	1	BL, E, Ecc, L, Ly, PA {Compare with *T. e. vagrans* and *T. s. sirtalis*. The body of available information indicate that *Thamnophis* spp. generally have no medical importance}	Nichols (1986)	C/D
Thamnophis sirtalis sirtalis Common garter snake; culebra de agua nomada comun; others depending on *T. sirtalis* sub-species (approximately 13) and locale (Plate 4.54A, D–J; note the subtle pattern/color variability of this common species; Plate 4.55A and B illustrate *T. radix*)	1 Note: The authors have observed or experienced many insignificant bites from this species, but these have not been formally documented	E, Ecc, L, Ly {Weed (1993) reported that 47 *T. sirtalis* bites reviewed in the northeastern USA were insignificant. Ernst and Barbour (1989) described development of hypersensitivity to *T. sirtalis* saliva as contact resulted in a "burning rash." A case of mild edema of the third phalanges and associated metacarpal region of the R hand was ascribed to a protracted bite from a snake tentatively identified as a *T. sirtalis sirtalis* (Lazkowski-Jones, 2009). As the identity of the specimen was not verified, this case is not included in the tally here}	Hayes and Hayes (1985)	C/D

Thelotornis capensis[b] (Plate 4.56A–C) Cape vine snake, Bird snake; Twig snake; voëlslang; kotikoti; others	7 (7)	ACP, BG, BL, CCo (DIC), CP, E, Er, F, H, HA, Hep, HT, L, P, PA, Thp, V {Atkinson et al. (1980) reported an anecdotal fatal case from "F. Muller." The victim was reportedly bitten on the tongue. This case is not included in the tally here. Although envenomations by *T. capensis* are rare, the hemorrhagic diathesis may be as severe as that of *D. typus*. See Section 4.3 for further discussion}	FitzSimons and Smith (1958); Broadley (1959); Blaylock (1960); Beiran and Currie (1967); Atkinson et al. (1980); McNally and Reitz (1987); Saddler and Paul (1988); Miguti and Dube (1998)	A
Thelotornis kirtlandii Kirtland's vine snake, bird snake; twig snake; ivissi; mbeya; gewone voëlslang; others	2 (2)	ARF, BG, BL, CCo (DIC), F, H, HA, He, L, LOC, Mel {In the case described by Mebs et al. (1978), dialysis did not ameliorate the anuria or improve the clinical course as it ultimately resulted in a fatal outcome. See Section 4.3 for further discussion}	Broadley (1957); Chapman (1968); Mebs et al. (1978)	A
Thrasops flavigularis Yellow-throated tree snake, Yellow-throated bold-eyed tree snake; Mduma	1	L, P, E {Reported also was a hematoma at the bite site. Edema and hematoma persisted for 5–6 days and minor pain/stiffness for a few additional days thereafter. See Section 4.3 for further details}	Ineich et al. (2006)	C/D
Tomodon spp. (species unidentified) Mock vipers; other names dependent on species and locale (Tribe Tachymeninii; three species)	1 (51)	L, P, "local hemorrhage" {Reported as part of a retrospective review (see text), original case documentation unavailable and species identification/verification are unknown}	Salomão et al. (2003)	C/D
Tomodon dorsatus (Plate 2.3A–F, p. 119) Mock viper; pampas snake; boipemi; corre-campo; cobra espada comum; others	1	E, P {The limited documented effects describe mild, transient local effects. Larger specimens may be capable of inflicting a painful local wound}	Warrell (2004)	C/D

(Continued)

Table 4.1 (*Continued*)

Taxa Frequent, Common Name(s)	Reports (Cases)	Reported Effects {Comments}	Reference	Evidence Rating[a]
Trimorphodon biscutatus (Plate 4.57) Lyre snake; limacoa nocturna de Sonora; codorniz; false nauyaca; others depending on reference to each of the approximately 6 sub-species of *T. biscutatus* as well as locale	1	E, P {Klauber (1928) reported no effects from the bite of *Trimorphodon* spp. A communicated anecdotal case that occurred in Costa Rica included discoloration and minor swelling. These cases are not included in the tally here}	Lowe et al. (1986); this study (Roy McDiarmid, personal verbal communication with DAW, September 2010)	C/D
***Tropidodryas* spp.** (species not designated) Serra snake (two species)	1 (13)	L, P {Reported as part of a retrospective review (see text), original case documentation unavailable and species identification/verification are unknown. Lacerations/puncture wounds reported in 55.6% of cases, and case series suggests mild local effects}	Salomão et al. (2003)	C/D
Waglerophis merremi (Plate 4.58) Wagler's snake; Merrem's snake; boipeva; boipeva comum; capitao do campo; cobra chata; false yarara; jararaca mbuva; jararacambeva; sapera; others	1 (122)	L, P, "local hemorrhage" {Data from a retrospective review (see Section 4.1 and previous entries for details). There are very few accounts of bites from this monotypic xenodontine species, and those in the referenced series were mild. De Carvalho and Nogueira (1998) reported that the majority of "nonvenomous" snake bites in Cuiba, Mato Grosso, Brazil, 1986–1993, were likely from *W. merremi* and *P. olfersii*}	Salomão et al. (2003)	C/D
***Xenodon* spp.** (Plate 4.59A and B) False fer-de lance; other names depending on species and locale (five species)	1 (75)	E, Er, L, P {Data from retrospective review (see above). There are also few data regarding bites from these xenodontines. Available data suggest insignificant or mild effects}	Salomão et al. (2003)	C/D

| *Xenodon severus* (Plate 4.59C) | 1 | E, P {Little detail provided. Symptoms reportedly persisted for 4 h. As noted in Section 4.3, there is an obscure report of a purported "fatality," that has been assigned to this species (Orcés, 1948). We have been unable to verify the details of this report, and further investigation is underway. Boulenger (1915) described the wide range maxillary rotation exhibited by this species. One specimen, while being held behind the head, attempted to inflict a bite by rotating the posterior enlarged maxillary teeth to a near vertical position} | Quelch (1893) | C/D |

Amazon false fer-de-lance; cuaima sapa; cururuboia; jararaca; jacanarana; pepeua; sapa; sapamanare; others

Abbreviations: ACP, abdominal cramping pain; AEM, abnormal erythrocyte morphology; ALFT, abnormal liver function tests; An, anemia; ARF, acute renal failure; BG, bleeding gums (gingivae/buccal mucosae); BL, bleeding; Bs, blisters, blebs; BV, blurred vision; Co, coagulopathy; CCo, consumptive coagulopathy; CK, creatine phosphokinase; CP, chest pain; D, dyspnea; DA, dysarthria; DIC, disseminated intravascular coagulation; Dp, dysphagia; DW, discharging wound; E, edema; Ecc, ecchymoses; Ep, epistaxis; Er, erythema; F, confirmed fatalities and/or bites can be life-threatening; FFP, fresh frozen plasma and/or cryoprecipitate; H, hemorrhage; HA, headache; He, hematemesis; HM, hematoma; Hep, hemoptysis; HT, hematuria; HUS, hemolytic-uremic syndrome; L, lacerations/puncture wounds; LOC, loss of consciousness; Ly, lymphadenopathy; Mel, melena and/or hematochezia; N, nausea; OL, oliguria; P, pain; PA, paresthesia/numbness; Pr, pruritis; PRBC, packed red blood cells; Pt, ptosis; Sh, shock; Thp, thrombocytopenia; Thr, thrombocytosis; V, vomiting; Ver, vertigo (this includes loss of balance as described in a given report, and may not have met the clinical criteria for true vertigo).

[a] Evidence is rated as a modified interpretation of some of the criteria in the Strength of Recommendation Taxonomy (SORT) system of Ebell et al. (2004): Level A: Multiple well-documented cases that contain thorough clinical detail and evaluation by a medical professional. Level B: Limited number of well-documented cases that contain thorough clinical detail and evaluation by a medical professional. Level C: Case report prepared/interpreted by nonmedically qualified author and/or contains limited clinical information (even if the case was prepared by a medically qualified individual). This level can also be assigned due to a lack of verified identity of the ophidian species responsible for the bite. Level D: Published report contains description of significant symptomology/signs without qualified clinical verification and/or supporting clinical details; report based on anecdotal information or second-hand account. IE: Insufficient evidence for basic, critical evaluation; only anecdotal information available.

[b] In the reported case or in one of the cases in a documented series, patient was treated with antivenom [usually anti-crotaline, e.g., anti-*Bothrops* spp., anti-*Crotalus* spp., and so on, or other polyvalent prepared against medically important species of the relevant region, e.g., South African Institute of Medical Research (SAIMR; now renamed, South African Vaccine Producers, SAVP)].

[c] The most parsimonious explanation for the clinical evolution in this case is fatal polyradiculitis from tetanus toxoid. See the cited reference and Section 4.4 for further details.

[d] In the reported case or in one or more of the cases in a documented series, patient(s) was (were) treated with monospecific antivenom against the envenoming species.

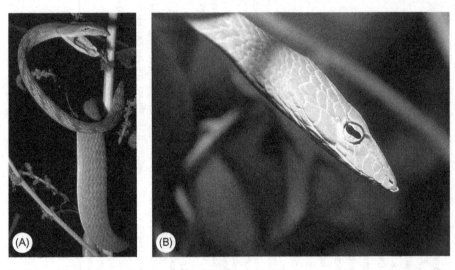

Plate 4.1 (A and B) Asian vine snake; as gulla (*Ahaetulla nasuta*). A slender, long-snouted, arboreal colubrine species with horizontal-key-hole eye pupils, *A. nasuta* feeds on lizards, nestling birds, and occasionally small fish. They are popular in private collections, and the few documented bites caused only mild local effects.
Plate 4.1A, photo copyright to David A. Warrell, Sri Lanka; Plate 4.1B, photo copyright to Julian White.

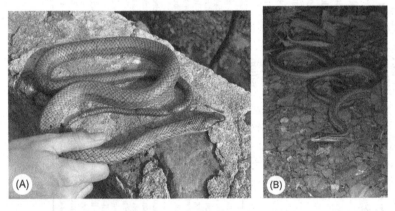

Plates 4.2, 4.3 West Indian, Caribbean or Central American, South American, and Galapagos racers (*Alsophis* spp.). These fast-moving, diurnal snakes belong to the family Dipsadidae, subfamily Xenodontinae, tribe Alsophiini, and also are commonly known by the useless name "racer," a name applied to many diverse species (e.g., see *Philodryas, Coluber, Platyceps,* and *Hemorrhois*). This group is taxonomically unstable and has recently been reviewed with many taxa re-assigned to either new or previously named genera (Hedges et al., 2009; see text, Section 4.2). Some limited insular *Alsophis* spp. populations are probably in danger of extirpation due to predation by rats. Some specimens exhibit damage to their posterior body/tail that has been presumed to be due to natural predatory attempts by soldier crabs (*Coenobita clypeatus*; Barun et al., 2007). Although there are very few documented medically significant bites by members of the Alsophiini, a handful of bites by *A. portoricensis*, and *A. cantherigerus* have caused

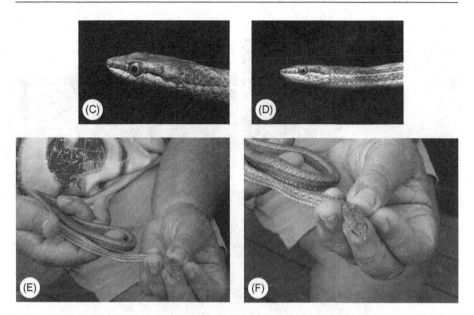

Plate 4.2, 4.3 (*Continued*) mild-to-moderate local effects (e.g., edema of varying severity, local bleeding, mild ecchymoses, and, uncommonly, minor blisters; see Tables 4.1 and 4.3, and Section 4.2).
Plate 4.2 (A–D) Puerto Rican racer, culebra corredora puertorriqueña [*Alsophis (Borikenophis) portoricensis*].
Plate 4.2 (E and F) Puerto Rican racer [*Alsophis (Borikenophis) portoricensis*] **responsible for the bite shown in Plate 4.4.**
Plate 4.2A, photo copyright to Gad Perry; Plate 4.2B–D, photos copyright to Robert Powell; Plate 4.2E and F, Mosquito Island, United States Virgin Islands, photos copyright to Kevel Lindsay.

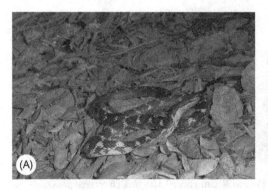
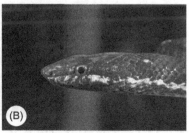

Plate 4.3 (A–C) Dominica racer, Antilles racer (*Alsophis sibonius***).** This species was previously considered a subspecies of *A. antillensis* (*A. a. sibonius* Cope), but was raised to a full species by Hedges et al. (2009). There are no documented cases of bites by this species.

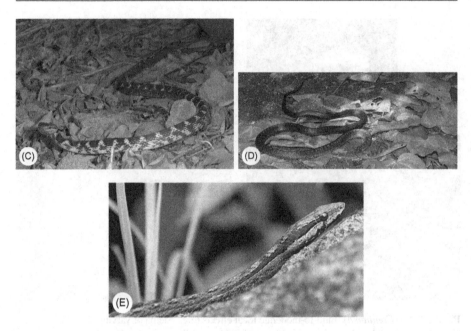

Plate 4.3 (D–E) (*Continued*) **Saba racer (*Alsophis rufiventris*).** There are no documented cases of bites by this species. Photos copyright to Robert Powell.

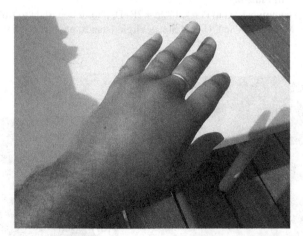

Plate 4.4 Local effects of a bite by the Puerto Rican racer [*Alsophis* (*Borikenophis*) *portoricensis*]. The specimen pictured in Plate 4.2E and F was responsible for the bite shown here (involving the distal and proximal phalanges, digit #2, L hand). The mild edema began to progress within 1 h of the bite, and the victim noted paresthesia, mild pain, stiffness, and mild ecchymoses. There were no sequelae, and the symptoms/signs persisted for several days, but resolved within 2 weeks (see Section 4.2 and Table 4.1). Photo copyright to Kevel Lindsay.

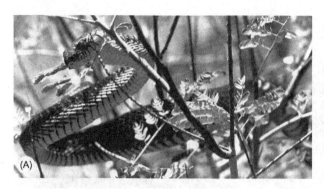
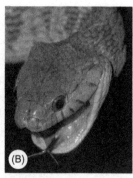

Plate 4.5 (A and B) Blanding's tree or cat snake (*Boiga* (*Toxicodryas*) *blandingi*). Attaining considerable body length (occasionally exceeding 3 m), and often sporting an open-mouthed threat display (Plate 4.5B), this western-sub-Saharan African species is viewed with suspicion by some authors. Although its Duvernoy's secretions contain a postsynaptic neurotoxin, there are no verified medically significant bites on record (see Table 4.1).
Plate 4.5A, Watamu, Kenya; Plate 4.5B, Kakamega Forest, Kenya; photos copyright to David A. Warrell.

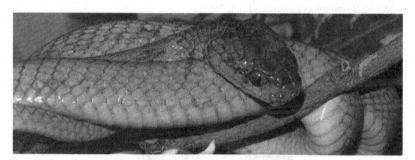

Plate 4.6 Green cat-eyed snake (*Boiga cyanea*), Thailand. *Boiga cyanea* is a common, primarily uniform green-colored colubrine species native to the forested zones of northeastern India, and Indo-China to Thailand. Their preferred prey consists of rodents, lizards, and nestling birds. Specimens appear relatively frequently in the commercial snake trade. The few reported bites from this species have included only mild, insignificant local effects (see Table 4.1).
Photo copyright to David A. Warrell.

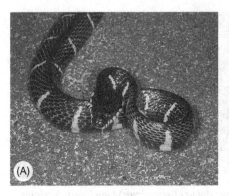
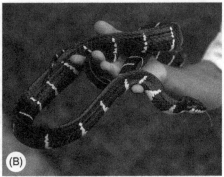

Plate 4.7 (A–D) **Mangrove cat snake or golden-ringed cat snake; ular tetak mas; bangkit** (*Boiga dendrophila*). Commonly maintained in captivity due to its ornate contrasting coloring and prominent barred pattern, bites documented to date have included only mild local effects. Cases have been posted on the Internet that illustrate more severe local effects, but these require formal medical confirmation. Large specimens are probably capable of inflicting bites that may cause more significant local pathology. This species produces an avian/saurian-specific postsynaptic neurotoxin; thus, its Duvernoy's secretion should be more accurately termed a "prey-specific venom" (see Table 4.1 and Appendix A).
Plate 4.7A and B, photos copyright to Julian White.

Plate 4.8 **Forsten's cat snake; naga; le mapila; naga mapila** (*Boiga forsteni*). The toxic potential of this species has been subject to speculation. The Sri Lankan populations have especially been feared locally, but there are no data supporting any significant danger from these snakes. Photo copyright to David A. Warrell.

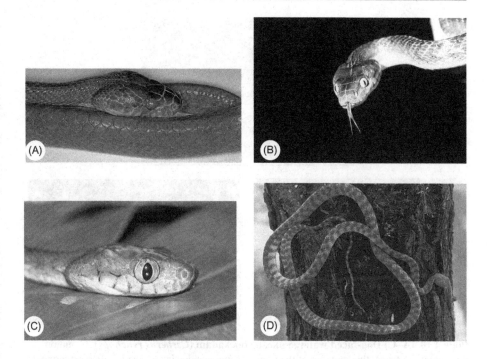

Plate 4.9 (A–D) Brown tree or cat snake (*Boiga irregularis*). The only snake species ever to be subjected to population control by an Act of the United States House of Representatives, this species has ecological and medical importance on Guam. Its spread through the Western Pacific island chains has been somewhat sensationalized, but its adaptability and fecundity still identify it as a species of ecological concern outside of its natural range (New Guinea and northeastern Australia). A handful of pediatric victims bitten by this species on Guam have reportedly exhibited systemic effects. However, the etiology of the described systemic effects remains inconclusive (see Section 4.4).

Plate 4.9A, photo copyright to David A. Warrell; Plate 4.9B and C, photos copyright to Gordon Rodda; Plate 4.9D, photo copyright to Julian White.

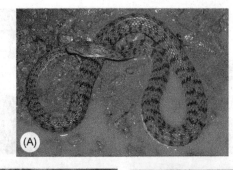

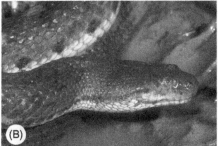
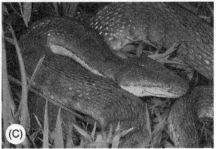

Plate 4.10 (A–C) Dog-faced water snake, or bockadam (*Cerberus rynchops*). Common throughout its range, this member of the family Homalopsidae is an aquatic, often estuarine inhabitant, and may be quick to bite when handled. However, to date, there are no documented medically significant cases.
Plate 4.10A, Phetchaburi, Thailand, photo copyright to Wolfgang Wüster; Plate 4.10B and C, Baucau, Baucau, Timor-Leste, photos copyright to Mark O'Shea.

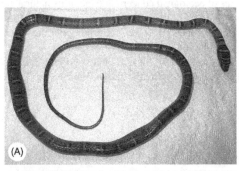

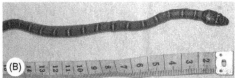

Plate 4.11 (A–D) Members of the genus, *Chrysopelea* (Asian tree or flying snakes). These colubrine snakes are inhabitants of the arboreal strata, and feed on lizards (a strong preference), birds, eggs, and small mammals. They are able to dorsoventrally flatten their bodies and exploit wind currents, thereby gliding between trees. This fascinating behavior has led to one of their

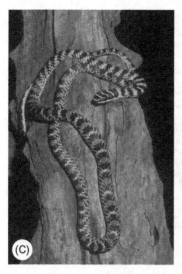
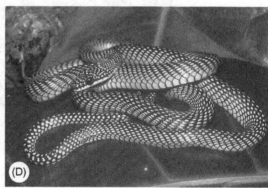

Plate 4.11 (A–D) (*Continued*) common names "flying snake" (as noted, "gliding snake" would be more accurate). Bites from members of this genus are usually insignificant. However, one well-documented alleged bite by *C. pelias* (twin-barred tree snake, see Plate 4.11A and B; Table 4.1) caused significant local edema and moderate pain.

(A and B) Twin-barred tree or flying snake (*Chrysopelea pelias*), Malaysia. The pictured specimen was killed shortly after presumably inflicting the bite described above. Although the bite was unobserved, the snake was found at the site immediately after the incident.

(C) Paradise tree or flying snake (*Chrysopelea paradisii paradisii*), Krakatau, Rakata Island, Indonesia. Anecdotally reported bites are medically insignificant, and usually only included minor punctures, brief bleeding, and mild erythema.

(D) Ornate tree or flying snake (*Chrysopelea ornata ornata*), Sri Lanka. This *Chrysopelea* spp. is relatively common in European, Asian, and North American private collections. As noted for *C. paradisii*, anecdotally reported bites are medically insignificant.

Plate 4.11A and B, photos copyright to Ahmed Khalil Ismail; Plate 4.11C and D, photos copyright to Mark O'Shea.

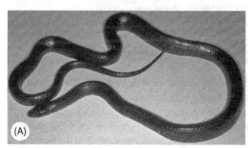
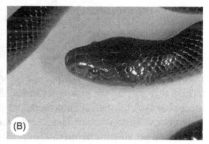

Plate 4.12 (A and B) Mussurana (*Clelia occipitoleutea*), Brazil. The common name is frequently applied to several *Clelia* spp. as well as other genera (occasionally used for *Boiruna* spp.). These dipsadids are included in the tribe, Pseudoboini. Most *Clelia* spp. are preferentially ophiophagous, but will accept rodents as well as lizards. The few documented bites have caused only mild-to-moderate local effects.

Photos copyright to David A. Warrell.

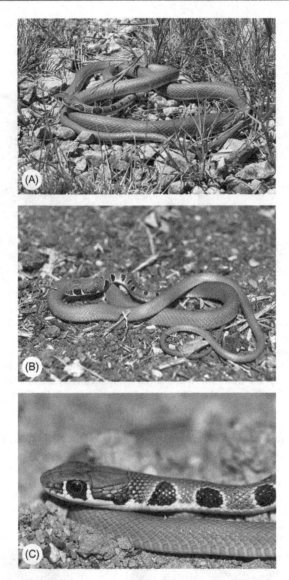

Plate 4.13 (A–C) Dahls' Whipsnake (*Platyceps najadum*). An active inhabitant of semiarid terrain, this species was previously included in the polyphyletic genus, *Coluber* (see text and other plates). Almost all documented, and anecdotally reported bites by this snake have been insignificant. However, one alleged case that occurred in Greece was presumptively implicated with a fatal progressive segmental neuropathy. This case is critically evaluated in Section 4.4. Photos copyright to Daniel Jablonski.

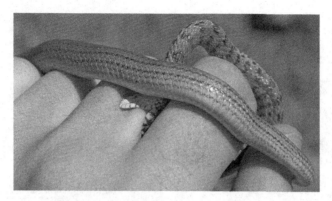

Plate 4.14 Jans' desert racer or cliff racer (*Platyceps rhodorachis*) inflicting a medically insignificant bite. *Platyceps rhodorachis* is a lengthy, agile species with widely variable, softly banded, coloration. It ranges from North Africa to the Arabian Peninsula, and into eastern Asia as far as India and Pakistan. Similar to other taxa previously clustered with the genus *Coluber*, it utilizes a range of microhabitats (desert, mountains, rocky areas, and biotopes with flowing water) within arid regions, and is considered semiaquatic. Its diet is generalized, consisting of tadpoles, toads, fish, other reptiles, birds, and small mammals. Although there is a report of two bites with elevated creatine phosphokinase (CK), thus far, bites have produced only mild local effects, and no systemic involvement.
Photo copyright to Alexander Westersröm.

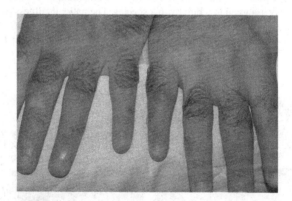

Plate 4.15 Minor local effects of a bite by the red-headed whipsnake (*Coluber rubriceps*), Israel. The victim was bitten on the proximal and distal phalanges of digit #5, right hand. There was brief, minor pain, scant bleeding and mild, transient erythema. The photo was taken approximately 10 h after the bite.
Photo copyright to Tomer Beker.

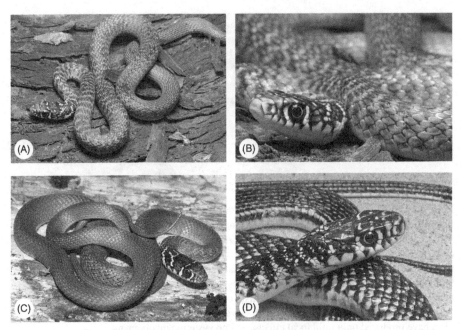

Plate 4.16 (A–D) Green or western whipsnake (*Hierophis viridiflavus*). A former
member of the genus *Coluber*, this common fast-moving species feeds on a generalized diet
consisting of lizards, small mammals, nestling birds, and amphibians. There is a single case of
neuropathy dubiously assigned to a bite by this species. The patient's illness was very likely
due to a far more common etiology (see Section 4.4; Table 4.1).
Plate 4.16A–C, Tuscany, Italy, photos copyright to Wolfgang Wüster; Plate 4.16D, photo
copyright to Maik Dobiey.

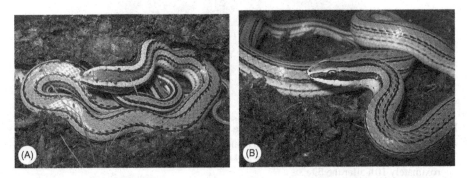

Plate 4.17 (A and B) Road guarder, guardo camino (*Conophis lineatus*). Several reports
have described mild local effects from bites by this species. One case was erringly ascribed
to the Central American blood snake, *Stenorrhina freminvillei*. This was later corrected via
examination of the photo accompanying the original report, and the case report re-assigned to
C. lineatus (see text).
Photos copyright to Maik Dobiey.

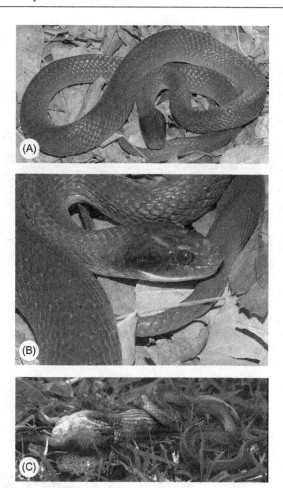

Plate 4.18 (A and B) Herald or red- or white-lipped snake; rooilipslang (*Crotaphopeltis hotamboeia*), olive phase, Kenya. Often found near bodies of water, these snakes favor aquatic prey. Although there are anecdotal reports of bites by *Crotaphopeltis* spp. that included moderate local effects, the single documented case was insignificant.
(C) *Crotaphopeltis hotamboeia* feeding on a bufonid toad, Zaria, Nigeria.
Photos copyright to David A. Warrell.

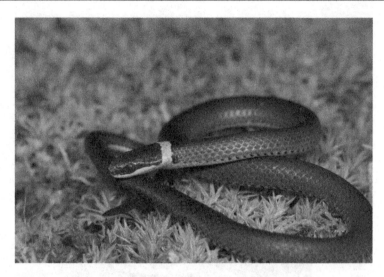

Plate 4.19 Northern ringneck snake (*Diadophis punctatus edwardsii*). A small, common semi-fossorial dipsadid found from Canada to Mexico and provisionally assigned to the subfamily, Heterodontinae, it feeds on small snakes, lizards, insects, and earthworms. Some observations suggest that *D. punctatus* uses Duvernoy's secretions to immobilize ophidian prey. Therefore, its Duvernoy's secretion may be best termed, "prey-specific venom"; its bite is medically insignificant. Photo copyright to Gary Sargent.

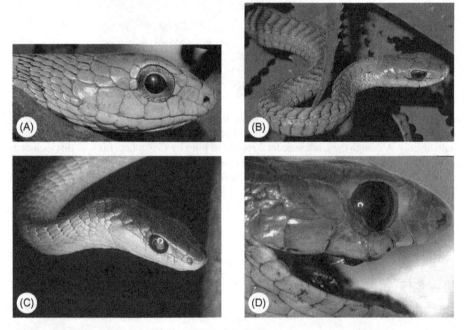

Plate 4.20 (A–D and L–O) Boomslang (*Dispholidus typus*). The most medically important non-front-fanged colubroid, *D. typus* is a hazard level 1 colubrid species that has inflicted

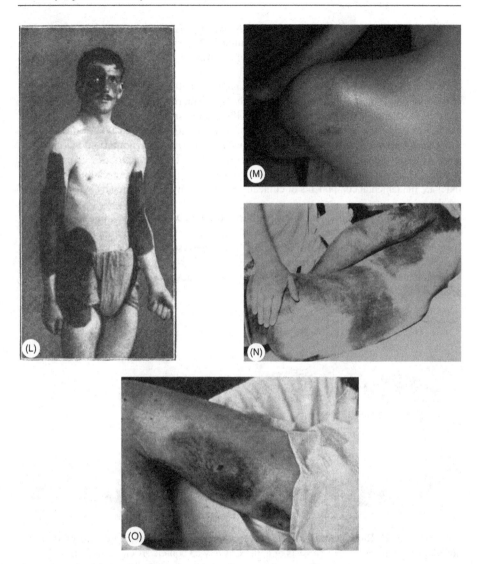

Plate 4.20 L–O (*Continued*)
a significant number of thoroughly documented life-threatening and fatal envenomations.
Monovalent anti-*D. typus* antivenom rapidly resolves envenomation-induced coagulopathy, but
is often difficult to obtain. These snakes are active and alert; note the large eyes (see Section 4.3
and Table 4.1).
(A) Kenyan specimen.
(B) *Dispholidus typus*, **green or "Jungle" phase, South Africa.** There are multiple
color phases of this species (see the following plates), and this can confuse identification,
particularly of dead specimens brought with a presenting snakebite victim to medical
personnel unfamiliar with snakes. There is sexual color dimorphism among some populations,
with males often green and females usually brown, but this is geographically variable.
(C) *Dispholidus typus.*

Plate 4.20 (A–D and L–O) Boomslang (*Dispholidus typus*). (*Continued*)
(D) *Dispholidus typus*, **male, Brown phase, Samaru, Nigeria.**
Plate 4.20A, B, and D, photos copyright to David A. Warrell; Plate 4.20C, photo copyright to Julian White.
(L) Illustration from FitzSimons (1912) with simulated effects of a Boomslang (*D. typus*) envenomation. FitzSimons (1909, 1912) was the first authority to carefully document the life-threatening potential of *D. typus* bites. The illustration simulates ecchymoses in order to emphasize the widespread effects that may occur after a serious envenomation by this species.
(M) Local ecchymotic effects of serious Boomslang (*D. typus*) envenomation. Victims who receive life-threatening envenomations may present without outward signs, or with extensive bruising, bleeding, and shock. Laboratory tests of hemostatic function (especially PT and INR) are fundamental components of clinically assessing any patient bitten by a dispholidine species.
(N and O) Photograph of ecchymoses from Boomslang (*D. typus*) envenomation. As shown here, extensive ecchymoses may be one of the signs of life-threatening consumptive coagulopathy caused by serious envenomation by *D. typus* (see Sections 4.3 and 4.6).
Plate 4.20M, photo copyright to Jimmy Thomas; Plate 4.20N, from EU Schmid Geneeskunde 4, 1962; Plate 4.20O, taken 20 days after the bite, from Mackay et al., 1960, all rights reserved.

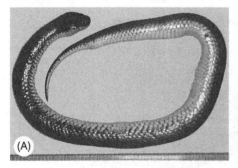

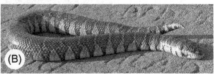

Plate 4.21 (A–C) Representative species of the Asian water snakes, genus *Enhydris*. The homalopsid genus, *Enhydris*, consists of approximately 23 aquatic species found primarily in riparian or estuarine biotopes. These snakes are often generalized feeders, and commonly take a variety of fish, amphibians as well as other small animals. Thus far, the few reported bites from *Enhydris* spp. included only mild local effects.
(A) Plumbeus water snake or common rice paddy snake; ngu pla (*Enhydris plumbea*), Thailand. Native to southern China, northern Vietnam, and Taiwan, this small (<0.75 m body length) very stout snake feeds primarily on fish and frogs. The term, plumbeus, refers to its lead-like coloration.
(B) Bocourts' water snake (*Enhydris bocourti*), Siem Reap, Cambodia. This species is a small (usually <1.0 m body length), stoutly built, striped water snake that has enlarged, grooved posterior maxillary teeth, and feeds on frogs and fish. It can be found throughout Thailand. It is heavily harvested for the snakeskin trade in Cambodia.

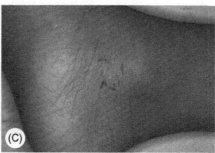

Plate 4.21 (*Continued*)
(C) Minor local effects from a bite by *Enhydris plumbea*, Thailand. Bite inflicted by the specimen shown in Plate 4.21A.
Plate 4.21A and C, photos copyright to David A. Warrell; Plate 4.21B, photo copyright to Laura Hermann.

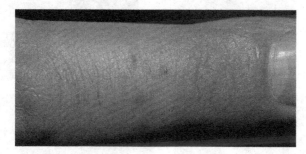

Plate 4.22 Minor local effects of a bite by the broad-banded South American water snake (*Helicops angulatus*). As in the minor bite pictured here, many "rear-fanged" colubroid snakes inflict bites that cause minor puncture wounds, lacerations, brief bleeding, locally reactive (minor) edema, and erythema. Tetanus prophylaxis should be considered in all cases of colubroid bites. Although the tetanus bacterium, *Clostridium tetani*, is uncommonly found in the ophidian oropharynx, wound contamination, and possible bacterial inoculation of the ophidian oral cavity via prey ingestion constitute a risk for tetanus.
Photo copyright to Zoltan Takács.

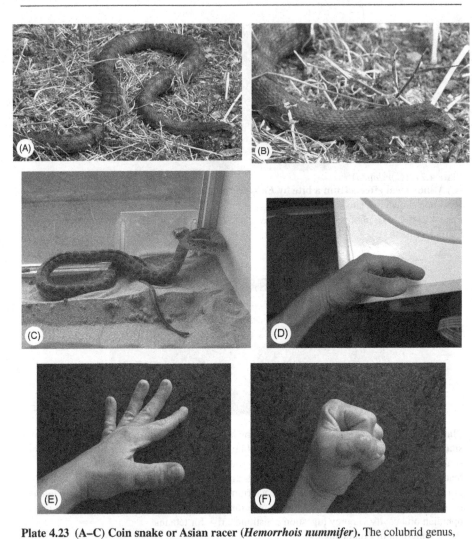

Plate 4.23 (A–C) Coin snake or Asian racer (*Hemorrhois nummifer*). The colubrid genus, *Hemorrhois*, consists of approximately four species that variously range from Europe and North Africa through the Middle East to northwest Asia and the Indian subcontinent. In parts of the Mediterranean (e.g., Cyprus) they are considered mimics of the blunt-nosed viper, *Macrovipera lebetina* (see Plate 4.72). All are fast-moving snakes, and can be found in dry, arid, sparsely vegetated terrain, especially rocky escarpments. Some taxa (e.g., *H. ravergieri*) are often found at elevations between 1200 and 3600 m. To date, reported bites by *Hemorrhois* spp., such as *H. nummifer*, have been medically insignificant (see Plate 4.23D–F).

(D–F) Mild local effects of a bite by a coin snake (*Hemorrhois nummifer*), Israel. The male victim was bitten while working with a captive specimen (see Plate 4.23C). The victim reported only transient mild pain, erythema, and brief, scant bleeding. These are the most commonly documented effects of bites by non-front-fanged colubroid snakes.

This victim also had brief induration at the wound site (D–F). Plate 4.23A and B, Symi, Greece, photo copyright to Matt Wilson; Plate 4.23C, Israel; Plate 4.23D–F, photos copyright to Tomer Beker.

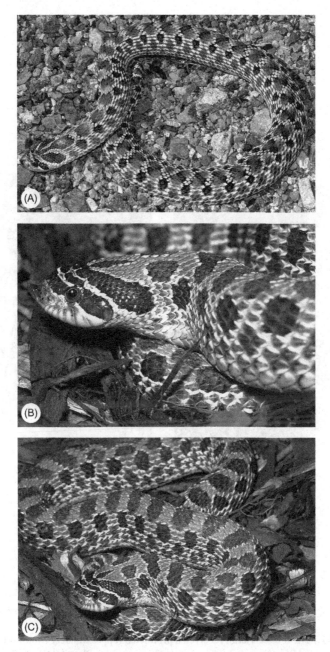

Plate 4.24 **(A) Western hognose snake (*Heterodon nasicus*), Tuscon, Arizona, USA.** A phlegmatic temperament and reluctance to bite contribute to the popularity of this species in private collections. Rare protracted bites by this species have caused significant local effects, and these have most often occurred while a captive specimen was offered food, or handled after the victim had prolonged contact with food items (see Section 4.1 and Table 4.1).
(B and C) *Heterodon nasicus nasicus* (see also Plate 4.91B–F).

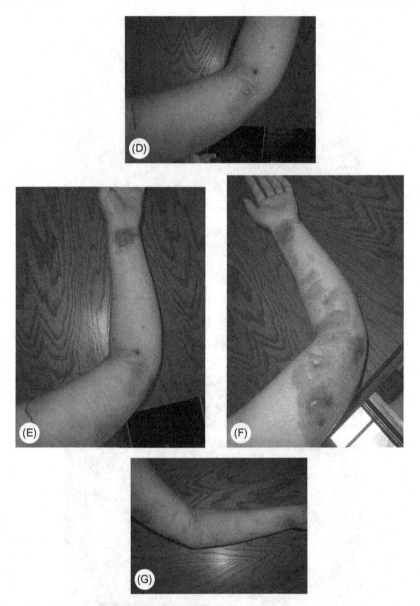

Plate 4.24 (*Continued*) **(D–J) Local effects of bites from the Western hognose snake, *H. nasicus*.**
(D–G, case #1.) The female victim received a protracted (approximately 3 min) bite on the left anticubital fossa while offering a mouse to a captive specimen. Plate 4.24D and E: 3 days after the bite, note the extensive ecchymoses, blistering, and edema. Plate 4.24F: 6 days postbite; Plate 4.24G: 16 days after the bite, note the resolving ecchymoses and blisters. The patient reported several months of pain and stiffness in the affected extremity.

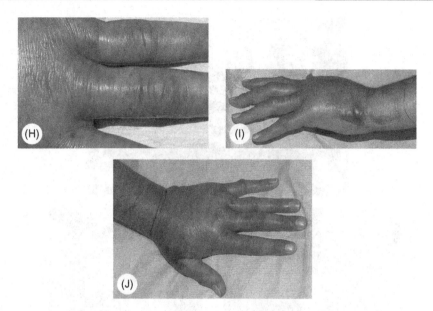

Plate 4.24 (*Continued*) **(H–J) Local effects of bites from the Western hognose snake, *H. nasicus*, case #2.**
The male victim also received a protracted bite on the proximal phalanx of digit #3 of the left hand from a captive specimen. There is significant edema, blistering, and ecchymoses.
Plate 4.24A, H–J, photos copyright to David A. Warrell; Plate 4.24B and C, photos copyright to Mark O'Shea; Plate 4.24D–G, photos copyright to Daniel E. Keyler.

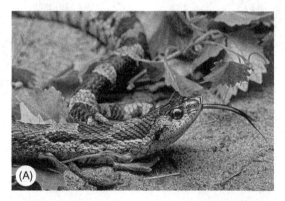

Plate 4.25 **(A–E) Eastern hognose snake (*Heterodon platirhinos*).** An anuran specialist with a strong preference for toads, *H. platirhinos* is well known for antipredator displays that include shamming death and neck flattening (see Plate 4.25C–E)—thus one of its common names, "spreading adder." There is only one well-documented medically significant bite by this species. It occurred accidentally while the snake's mouth was agape during shamming death behavior. Hognose snakes should not be considered "venomous" or "dangerous." Care should be taken when offering food to captive specimens (see Section 4.1).

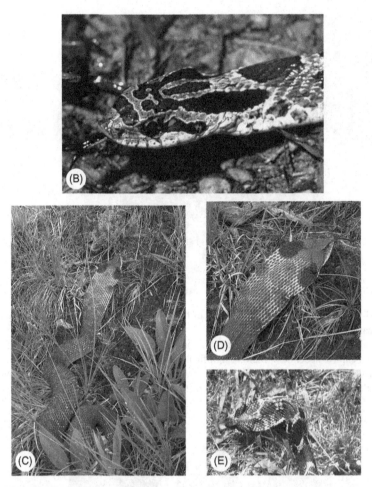

Plate 4.25 (*Continued*) Plate 4.25A, photo copyright to Gary Sargent; Plate 4.25B and E, photos copyright to Mark O'Shea; Plate 4.25C and D, photos copyright to Barney Oldfield.

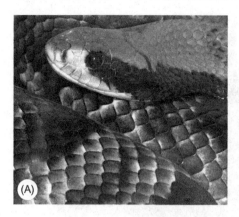
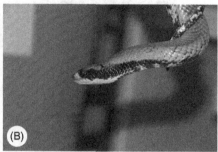

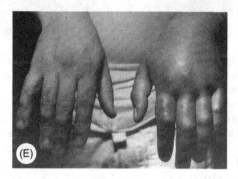

Plate 4.26 (A–B and E) **False-water cobra (*Hydrodynastes gigas*).** This large, heavy-bodied xenodontine species is commonly maintained in private collections, and when disturbed will often flatten its neck. It is capable of inflicting a locally painful wound. Large specimens may cause more severe local effects. A well-documented case described notably delayed symptoms including premature atrial contractions that were likely associated with anxiety (see text).
(E) Effects of a bite by the South American false-water cobra (*Hydrodynastes gigas*). Large specimens of *H. gigas* may inflict painful bites that include moderate local edema, as shown here (left hand). Although there are no documented cases that provide clinically reliable evidence of systemic effects from bites by this species, large specimens have produced relatively large volumes of Duvernoy's secretions that have strong proteolytic activity. Therefore, these snakes should always be handled with care.
Plate 4.26A, Brazilian specimen, photo copyright to David A. Warrell; Plate 4.26B, photo copyright to Kim McWhorter; Plate 4.26E, photo copyright to Dave Ball.

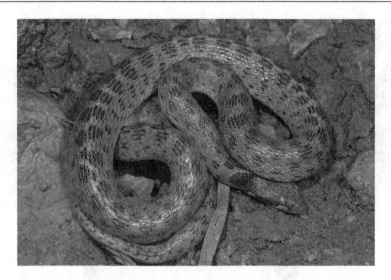

Plate 4.27 Spotted night snake (*Hypsiglena torquata ochrorhyncha*); Culebra nocturna manchada. A denizen of rocky foothill terrain, this dipsadid is found in the southern Baja Peninsula. Average adult specimens of *Hypsiglena* spp. may attain a length of approximately 0.35 m, and prey includes lizards, squamate eggs, frogs as well as occasionally snakes, amphibaenians (worm lizards), and insects. As with many non-front-fanged colubroids, the taxonomic status of *H. torquata* is uncertain, and several subclades are recognized with *H. t. ochrorhyncha* included in the coast clade. A recent phylogeographic and molecular systematics investigation (using mitochondrial DNA) recognized six species that were previously *H. torquata*, a taxon that consisted of approximately 17 subspecies (Mulcahy, 2008). Vest (1988) reported a murine s.c. LD_{50} of 26.0 mg/kg for *H. t. texana* Duvernoy's secretion. These snakes are reluctant to bite, and only one scantily documented case of a bite by *H. t. texana* reported only mild, transient local pain. The semi-fossorial nature, low experimental toxicity, and reluctance to bite, all are indicative of the medical insignificance of this species (see Table 4.1).
Photo copyright to Robert and Ann Simpson.

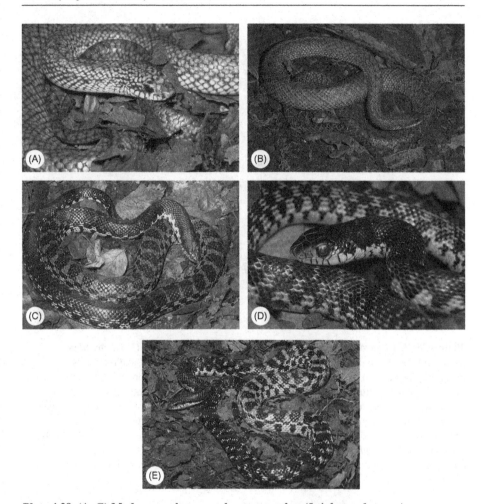

**Plate 4.28 (A–G) Madagascar brown or hognose snakes (*Leioheterodon* spp.),
Madagascar.** Members of this genus of the family, Lamprophiidae, subfamily,
Pseudoxyrhophinae, have become increasingly popular in some private collections. Although
often called by its popular common name, "hognose," it is unrelated to North American
Heterodon spp. and their allies (South American, or tricolored hognose snakes, *Lystrophis*
spp., see Plate 4.28H). A few documented bites by *Leioheterodon* spp. have included only
mild local effects (see Table 4.1).

(A and B) Madagascan speckled hognose or brown snake (*Leioheterodon geayi*). This
species is occasionally maintained in amateur collections. In the wild it feeds on amphibians,
lizards, and snakes, but will accept small rodents in captivity. Although rumored to be capable
of inflicting a medically significant bite, there is insufficient documented information for an
assessment of the possible medical risks of this species.

(C–E) Malagasy giant hognose or brown snake (*Leioheterodon madagascariensis*).
Popular in amateur collections, this species has been extensively exported to the USA and
Europe. Generally reported to be mild tempered, they will flatten their neck (appearing as a
hood) and hiss if disturbed. The few documented cases of bites by this species report only
mild local effects (see Table 4.1).

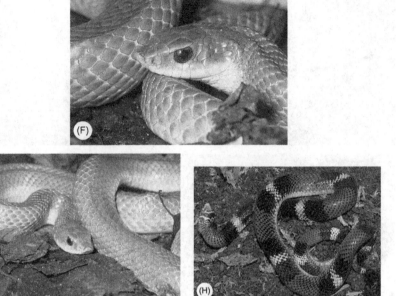

Plate 4.28 (*Continued*) **(F and G) Malagasy blonde hognose snake (*Leioheterodon modestus*).** *Leioheterodon modestus* has also been extensively exported, and is the least commonly available in the commercial snake trade. Thus, over-collection, in addition to extensive habitat destruction, has raised the question of potential extinction of wild populations. **(H) Ringed hognose snake; boicora, nariguda falsa coral (*Lystrophis semicinctus*).** Some members of the xenodontine dipsadid genus, *Lystrophis*, are popular in private collections, and often termed "tricolor hognose snake," or "South American hognose." Zaher et al. (2009) synonymized *Lystrophis* with *Xenodon*. There are no documented bites from this species. Plate 4.28A–G, photos copyright to Mark O'Shea; Plate 4.28H, photo copyright to David A. Warrell.

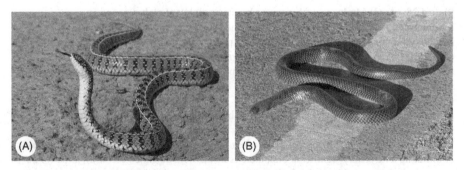

Plate 4.29 Central and South American ground snakes (*Liophis* spp.). The genus *Liophis* consists of some 40+ species of xenodontine dipsadids that range throughout Central and South America. Several taxonomic investigations have recommended differing reassignments for these snakes (Curcio et al., 2009; Pinou et al., 2004; Vidal et al., 2010; Zaher et al., 2009). The genus has been intermittently classified as *Leimadophis*, but recent review has recognized

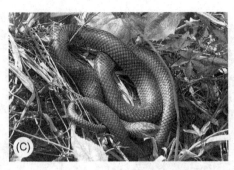

Plate 4.29 (*Continued*) *Liophis* (Vidal et al., 2010). Most species have a strong preference for anuran prey (e.g., hylids, bufonids; Michaud and Dixon, 1989; Pinto and Fernandes, 2004; Vitt, 1983), but will take other small vertebrates opportunistically. Some observations suggest that some *Liophis* spp. may have notable tolerance for anuran skin toxins that are among the most potent biological toxins characterized to date (e.g., the voltage-gated Na+ channel mixed agonist/antagonist, batrachotoxin, murine i.v. LD_{50}—$0.2\,\mu g/kg$). *Liophis epinephelus* has been identified as a potential predator of the golden poison arrow or dart frog, *Phyllobates terribilis* (Myers et al., 1978). Thus, this species may have molecular adaptations (altered toxin-binding sites per amino acid substitutions) to an otherwise little-exploited prey species such as in garter snakes (*Thamnophis* spp.) that feed on newts (including the rough-skinned newt, *Taricha granulosa*) without any toxic effects (these newts contain the potent voltage-gated Na+ channel antagonist, tetrodotoxin), but with a cost to performance caused by changes in the biophysical properties, and ion selectivity of the toxin-resistant Na+ channels (Geffeney et al., 2005; Lee et al., 2011). *Liophis melanotus* is called "doctor snake" in Trinidad and Tobago, as it is believed to have the ability to heal other snakes (Boos, 2001). As noted by Mole (1924) and Boos (2001), this belief has occurred elsewhere, and may be derived from the Greek myth describing the resuscitation/reanimation of *Glaucus* by *Polydus* after observing a dead snake revived by another using leaves. There are only a handful of well-documented bites by *Liophis* spp. (Section 4.1; Table 4.1), and the symptoms/signs consisted of mild-to-moderate local effects. A majority of retrospectively reviewed cases reported by Salomão et al. (2003) consisted of only mild local effects, but many of these cases lacked verified identification of the precise species responsible for the bite. This emphasizes the importance of verifying the species responsible for a reported snakebite. The confirmation of the most recent taxonomic status of any snake involved in a medically significant case is similarly valuable as this can influence management of medically significant bites by species of unknown medical importance. This is especially applicable to members of a taxonomically unstable genus such as *Liophis* as this group will very likely be subjected to considerable re-arrangement in the future.

(A) Goldbauchnattar; culebra listada, culebra ranera (*Liophis anomalus*), Magdalena, Buenos Aires, Argentina. This species is found in Paraguay, Uruguay, Argentina, and Brazil. There are no documented bites by this species.

(B) Military swamp snake, military ground snake; cobra d' agua (*Liophis miliaris*), Ribera Norte, Acassuso, Buenos Aires, Argentina. A widely ranging, semiaquatic South American species, it attains an average adult total length of approximately 0.7 m. It favors anuran and piscine prey, but will take small mammals. The few well-documented cases of bites by this species have included mild-to-moderate local effects. As in some cases of bites by non-front-fanged colubroids (especially South American species), occasional victims bitten by *L. miliaris* with moderate local effects have been inappropriately treated with antivenom (see Section 4.1; Table 4.1).

(C) Military ground snake; cobra lisa pampeana, cobra preta de banhad (*Liophis miliaris semiaureus*), Entre Rios, Argentina. This taxa has been raised to a full species (*L. semiaureus*) by Giraudo et al., 2006. Plate 4.29A–C, photos copyright to Alec Earnshaw.

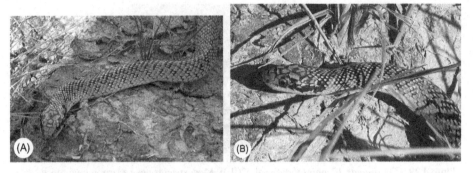

Plate 4.30 (A and B) Stripe-bellied water snake; culebra verdinegra (*Liophis poecilogyrus sublineatus*), Ceibas, Entre Rios, Argentina. There is a single documented case of a brief bite by one of these snakes. The victim-author reported local and referred pain that persisted for about 3 days. The bite also caused minor ecchymoses and mild edema. This is similar to a reported case of a bite by a presumed nominate *L. poecilogyrus* (see Table 4.1).
Photos copyright to Alec Earnshaw.

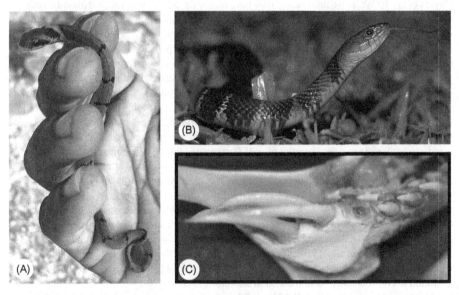

Plate 4.31 (A–C) The keel-backs, keel-back water snakes, or Asian false vipers, genus *Macropisthodon*. The four known semiaquatic species of *Macropisthodon* range variously in northern-western Asia, Southeast Asia, and/or the Indian subcontinent. The genus name describes their markedly enlarged posterior maxillary teeth. There are only a few documented bites from these natricid snakes. Aside from a single reported case critically analyzed in Section 4.5, *Macropisthodon* bites have been medically insignificant.
(A) Green keel-back (*Macropisthodon plumbicolor palabariya*), Kandalama, Sri Lanka. This species also possesses a series of dorsally located glands that are similar to those found in some members of the genus *Rhabdophis* (the like-named, Asian keel-backs, or flower snakes). The nuchal gland of *R. tigrinus* produces several novel polyhydroxylated steroid toxins, the bufadienolides. Unlike the toxins present in Duvernoy's glands, these toxins are formed from

(Continued)

◄ dietary precursors. The function/products of the dorsal-nuchal glands of *M. plumbicolor* are unknown (see Figure 4.2).

(B) Orange-necked keel-back (*Macropisthodon flaviceps*), Pangkalan, Bun Tanjung Putting National Park, Central Kalimantan. This species is found in Southeast Asia, and little is known of its natural history.

(C) Close-up of enlarged posterior maxillary teeth of the red keel-back or false habu (*Macropisthodon rudis*), Fukien, Chungan Hsien, China. *Macropisthodon* were of particular interest to Malcolm Smith (1875–1958), the physician-herpetologist who served as physician to the Royal Court of Siam, and was the founding president of the British Herpetological Society. His contributions notably increased knowledge of the Malaysian herpetofauna as well as that of Southeast Asia at large. Smith questioned the ability of these snakes to employ their enlarged teeth due to their seemingly disproportionate size. As noted previously, tooth size alone should not be considered a marker of potential hazard (e.g., see Plates 2.11A and B, and pp. 20-21). The potential hazards posed by any species must be considered in relation to their oral secretion properties, prey specificity of toxins, if any, and the associated delivery apparatus.

Plate 4.31A, photo copyright to David A. Warrell; Plate 4.31B, photo copyright to Peter Ellen; Plate 4.31C, AMNH specimen #34513, photo copyright to Arie Lev.

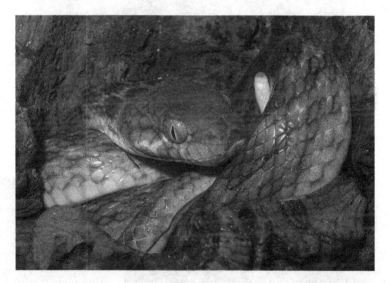

Plate 4.32 Malagasy cat-eyed or night snake (*Madagascarophis meridonalis*). The genus *Madagascarophis* contains four species of little-known, nocturnal pseudoxyrhophiine lamprophiid snakes that are widespread on Madagascar, and often occur close to human domiciles. Recent taxonomic study has identified at least six clades (and perhaps an additional species) of *Madagascarophis* (Nagy et al., 2007). There are two documented bites by *M. meridonalis* that included only minor local effects. Photo copyright to Maik Dobiey.

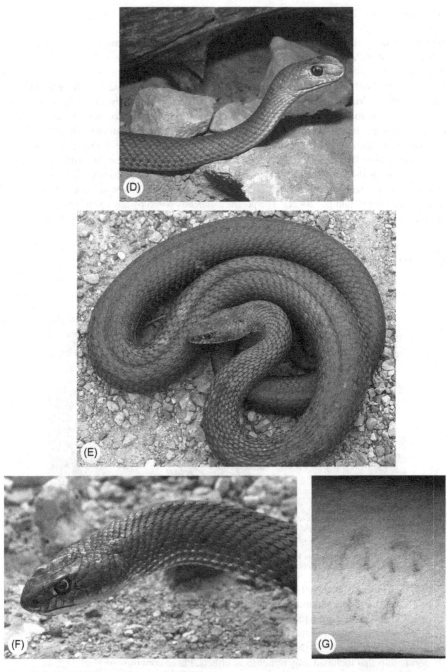

Plate 2.4 (D–F) Montpellier snake (*Malpolon monspessulanus*). Now considered by most authorities as a member of the subfamily Psammophinae, family Lamprophiidae, this snake is a fast-moving, alert species. It widely ranges from southern Europe to the Middle East, and Northern Africa. Many documented accounts of bites attributed to this species lack verified

(*Continued*)

◄ identification of the snake responsible for the reported injury. Although most recorded bites were insignificant, there is at least one confirmed bite that resulted in cranial nerve (CN III, IV, and VI) palsies (see Section 4.4).

(D and F) Montpellier snake (*Malpolon monspessulanus*). Plate 2.4D, locality unknown; Plate 2.4E and F, male specimen, Cartagena, Spain.

(G) Bite from *Malpolon monspessulanus*. As reported in most verified cases, this species most commonly causes only mild puncture wounds, lacerations, and brief bleeding. However, these snakes must be considered dangerous as there is at least one confirmed systemic envenoming that included cranial nerve palsy as noted above.

Plate 2.4E and F, photos copyright to Matt Wilson; Plate 2.4G, photo copyright to Zoltan Takács; Plate 2.4D copyright to Julian White.

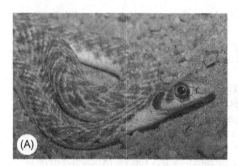 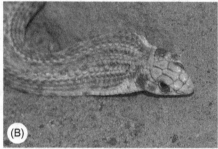

Plate 4.33 (A and B) Moila's snake or hooded malpolon [*Malpolon (Scutophis) moilensis*]. Although its congener, *M. monspessulanus*, has inflicted a verified neurotoxic envenomation, the few reported bites (only one formally documented) from *M. moilensis* have been medically inconsequential. When agitated, like *Heterodon* spp., *W. merremi*, and *Hydrodynastes gigas*, this snake will display by flattening its neck into a "hood" as shown in Plate 4.33B.
Photos copyright to Maik Dobiey.

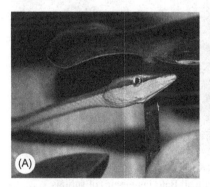 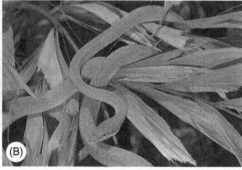

Plate 4.34 (A–D) The vine snakes, genus *Oxybelis*. The colubrine genus *Oxybelis* contains approximately four species of slender, sharply snouted, arboreal snakes that occur from northern Mexico (with some populations in the extreme southwestern USA) to South America. There are a few anecdotal accounts of mild local effects from bites by members of this genus, including *O. fulgidus*. A recent report has described the rapid immobilization of avian prey when grasped by *O. fulgidus*, but lizards may be less rapidly affected. Such observations may support use of the proposed term, "prey-specific venom" (see text).

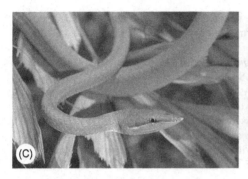
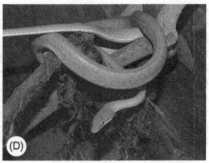

Plate 4.34 (*Continued*) **(A) Brown vine snake or Mexican vine snake; Bejuquilla Parda** (*Oxybelis aeneus*). This slender arboreal snake reaches up to 1.5 m in length, and is found from southern Arizona in the USA down through Mexico, Central America, and into northern South America. Its preferred prey is lizards, but also accepts frogs and birds. Bites by this species cause only mild local effects.
(B–D) Green vine snake (*Oxybelis fulgidus*). This arboreal snake is a long (it may attain 1.5–2.0 m body length), slender, arboreal species, native to Central and South America. It typically will grasp its prey (primarily lizards and birds) with a protracted grip prior to deglutition. Some limited observations suggest that birds are relatively rapidly subjugated with such a protracted grip, while grasped lizards appear less affected, and require a longer period of time for immobilization. Human victims who are bitten by this species experience only mild local effects.
Plate 4.34A and D, photos copyright to Julian White; Plate 4.34B and C, photos copyright to Maik Dobiey.

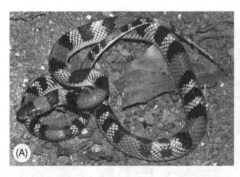
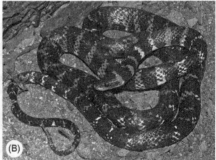

Plate 4.35 False-coral snakes, genus *Oxyrhopus*. Several genera of non-front-fanged colubroids are known by this common name as they are all Batesian mimics of various species of the elapid genus, *Micrurus* (see Table 4.1). Retrospective studies of snakebites in Brazil have reported mild-to-moderate local effects from bites by the xenodontine dipsadids, *Oxyrhopus* spp., although specifically verified identity is lacking in a number of these cases.
(A) Brazilian false-coral snake; boicora; cobra-coral, others (*Oxyrhopus trigeminus*), Northeastern Brazil.
(B) Dumeril's false-coral snake; falsa coral serrana; falsa coral laranja, others (*Oxyrhopus clathratus*), **Juquitiba, Brazil.**

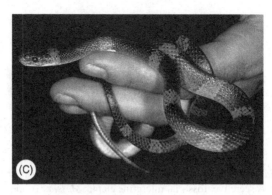

Plate 4.35 (*Continued*) **(C) Forest flame snake; calico false-coral snake; cobra-coral; falsa coral de calico, others (*Oxyrhopus petola*), Ecuador.**
Plate 4.35A–C, photos copyright to David A. Warrell.

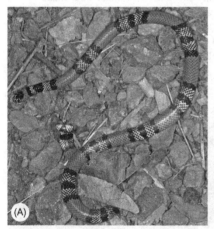
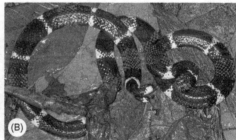

Plate 4.36 (A) Brazilian coral snake; Southern coral snake; boipinima; coral venenosa; mboi-chumbe-guazo; others (*Micrurus frontalis*), Brazil. This micrurine elapid has highly toxic venom and is a medically important species in Brazil. The venom contains postsynaptic neurotoxins and myotoxins. Serious envenomations are life threatening, and fatalities are well-documented. Several genera of non-front-fanged colubroids (e.g., *Oxyrhopus*, *Erythrolamprus*, *Pliocercus* as well as some *Lampropeltis* and others) are mimics of some taxa of micrurines (see Table 4.1).
(B) Surinam coral snake; boichumbeguacu; coral de agua; naca naca de agua; others (*Micrurus surinamensis*), Mita Vaupes, Colombia. This unusual aquatic coral snake is a large, relatively heavy-bodied micrurine elapid. Although it is known to inhabit slow-moving streams, and favors fish as prey, its natural history is poorly known.

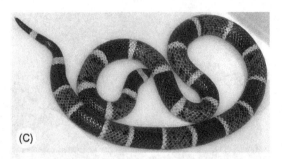

(C)

Plate 4.36 *(Continued)* **(C) Texas coral snake; coralillo tejano (*Micrurus tener*), Kingsville, Texas.** A secretive, fossorial micrurine elapid, *M. tener* is one of three species of micrurine elapids found in the USA. It favors other fossorial reptiles (e.g., the worm snake, *Carphophis amoenus*) as prey, and occasionally figures in snakebites. In contrast to envenomation by the eastern coral snake (*Micrurus fulvius*), bites by *M. tener* can result in significant pain. Some of these occur as a result of intentional contact with these snakes, but bites may happen as the victim accidentally uncovers the snake during work that involves turning of soil, or other landscaping. The uncommonly encountered Arizona coral snake (*Micruroides euryxanthus*) is reluctant to bite even when restrained. However, there is a documented case of transient paralytic effects after a *M. euryxanthus* bite that was delivered to the interdigital folds of the respective victim's hand.
Plate 4.36A–C, photos copyright to David A. Warrell.

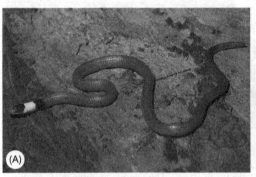
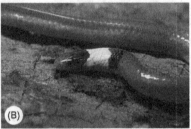

(A)   (B)

Plate 4.37 (A–C) Diadem or tricolored burrowing snakes (*Phalotris* spp.). This little-known South American (found in Brazil, Paraguay, Argentina, and Bolivia) group of approximately 12 taxa of fossorial xenodontine snakes are of unsettled taxonomic status as are the allied genera, *Apostolepis* (the burrowing snakes), and *Elapomorphus* (also known as diadem snakes). There are only a few reports describing the effects of bites by *Phalotris* spp. and *Elapomorphus* spp. Most of these cases have been poorly documented, and thus are not amenable to evidence-based analysis. These have reported only mild local effects. One report of a bite by *Phalotris trilineatus* (Argentine black-headed snake) included alleged systemic symptoms/signs. This case is critically reviewed in Section 4.5, and the limited available evidence does not support any significant medical hazard posed by these snakes.
(A and B) *Phalotris tricolor*, Tupi Paulista, Brazil.

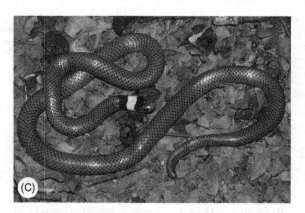

Plate 4.37 (*Continued*) (C) *Phalotris mertensii*, **Gertrudes São Paulo, Brazil.**
Plate 4.37A–C, photos copyright to Wolfgang Wüster.

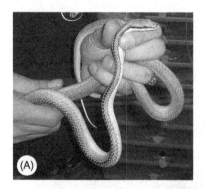 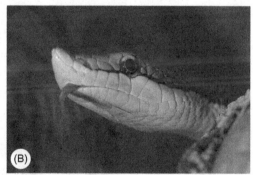

Plate 4.38 (A) Baron's racer; culebra verde; culebra narigona; others (*Philodryas baroni*),
blue phase. This is an active South American species that is popular in private collections. The
few reports of bites by this species have described only mild local effects. It has multiple color
phases that may confuse its identification.
(**B**) *Philodryas baroni*, **green phase.**
Plate 4.38A, photo copyright to Daniel E. Keyler; Plate 4.38B, photo copyright to Maik
Dobiey.

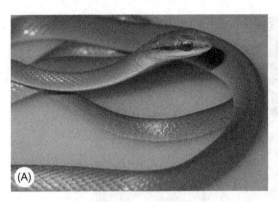
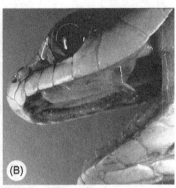

Plate 4.39 (A and B) South American green racer (*Philodryas olfersii*). The non-front-fanged colubroid species with the greatest number of well-documented bites in Brazil, its bite often produces only mild-to-moderate local effects (see Section 4.1 and Table 4.1). However, occasional cases may have systemic effects (e.g., extensive/widespread ecchymoses; see Plate 4.40A and B). An oft cited "fatal" case contains no documented support for such an outcome, rather contains an anecdotal report accompanied by public health advice for the management of colubroid bites with emphasis on potential pediatric victims (see text).
Photo copyright to David A. Warrell.

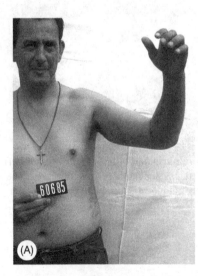
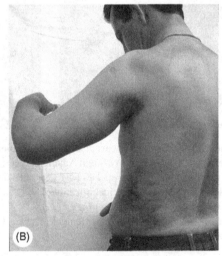

Plate 4.40 (A and B) Widespread ecchymoses from a bite by *Philodryas olfersii*, Instituto Butantan, Brazil. As the bite of this species may cause extensive ecchymoses distant from the bite site, it must be considered capable of inflicting a systemic envenomation. To date, there are no documented cases conclusively demonstrating coagulopathy after bites by any *Philodryas* spp., including *P. olfersii* (however, see Section 4.1 and Plate 4.41)
Photos copyright to Javier José Carrasco Araújo.

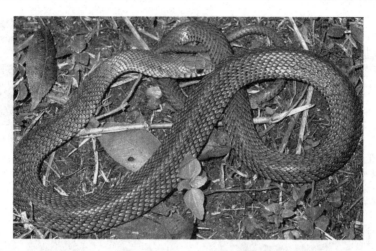

Plate 4.41 Patagonian racer (*Philodryas patagoniensis*), Brazil. Several series of bites by this species have been well-documented and analyzed. This species has medical importance in parts of South America similar to that of *P. olfersii*. The majority of bites produce only mild local effects. There are no documented systemic effects from bites of this species, although it produces Duvernoy's secretions that contain fibrinogenolytic enzymes, and the possibility of a coagulopathic envenomation must be considered (see Section 4.1 and Table 4.1).
Photo copyright to David A. Warrell.

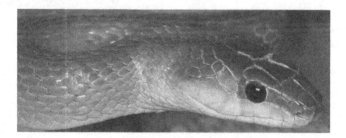

Plate 4.42 Common green racer or green palm snake; boiobu; boiobi; cobra cipo; tucanaboia; lora verde; others (*Philodryas viridissimus*), Manaus, Brazil. Another active South American "racer," there are few reports of bites by this species. One case, in which medical documentation is lacking, involved a bite from a captive specimen and included progressive edema as well as surgical intervention (fasciotomy; see Section 4.1 and Table 4.1).
Photo copyright to David A. Warrell.

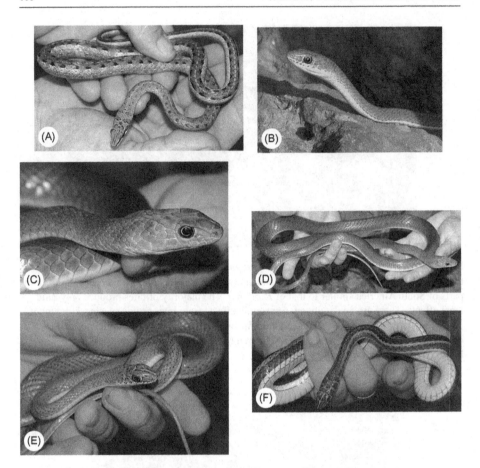

Plate 4.43 (A–I) African grass or sand snakes (*Psammophis* spp.). The type genus *Psammophis*, of the family Lamprophiidae, subfamily Psammophinae, is a complex group of African snakes with uncertain taxonomic status. Kelly et al. (2008) divided the *Psammophis sibilans* complex into two monophyletic entities, provisionally named the "*phillipsii*" and "*subtaeniatus*" complexes, and supported the status of many recognized *Psammophis* spp., but did not uphold any distinction between *P. p. phillipsii* and *P. mossambicus*. There are few well-documented bites by *Psammophis* spp., and these include only mild local effects.

(A) Link-marked sand snake; two-striped sand racer; mararinga; kitlaku, others (*Psammophis biseriatus*), Kenya.

(B) Olive grass snake or racer; joppaguri (*Psammophis phillipsii*), Gambia.

(C and D) Olive whip snake or sand snake; hissing sand snake (*Psammophis mossambicus*), Kenya.

(E) Link-marked sand snake; two-striped sand racer; mararinga; subhainyu (*Psammophis orientalis*), Kenya.

(F) Sudan sand snake or racer (*Psammophis sudanensis*), Kenya.

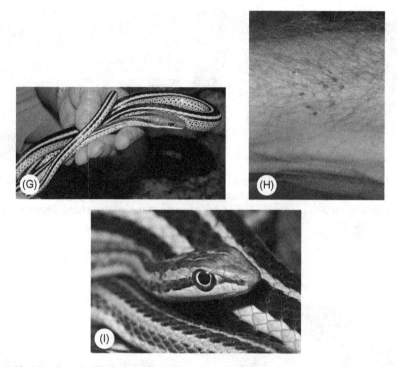

Plate 4.43 (*Continued*) **(G) Speckled sand snake; ekrace, ndasiangombe (*Psammophis punctulatus*), Kenya.**
(H) Minor local effects of a bite by *Psammophis punctulatus* (Kenya).
(I) Olive grass or sand snake; olyfkleurige grasslang (*Psammophis sibilans*).
Plate 4.43A–H, photos copyright to David A. Warrell; Plate 4.43I, photo copyright to Maik Dobiey.

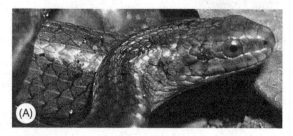

Plate 4.44 (A) South American fanged water snake (*Ptychophis flavovirgatus*), São Vicente de Minas, Brazil. Aside from lacking sexual dimorphism, and having reproductive patterns somewhat predictably linked to dry and rainy seasons (Scartozzoni and Marques, 2004), there is scant information about the natural history of this little-known aquatic member of the tribe, Tachymenini (Plate 4.44A).

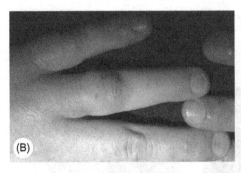

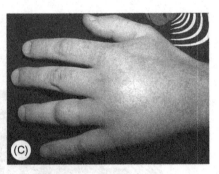

Plate 4.44 (*Continued*) It can deliver a locally painful bite, as shown in Plate 4.44B and C. The male victim was bitten on the proximal phalanx of the left fourth digit with subsequent development of mild-to-moderate local edema and pain of the involved hand. Photos copyright to Marcelo Duarte.

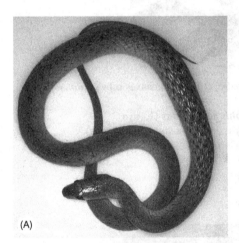

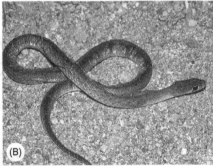

Plate 4.45 (A and B) Red-necked keel-back (*Rhabdophis subminiatus*), Thailand. Although there are no fatal cases yet recorded, envenomations by this hazard level 1 natricid may be life threatening. The pathophysiology of envenoming is identical to that of its congener, *R. tigrinus*. There is no monospecific antivenom against this species, but laboratory data suggest paraspecific protection against this species by anti-*R. tigrinus* antivenom.
Plate 4.45A, photo copyright to David A. Warrell; Plate 4.45B, photo copyright to Julian White.

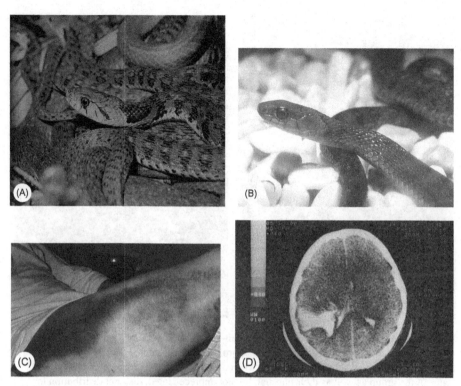

Plate 4.46 (A and B) Tiger keel-back, or yamakagashi (*Rhabdophis tigrinus*), Japan.
Although all of the fatal or life-threatening envenomations from this hazard level 1
colubroid species have occurred in Japan, there are occasional concerns regarding confused
identification of this natricid species with Asian garter snakes (also known as keel-backs),
Amphiesma spp., in the commercial snake trade. As noted in envenomations caused by other
hazard 1 colubroids, acute renal injury with renal failure poorly responsive to dialysis may
occur after bites from this species. There is a limited supply of antivenom against this species.
(C and D) Clinical effects of life-threatening *R. tigrinus* envenomation. The extensive
ecchymoses that may develop after envenomation by *R. tigrinus* is shown in Plate 4.46C. Plate
4.46D illustrates the results of a computerized axial tomographic (CAT) scan of the brain of
the victim of a fatal envenomation by *R. tigrinus*. There is a large brain hemorrhage involving
the left temporal and occipital lobes with intraventricular perforative involvement.
Plate 4.46A, photo copyright to S. Mishima; Plate 4.46B, photo copyright to Julian White;
Plate 4.46C and D, photos copyright to the estate of the late Yoshio Sawai.

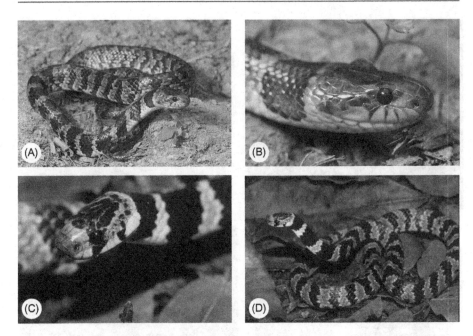

Plate 4.47 (A–D) South American tree or snail-eating snakes (*Sibynomorphus* spp.). The dipsadid genus, *Sibynomorphus*, consists of approximately 12 species. The systematics of the genus were reviewed by Cadle (2007), who commented on the taxonomically unsettled status of the group as well as their unusual, but not unprecedented, disjunct distribution in western South America. He also noted the marked pattern polymorphism in several species, and considered possible mimicry of crotalines among some *Sibynomorphus* spp. Although Salomão et al. (2003) reviewed a series of 74 alleged cases of bites from *Sibynomorphus* spp., these cases lacked any specific documentation, and verified identification of the snakes deemed responsible for the bites. There is only a single verified case of a bite by *S. mikanii* that documented only mild local effects, but one unverified case purportedly included "mild coagulopathy" (Table 4.1). There is very limited information about bites from other gastropod specialists, such as the genera (note the frequently shared common and general names): *Duberria* (African slug-eating snakes; two species; sub-Saharan Africa), *Asthenodipsas* (slug-eating or snail snakes; three species; Southeast Asia), *Aplopeltura* (blunt-headed slug or tree snake; monotypic; Southeast Asia), *Pareas* (slug-eating snakes; approximately 11 species; northern and Southeast Asia); *Atractus* (ground snakes; approximately 112 species; Central and South America, see Table 4.1), *Sibon* (snail-eating or snail-sucker snakes; approximately 15 species; Central and South America), *Dipsas* (snail-eating or thirst snakes; at least 33 species; Central and South America), and *Tropidodipsas* (snail-eating or snail-sucker snakes; approximately three species; Central America). Other species that favor molluscan prey include some Brazilian populations of the mock viper, *Tomodon dorsatus* (see later, Plate 2.3E and F), the North American dipsadid, *Contia* (sharptail snakes; two species; no documented bites), and some Thamnophiines (typically medically insignificant with an occasional protracted bite causing mild-to-moderate local effects; see Table 4.1).
(A and B) William's tree or snail-eating snake (*Sibynomorphus williamsii*).
(C and D) South American tree or snail-eating snake; dormideira preta (*Sibynomorphus mikanii*), São Paulo State, Brazil.
Plate 4.47A and B, photos copyright to Maik Dobiay; Plate 4.47C and D, photos copyright to Wolfgang Wüster.

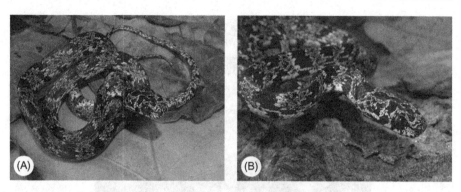

Plate 4.48 (A and B) Cloudy snail-sucker, speckled snail-sucker, cloud snail-eating snake; Culebra Jaspeada, Caracolera, Dormideira, Cobra-Cipo, and others (*Sibon nebulata*). Photos copyright to Jackson Shedd.

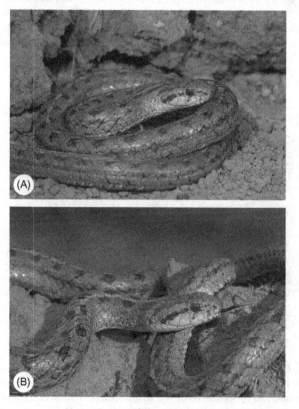

Plate 4.49 (A and B) Peruvian slender snake (*Tachymenis peruviana*). The Tribe Tachymenini is a viviparous group of seven dipsadid genera (*Calamodontophis*, *Gomesophis*, *Pseudotomodon*, *Ptychophis*, *Tachymenis*, *Thamnodynastes*, and *Tomodon*; Zaher et al., 2009). One of these, the genus *Tachymenis*, contains approximately six species of little-known South American nocturnal snakes. *Tachymenis peruviana* is an uncommon species that has been incorrectly associated with a fatal bite that did not in fact occur. There is no documented information that supports any significant risk from this species (see text and Table 4.1). Plate 4.49A and B, photos copyright to Maik Dobiey.

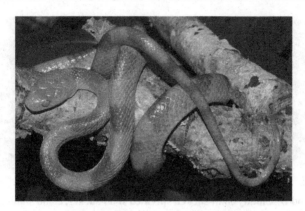

Plate 4.50 African tiger snake (*Telescopus semiannulatus*), Kenya. The colubrine genus
Telescopus contains approximately 12 species. *Telescopus semiannulatus* is a small (<90 cm
in length) colorful snake most commonly found with a cross-barred pattern that is native
to central, eastern, and southern Africa (Congo, Tanzania, South Africa). Although *in vitro*
studies of its Duvernoy's secretion have detected postsynaptic neurotoxic activity, to date,
bites have resulted in only mild local effects (e.g., minor pain and swelling).
Photo copyright to David A. Warrell.

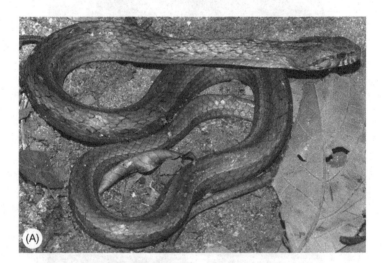

**Plate 4.51 (A–C) South American house snake (*Thamnodynastes strigilis*), Instituto
Butantan, São Paulo, Brazil.** This crepuscular semiarboreal tachymenine species feeds
on lizards, anurans, and opportunistically on small mammals. Most documented bites by
members of this genus have described only mild local effects. However, one case included
more extensive edema and pain (see Table 4.1). Plate 4.51C shows an enlarged posterior
maxillary tooth in a *T. strigilis* specimen.

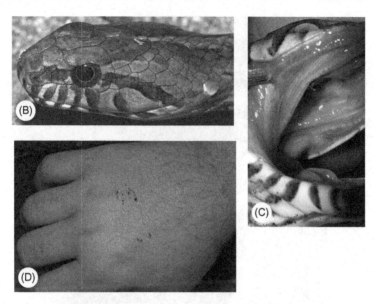

Plate 4.51 (*Continued*) **(D)** Bleeding puncture marks immediately after a medically insignificant bite by *T. strigilis*, Instituto Butantan, São Paulo, Brazil. Plate 4.51A–D, photos copyright to David A. Warrell.

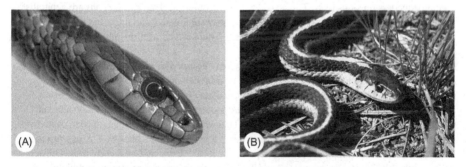

Plate 4.52 (A) Coast garter snake (*Thamnophis elegans terrestris*), Western USA. This natricid is a diurnal, active species that has a strong prey preference for slugs. Its diet may also include other invertebrates such as earthworms, and occasionally small vertebrates such as nestling mice. The few documented bites have included only mild local edema and minor ecchymoses. Most bites are medically insignificant.

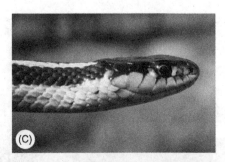

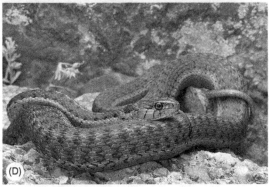

Plate 4.52 (*Continued*) **(B and C) Mountain garter snake (*Thamnophis elegans elegans*), Lake Tahoe, California, USA.** Some members of the *T. elegans* complex are considered specialist feeders on slugs (e.g., *T. e. terrestris*), while others such as *T. e. elegans* are generalist feeders. *Thamnophis elegans* may use coiling to partly subjugate small mice, but these prey are still usually swallowed alive (Gregory et al., 1980). There are no well-documented medically significant bites by *T. e. elegans*.
D. Wandering or Western terrestrial garter snake (*Thamnophis elegans vagrans*). *Thamnophis e. vagrans* are found in a variety of biotopes (e.g. near brooks or creeks in coniferous forest, meadows, rocky outcrops and mixed woodlands), and may be found at sea level as well as at elevations of 3200 m. These snakes are generalist/opportunistic predators, and feed on a broad variety of small vertebrate and invertebrate prey. They will readily accept small mice in captivity. Although they are medically insignificant, there are a few documented bites by *T. e. vagrans* that included local pain, development of mild to moderate local edema, and mild ecchymoses/blisters limited to the bite site. (see section 4.2.3 and Table 4.1; photo copyright to Barney Oldfield). Plate 4.52A-C, photos copyright to Mark O'Shea.

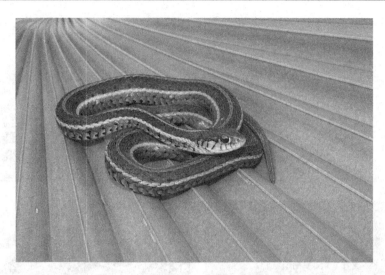

Plate 4.53 Blue-striped garter snake (*Thamnophis sirtalis similis*), Dixie County, Florida, USA. A specimen of *T. s. similis* inflicted a bite that reportedly caused mild ecchymoses and lymphadenopathy. This species is endemic to Florida, and is reasonably popular among *Thamnophis* collectors (see Section 4.2 and Table 4.1).
Photo copyright to Jake Scott.

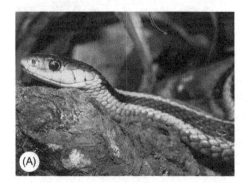
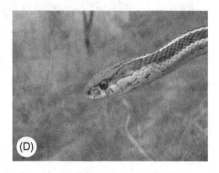

Plate 4.54 (A, D–J) Common garter snake (*Thamnophis sirtalis sirtalis*). One of the most popular "pet" snakes in North America, many natural scientists and amateur collectors began exploring their interests by maintaining specimens of *T. sirtalis*. These profiles of representative specimens show their variability in color and subtle pattern features. Although there are several documented cases of mild local effects caused by bites from members of the genus, particularly *T. elegans vagrans*, their bites are most often medically insignificant.
Plate 4.54A, photo copyright to Julian White; Plate 4.54D–F, photos copyright to Christopher E. Smith; Plate 4.54G–J, photos copyright to Jeffrey B. LeClere.

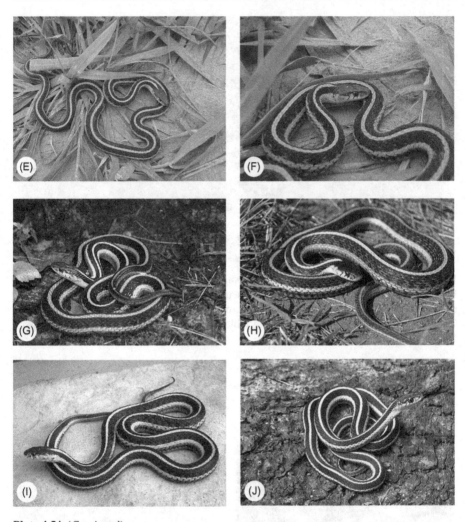

Plate 4.54 (*Continued*)

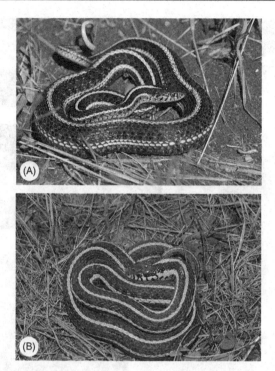

Plate 4.55 (A and B) Plains garter snake (*Thamnophis radix*). Found in the central USA and ranging into central-western Canada, this common species may be found in urban park grounds. It often favors moist grasslands and the banks of streams, bogs, or lakes. It is a generalist feeder, and will take leeches, earthworms, fish, frogs, and on occasion, nestling rodents. There are no documented bites by this species.
Photos copyright to Christopher E. Smith.

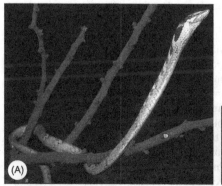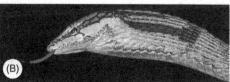

Plate 4.56 (A–I) African twig, bird or vine snakes (*Thelotornis* spp.). Serious envenomations by *Thelotornis* spp. and *D. typus* cause consumptive coagulopathy, disseminated intravascular coagulation, subsequent bleeding, and acute kidney injury. A specimen of *T. kirtlandii* was maintained in a home vivarium by the prominent herpetologist, Robert F.W. Mertens. He received a "dry bite" some weeks prior to being fatally envenomated by the same snake.

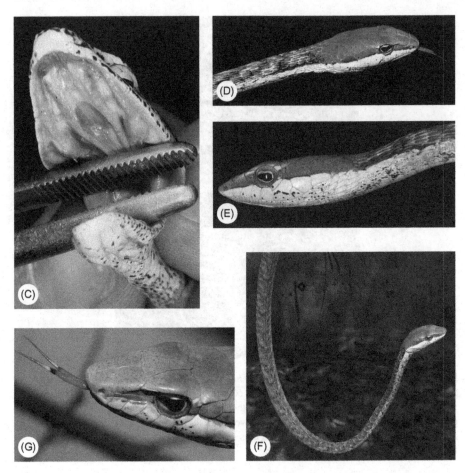

Plate 4.56 (*Continued*) **(A–C) Cape twig, bird or vine snake (*T. capensis*).** The specimens shown in Plate 4.56A and B are poised in defensive threat displays that are accomplished by inflation of the throat. Incorrect assumptions about this hazard level 1 colubrid species such as it being "harmless" or "mildly toxic" may have contributed to some of the fatal or life-threatening envenomations by this species. There is no commercial antivenom for bites from this species, and envenomations are treated with replacement therapy only (see Sections 4.3 and 4.6).
(A) *Thelotornis capensis*, **South Africa.**
(B) Oates' twig, bird or vine snake; Oates' savannah twig snake (*T. capensis oatesii*), northern Zimbabwe. Although there are few published reports of bites from subspecies of *Thelotornis*, a well-documented envenomation by *T. c. oatesii* resulted in bleeding complications, defibrination, prolonged prothrombin, and partial thromboplastin times.
(C) Enlarged posterior maxillary teeth in a living specimen of *T. capensis*, South Africa. As noted in *D. typus*, these enlarged teeth have deep grooves running almost the entire length, and sharp lateral ridges.
(D–G) Mozambique twig, vine or bird snake (*T. mossamibicanus*), Gede, Kenya. Although there are no documented envenomations by this taxon, it is likely to be as dangerous as *T. capensis* and *T. kirtlandii*. This species is infrequently illustrated.
Plate 4.56A–G, photos copyright to David A. Warrell.

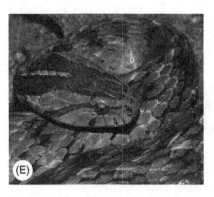 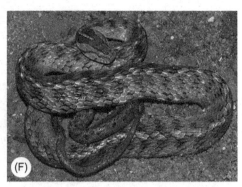

Plate 2.3 (E and F) Pampas snake, false viper or mock viper (*Tomodon dorsatus*), Ibiuna, Brazil. There are three species of *Tomodon*, one of the seven genera included in the tribe Tachymenini. Some investigators have reported that southeastern Brazilian populations of *Tomodon dorsatus* have a strong preference for gastropod prey (e.g.veronicellid slugs; Bizerra et al., 2005). To date, the few documented bites by these dipsadids have included only mild, transient local effects.

For more information, see legend of Plate 2.3A–F in Chapter 2. Photos copyright to David A. Warrell.

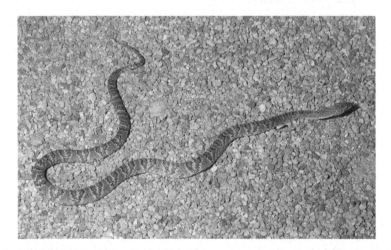

Plate 4.57 Sonoran lyre snake; Limacoa Nocturna de Sonora (*Trimorphodon biscutatus lambda*). Ranging from the southwestern USA through western Mexico to Panama, this secretive nocturnal colubrine species feeds on lizards, small mammals and, occasionally, bats. Devitt et al. (2008) recommended recognition of *T. b. lambda* as a full species, *T. lambda*. A number of non-front-fanged colubroids such as *T. biscutatus* have Duvernoy's secretions that contain post-synaptically active neurotoxins. Aside from *Malpolon monspessulanus*, to date, these do not have any clinical significance.

Photo copyright to Robert and Ann Simpson.

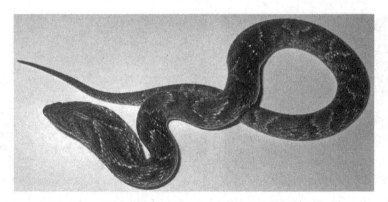

Plate 4.58 Wagler's snake or Merrem's snake (*Waglerophis merremi*), Brazil. Also referred to as "mock vipers" (a common name used for a variety of species in South America and Asia) these are large, robust, monotypic snakes that have enlarged, nongrooved, posterior maxillary teeth. In a recent taxonomic review of the Dipsadidae, Zaher et al. (2009) synonymized *Waglerophis* with *Xenodon*. This is a species that should be handled cautiously. Although little documentation of bites is available, a glancing finger bite resulted in sharp pain and freely bleeding tooth puncture wounds; however, a retrospective review reported only mild effects (see Table 4.1).
Photo copyright to David A. Warrell.

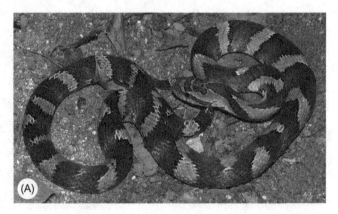

Plate 4.59 (A and B) False-Fer-de-Lance; Falsa Coitara (*Xenodon neuwiedii*), Cajamar, Brazil. The xenodontine dipsadid genus, *Xenodon*, contains approximately five neotropical species. These snakes are sometimes mistaken for lance-headed vipers (*Bothrops* spp.), although their mimicry of these may be questionable.

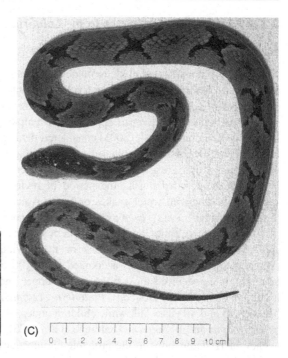

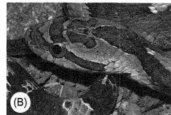

Plate 4.59 (*Continued*) **(C) False-Fer-de-Lance; Cuaima Sapa (*Xenodon severus*), Porto Velho, Brazil (found dead on road).** There is an obscure anecdotal report that allegedly reports a *X. severus* bite with a fatal outcome. This report has not yet been reviewed, and there is no available evidence that supports any significant hazard associated with this species. The single documented case consisted of only mild local effects (see Section 4.3 and Table 4.1). Plate 4.59A–C, photos copyright to David A. Warrell.

Many of these minor cases received combined evidence rankings between levels C and D due to: very limited documented reports (frequently only single reports); numerous accounts authored by medically unqualified observers; limited information in the report, or secondhand accounts; the very mild effects of bites inflicted by the species involved, as well as the possible influence on signs and symptoms of first-aid treatments, and acquired hypersensitivity to venom or other ophidian products (salivary proteins, shed skins, etc.). Bites from many of these species (e.g., the garter and ribbon snakes, *Thamnophis* spp., and the Asian racers, *Hemorrhois* spp.) produce mild local reactions typically featuring erythema, puncture wounds/lacerations, mild pain, and, occasionally, ecchymoses, lymphadenitis/lymphangitis (Hayes and Hayes, 1985), and hemorrhagic vesicles (Gomez et al., 1994; Table 4.1). Some of these accounts suggest significant distress and anxiety due to the unexpected nature of *any* uncomfortable effects from what was perceived as a "harmless" or "nonvenomous" species.

4.1.1 Epidemiology of Bites from "Colubrid" Snakes

4.1.1.1 South America

There are few documented epidemiological studies of bites from members of the former colubrid assemblage. The largest volume of information regarding epidemiological features of colubrid bites has been gathered from cases involving South American species, particularly *Philodryas* spp. As an example of a study addressing this challenging task, Salomão et al. (2003) considered data regarding snakebite admissions to Hospital Vital Brazil at the Instituto Butantan in São Paulo, Brazil, from 1959 to 1999. They reported that 26 genera of "mildly venomous" colubrid snakes were involved in snakebites recorded during the period of review. In descending order, *Helicops* spp. (South American water snakes or South American keel-backs), *Philodryas* spp. (South American racers), *Liophis* spp. (Central and South American ground snakes), *Oxyrhopus* spp. (Central and South American false-coral snakes), *Thamnodynastes* spp. (South American house snakes or mock vipers), and *Waglerophis merremi* (Wagler's or Merrem's snake) accounted for >100 cases each (Table 4.1). Not surprisingly, bites occurred most often on the upper and lower extremities. The majority of patients bitten by *Helicops*, *Philodryas*, *Liophis*, and *Thamnodynastes* spp. were between 15 and 40 years old, while children under 14 years old were most often bitten by *Oxyrhopus* and *W. merremi* (Salomão et al., 2003). The authors related the high frequency of *Helicops* bites to the probable circumstance of encountering these aquatic snakes during water-related human activities (particularly fishing), as the victim's lower extremities would be most likely unprotected against inflicted bites (Salomão et al., 2003). Truncally inflicted bites from genera such as *Erythrolamprus* spp. (also known as false-coral snakes), *Tomodon* spp. (Pampas snakes, also called mock vipers), and others were correlated with the victim lying in bed or in a bath. As discussed later, the absence of taxon-specific identification reduces the value of this survey containing a large sampling of bites by members of these genera.

Salomão et al. (2003) also associated *Helicops* bites with reported defensive behavior of these snakes, as well as a frequent lack of footwear among farm workers and others who commonly encounter them. These authors considered the role of cryptic coloration of *Liophis* spp., *Helicops* spp., and several other genera in contributing to the frequent involvement of these species in snakebites. Conversely, many patients reportedly bitten by genera with attractive patterns/coloration (*Philodryas* spp., *Erythrolamprus* spp., etc.) stated that they were bitten while attempting to collect or handle the snake (Salomão et al., 2003). Seasonal associations between bites inflicted by *P. olfersii* and *P. patagoniensis* were reported by Fowler and Salomão (1994) and de Medeiros et al. (2010). Bites from *P. olfersii* were most frequent from late winter (August) to early autumn (April). Bites from *P. patagoniensis* occurred most commonly mid-summer (January). Bites from *P. aestivus* (Brazilian green racer, boiobu, cobra verde, and others) were less common than from either *P. olfersii* or *P. patagoniensis* (Fowler and Salomão, 1994). Although the *n* was relatively small, these authors also reported that a greater number of female *P. patagoniensis* and male *P. olfersii* were respectively involved in reported bites. Bites from these species were more frequent between 1100 and 1600 h (Fowler and Salomão, 1994). These investigators also noted that the arboreal nature of *P. olfersii* was reflected by the occurrence of a sampling of bites while the victim was "off of the ground" (presumably, in an elevated dwelling/ domicile or low-lying tree), while all of the bites from *P. patagoniensis* occurred with the victim on level ground.

Similarly, Ribeiro et al. (1999) reported that *P. olfersii* bites occurred in Brazil most frequently during the hottest months, with a peak incidence in January (23.3% of diagnosed *P. olfersii* bites recorded at Instituto Butantan, 1982–1990). Of 43 patients reviewed in their retrospective study, 74.4% were male, and most victims were bitten between 2400 and 0600h (58.1%) and between 0600 and 1200h (27.9%). Forty-one snakes involved in these cases were measured, and the overwhelming majority (90.2%) were >50cm in length (Ribeiro et al., 1999). The measured lengths of 21 specimens were recorded with a mean length of 87.7cm. Twelve snakes were sexed; 10 were female, two male (Ribeiro et al., 1999). Twelve of the victims were handling the snake when bitten, while 12 reported being bitten while working, and eight children were bitten while playing. The authors indicated that it was unclear if any of the children were handling or trying to capture the snake when bitten. Of the remaining victims, only two reported being bitten while sleeping. This is in contrast with many reported bites from brown tree snakes (*B. irregularis*) on Guam (see later, and in Section 4.4). Not surprisingly, victims were most commonly bitten on the hands (72.1%) or feet (20.9%). Twenty-seven victims (62.8%) exhibited symptoms that may have resulted from the bite, while 16 (37.2%) were asymptomatic and showed no evidence of envenoming (Ribeiro et al., 1999).

Between 1959 and 2008, 297 cases of bites by *P. patagoniensis*, proven by qualified examination of the dead snake, were admitted to Instituto Butantan's Hospital in São Paulo, Brazil (de Medeiros et al., 2010). It is relatively uncommon and noteworthy that the identity of the offending snakes was formally verified in all cases included in their study. Snakes' lengths (snout–cloaca [vent]) ranged 160–1080mm, and 61.3% of the snakes were female. Most (89.1%) had empty stomachs. As reported by Fowler and Salomão (1994) and Ribeiro et al. (1999) in regard to bites from *P. olfersii* and/ or *P. patagoniensis* in Brazil, most of the bites (66%) occurred during spring and summer (October–March) during warmer periods of the day (likely reflecting the diurnality and periods of heightened activity of these taxa; 1000–1600h); 34% occurred during autumn and winter (April–September; de Medeiros et al., 2010). The mean age of bite victims was 24.1 ± 15.1 years and, as noted in previous studies, the majority of the victims were male (69.4%). There were no significant differences per distribution of bites by age group according to gender (de Medeiros et al., 2010). Most of the victims (92%) sought medical attention within 6h of being bitten, and the majority of bites were inflicted on the feet and hands (69%). Symptoms included pain (50.8%), transient bleeding (36%), erythema (16%), and edema in the absence of a tourniquet (13%). None of the victims exhibited ecchymoses. Seven patients reported mild dizziness, and the authors commented on the likely anxiety-driven etiology for this complaint (de Medeiros et al., 2010). None had incoagulable blood, but eight (2.7%) were given *Bothrops* antivenom before referral to Butantan. The minor nature of most of these bites is demonstrated by the minimal number of patients (13.4%) who received any treatment, limited to antihistamines and/or analgesics. Eighty-eight (29.6%) of

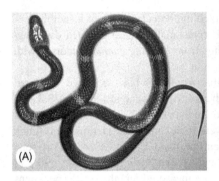 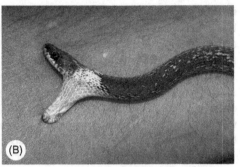

Plate 4.60 (A and B) Indian wolf snake or ular tana (*Lycodon aulicus*). There are approximately 29 species of *Lycodon* that occur in North and West Asia, Southeast Asia, and the Indian subcontinent. One species, the northern wolf snake (*Lycodon striatus*), is also found in the Middle East. These colubrine snakes are semiarboreal, nocturnal, and have dentition (enlarged anterior and posterior maxillary teeth that lack grooves) that may be specialized for their preferred prey: skinks and geckos. Bites by these snakes are typically medically insignificant.
(A) *Lycodon aulicus*, Sri Lanka.
(B) *Lycodon aulicus*, India, inflicting a medically insignificant bite.
Photos copyright to David A. Warrell.

those bitten had no evidence of envenoming (de Medeiros et al., 2010). Ten percent had received a tourniquet before arriving at the hospital, and tourniquet use was significantly associated with local edema. Secondary infection was reported in only 1% of patients. These investigators concluded that *P. patagoniensis* bites may cause mild local effects, and correct diagnosis is crucial in order to avoid the unnecessary use of antivenom (de Medeiros et al., 2010).

In Cuiaba, Mato Grosso, Brazil, two-thirds of medically unimportant snakebites are inflicted by *P. olfersii* (De Carvalho and Nogueira, 1998).

4.1.1.2   India

In a retrospective study conducted in three districts of West Bengal, Saha and Hati (1998) described patterns of nonvenomous snakebites inflicted by *Cerberus rhynchops* (dog-faced water snake or bockadam; Plate 4.10A–C), *Lycodon aulicus* (common or Indian wolf snake or ular tana; Plate 4.60A and B), and *Ptyas mucosus* (Indian or oriental rat snake, dhaman; rope snake; Plate 4.61). They reported that 31 of 157 (19.7%) non-venomous bites occurred in victims between 20 and 24 years old, and the lowest incidence (8 of 157; 5.0%) was in victims between 5 and 9 years old. In comparison, bites from venomous species such as *Daboia russelii* (Western Russell's viper, or in Sinhala, "tit polôngã"; Plate 4.62), *Naja naja* (Indian cobra, spectacled cobra, Asian cobra, gokhura, nag, and many others; Plate 4.63A and B), and *Bungarus caeruleus* (common, Indian or blue krait, kalaz, domna chitti, and many others; Plate 4.64) were most common in victims between 30 and 34 years old (15 of 88; 17%) and least frequent (1 of 88; 1.1%) in victims 0 to 4 years old (Saha and Hati, 1998). Although the specific

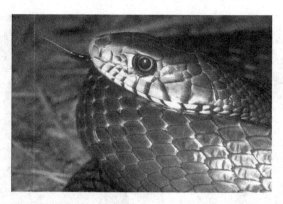

Plate 4.61 Indian rat snake, or dhaman (*Ptyas mucosus*), Bardia National Park, Bheri, Nepal. The genus *Ptyas* contains approximately nine species of colubrine snakes of appreciable body length that range throughout northern and western Asia, Southeast Asia, and the Indian subcontinent. In a study investigating the basic biology of *Ptyas mucosus* in central Java, Boeadi et al. (1998) measured 174 specimens, and reported a mean snout–vent length of 1.41 m. These snakes can reach in excess of 3 m, and a 3.58 m specimen has been recorded. They are commercially exploited for their skin and also are a common prey item for the king cobra (*Ophiophagous hannah*). They have a reputation for their irascible temperament when disturbed, but there are no medically significant bites documented to date. Although *Ptyas mucosus* has serous Duvernoy's glands (Taub, 1967), it lacks any notably modified dentition. Photo copyright to Mark O'Shea.

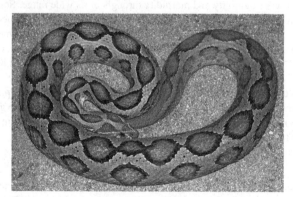

Plate 4.62 Russell's viper (*Daboia russelii*), India. This viperine viperid has long, distensible fangs ("solenoglyphous") and a large reservoir of highly toxic venom. Commonly found near populated rural locations in northern and western Asia, through Southeast Asia, and the Indian subcontinent, it is one of the world's most medically important venomous snakes. Envenomations from this species may cause acute kidney injury similar to that caused by hazard level 1 colubrids. A nephrotoxin has been identified in *D. russelii* venom. Photo copyright to David A. Warrell.

percentage of bites from individual species of nonvenomous snakes was not included, males were bitten more than twice as frequently as females (68.8% and 31.2%, respectively). There was a strong preponderance of cases during the rainy season

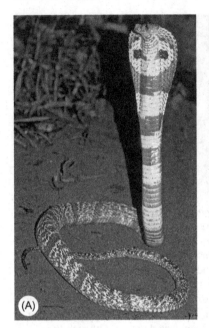 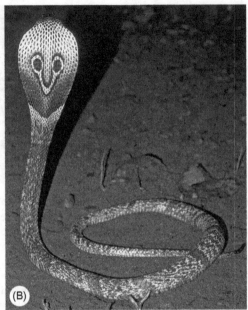

Plate 4.63 (A and B) Common Asian cobra, spectacled cobra, or Indian cobra; nag (*Naja naja*), Sri Lanka. The world's most medically important elapid snake, *N. naja* is responsible for a large proportion of mortality and morbidity throughout its wide range. Some populations produce postsynaptic neurotoxins, others necrotic cytotoxins, and a few produce a mixture of the two. Therefore, envenomated patients may present with paralytic features/respiratory failure, with severe locally necrotic disease, or, less commonly, a combination of these. The weak hemolysin, "direct lytic factor," synonymous with "cardiotoxin," occurs in venoms of some populations. Cardiotoxic effects are uncommonly documented, but have occurred in some patients envenomated by this species, particularly in Malaysia. Various phases of this species are popular in private collections. The long-confused taxonomy of the genus *Naja* has been subjected to recent review, and continuing reassignments in this group are likely. Photos copyright to David A. Warrell.

(June–September; 55.4%), and a notable decrease during the winter season (October–January; 18.4%). This is similar to the data reported by De Silva (1976a) and parallels the data reported for incidence of *P. olfersii* bites in Brazil (e.g., Ribeiro et al., 1999). Peak incidence of bites occurred between 1700 hours and 2400 hours (42%), and the least number of cases were recorded between 0100 and 0800 hours (9.55%; Saha and Hati, 1998). As noted in the other few epidemiological studies of non-front-fanged colubroid snake ("rear-fanged colubrid") bites, in the West Bengali region the majority of bites were inflicted on the victims' extremities; in this survey, the lower extremities were most commonly affected (77.7%; Saha and Hati, 1998). Unfortunately, Saha and Hati (1998) did not include any clinical detail of the presentations. They reported no significant effects from the nonvenomous bites recorded in the study, but a 6.81% mortality rate for the venomous bites. One of the authors previously reported an average

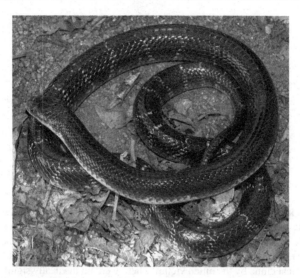

Plate 4.64 Blue or common krait (*Bungarus caeruleus*), India. These secretive semifossorial elapids often search for prey (e.g., other snakes, small mammals) inside human dwellings. In the Indian subcontinent, these snakes are an important cause of life-threatening snakebites. Victims may be bitten while asleep, an epidemiological feature in common with that of some bites inflicted by brown tree snakes (*Boiga irregularis*) on Guam. Photo copyright to David A. Warrell.

of 16.40 fatalities/10 years from venomous snakebites in Burdwan District of West Bengal (Hati et al., 1992). The authors emphasized the need for increased awareness among medical professionals of the difference between nonvenomous and venomous snakebites in order to avoid the inappropriate use of antivenom. They noted also the significant role of fear in most presented cases of snakebite inflicted by any species (Saha and Hati, 1998; see Section 4.5). The effects of fear were also described by the perceptive Frank Wall (1913) who described several cases of prolonged stupor or even death following bites by checkered keel-backs, *Xenochrophis* (*Tropidonotus* Boulenger 1896) *piscator* Schneider, 1799 (Plate 4.65), wolf snakes, *L. aulicus*, and several species of unidentified lizards, all presumed to be harmless. The survey by Sata and Hati (1998) suggests that the non-front-fanged colubroid snakes included in the study produced medically insignificant bites. This is concordant with the anecdotal information regarding these species, as there are no formally well-documented cases involving these taxa (e.g., *C. rhynchops*; Table 4.1).

4.1.1.3 Bangladesh

In Chittagong, 534 patients out of 884 who had been bitten by snakes developed no systemic envenoming and negligible or no local envenoming (Harris et al., 2010). Their average age was 26.4 years, and more than 95% had been bitten on the lower limbs. The incidence of nonenvenomed bites increased during the hot dry period of April and May to peak during the monsoon period of May–July. Thereafter, the

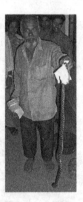

Plate 4.65 Checkered or painted keel-back (*Xenochrophis piscator*), Chittagong, Bangladesh. The *X. piscator/Xenochrophis flavipunctatus* complex is a group of natricids that widely range in Asia. The complex has been subject to repetitive taxonomic revision (Vogel and David, 2006), and may contain eight or more species. The pictured specimen was brought to a medical clinic by the bitten victim. There were no medically significant effects. Harmless species such as *X. piscator* are greatly feared in some communities as bites from any snake may be considered tantamount to a death sentence. Such fears may contribute to the somatic amplification of mild local effects or exacerbations of the victim's preexisting medical conditions (see Section 4.5). Photo copyright to Richard Maude.

incidence decreased except for a brief secondary peak during October. There were two peaks of biting incidence during the day, at 0800–1200 h and at 1800–2100 h. Only 2% of bites involved sleeping subjects. Eighteen of the snakes brought for identification were non-front-fanged colubroids: one *X. piscator*, four *C. radiatus*, and 13 *L. aulicus*. All four *C. radiatus* bites were on the feet during the evening and caused pain and bleeding at the bite site. Ligatures had been applied to all four victims, and they reached the hospital between 1.5 and 4 h (mean 3 h) after the bite. Fifty-five percent of bites by *L. aulicus* involved the feet, and 45% involved the hands. Sixty-six percent occurred indoors. All subjects experienced pain and bleeding at the bite site, and ligatures were used in all cases. All patients were admitted to the hospital between 1.5 and 6 h (mean 4 h) after the bite (Harris et al., 2010).

4.1.1.4 Thailand

A national survey of cases of snakebites in which the snakes were available for identification collected 1,631 snakes responsible for bites, of which 490 were neither elapids nor viperids (Viravan et al., 1992). Twenty-two non-front-fanged colubroid species were involved, including *Rhabdophis subminiatus*, *C. radiata*, *Homalopsis buccata* (Plate 4.66), *Oligodon* (Plate 4.67A and B, kukri snakes), *Lycodon*, *Boiga*, and *Enhydris* spp. (Plate 4.21A and B). None of the patients developed any significant signs of local or systemic envenoming, but in 22 cases medical staff misidentified the snakes as venomous, leading to inappropriate use of antivenom. The five patients bitten by *R. subminiatus* had accidentally trodden upon or touched the snake. Apart from bleeding from the bite wound, there were no adverse effects (Table 4.1).

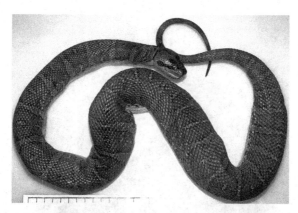

Plate 4.66 Masked or puff-faced water snake; ular kadut (*Homalopsis buccata*), Thailand. These snakes are members of the family, Homalopsidae, and range fairly widely in the Indian subcontinent and Southeast Asia. They favor aquatic or semiaquatic habitats, and are often found in estuarine habitats. The specimen shown was killed by the bitten victim who suffered no medically significant effects.
Photo copyright to David A. Warrell.

4.1.1.5 Sri Lanka

In a national survey of snakebite in Sri Lanka, the dead or living snake responsible was brought to the hospital by 860 bitten patients (Ariaratnam et al., 2009). In 94 cases (11% of the total) the snakes were nine non-front-fanged colubroid species: 48 wolf snakes (15 *Lycodon striatus sinhalayus* and 33 *L. aulicus*), 10 green vine snakes (*Ahaetulla nasuta*), 14 cat snakes (eight *Boiga forsteni*, four *Boiga trigonata trigonata*, and two *Boiga ceylonensis*), 11 rat snakes (*Ptyas mucosus*), six kukri snakes (*Oligodon arnensis*), one trinket snake (*Elaphe helena*), three *X. piscator*, and one ornate tree or flying snake (*Chrysopelea ornate ornata*). None of these bites was associated with systemic or significant local envenoming. Cat snakes [*Boiga ceylonensis* (Sri Lankan or Ceylon cat snake; nidi mapila), and *B. trigonata trigonata* (Gamma or common cat snake; ran mapila)] were twice misidentified as hump-nosed pit vipers (*Hypnale hypnale*; Plate 4.68), as were Russell's vipers (*Daboia russelii*) three times, and as was a saw-scaled viper (*Echis carinatus*; Plate 4.69A and B) once. Wolf snakes (*L. aulicus* and *L. striatus sinhalayus*) were misidentified as common kraits five times, and rat snakes as cobras twice. Antivenom was given inappropriately on 13 occasions because a nonvenomous species or a *H. hypnale* had been mistaken for one of the four species covered by Indian polyspecific antivenom (Ariaratnam et al., 2009). In Sri Lanka, *B. forsteni* (in Sinhala, naga or le mapila) is feared because of the myth that they hang down from the ceiling and suck the blood of sleeping humans. However, effects of bites are mild and localized. Similarly, the green vine or whip snake, *Ahaetulla nasuta* (in Sinhala, ahaetulla/ahata gulla/as gulla—meaning "eye plucker") is reputed to pluck out the eyes of humans, as first alluded to by a Portuguese traveler João Ribeiro in 1685 (Ribeiro, 1989). Its bite causes only mild local effects (De Silva and Aloysius, 1983; Table 4.1).

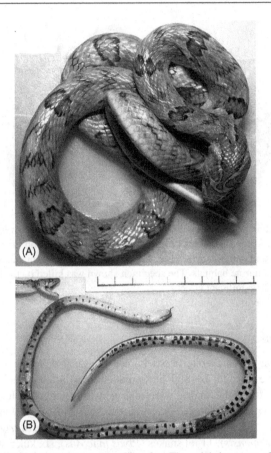

Plate 4.67 (A and B) Kukri snakes, genus *Oligodon*. The colubrine genus *Oligodon* contains approximately 68 species that feed on small vertebrates (e.g., birds, lizards) and their eggs as well as large insects (dietary preferences vary according to species). *Oligodon* spp. have a wide range in northern to western Asia, Southeast Asia, and the Indian subcontinent. *Oligodon* spp. are a common cause of snakebites, but only mild local effects have been documented. An *O. arnensis* bite reported by the famous British herpetologist and physician, Frank Wall (1868–1950), allegedly resulted in death. However, review of this case reveals Wall's own doubts regarding the etiology of the fatal outcome. This case is critically reviewed in Section 4.3.
(A) Common or Cantor's kukri snake (*Oligodon cycluris*), Thailand. After being bitten, the victim brought this specimen to the medical clinic. The bite was medically insignificant.
(B) Loos snake or striped kukri snake (*Oligodon taeniatus*), Thailand. Another specimen killed after inflicting a medically insignificant bite, the enlarged posterior maxillary teeth are also shown in profile (upper left corner).
Photos copyright to David A. Warrell.

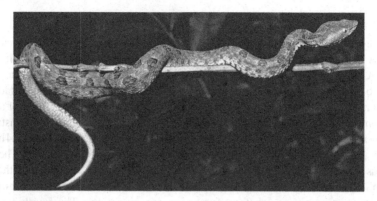

Plate 4.68 Merrem's hump-nosed viper or pit viper; Polonthelissa, Kunakatuwa (*Hypnale hypnale*). This medically important crotaline viperid is found in southwestern India and Sri Lanka. Envenomations from this species may cause consumptive coagulopathy and acute kidney injury similar to that caused by hazard level 1 colubrids.
Photo copyright to David A. Warrell.

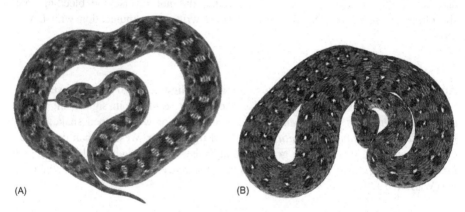

(A)   (B)

Plate 4.69 (A and B) Saw-scaled vipers (*Echis* spp.). There are approximately 12 species of *Echis* that range from Western Asia through the Indian subcontinent, the Middle East, and Africa. Their name is based on their making tight, figure-eight or C-shaped coils, with the loops producing friction from the contact between scales that are rubbed together, and thereby yield a loud, rasping-steam sound. Saw-scaled vipers are among the world's most important venomous snakes, and are responsible for a large proportion of the snakebite-related morbidity as well as mortality throughout their range. In particular, there are a large number of cases involving agricultural workers in rural communities in Africa and the Indian subcontinent where these snakes constitute a serious public health risk. Serious envenomation by *Echis* spp. includes consumptive coagulopathy similar to that caused by hazard level 1 colubrids. In some rural communities, several non-front-fanged colubroid species may be misidentified as viperine viperids such as *Echis* (see text).
(A) Sochurek's saw-scaled viper; Eastern saw-scaled or carpet viper; phoorsa (*Echis carinatus sochureki*). *Echis c. sochureki* are native to Bangladesh and Pakistan.
(B) West African saw-scaled viper or carpet viper; ocellated carpet viper (*Echis ocellatus*), Nigeria. This species is native to the savannahs of West Africa and similar in behavior to other *Echis* spp.
Photos copyright to David A. Warrell.

4.1.1.6 Kenya

On the coast of Kenya (between Kilifi and Malindi), there have been four cases of *D. typus* bite since 2006 (Sanda Ashe, personal written communication with DAW, 2010). A snake collector who was bitten twice on the forearm by a *D. typus* while trying to bag the snake developed hematemesis, bloody diarrhea, and intracranial hemorrhage about 36 hours after the bite and died while awaiting the arrival of antivenom from South Africa. A second snake collector, bitten under similar circumstances, was already vomiting and passing blood when he was first seen less than 24 h after the bite. He was treated with boomslang antivenom and recovered rapidly. The third case was a child who had put his hand into a bird's nest and was bitten at the base of his middle finger by a juvenile *D. typus*, which was brought for identification. He was treated with antivenom before developing any symptoms. The fourth case was a 6-month-old female infant bitten on the sole of the foot in Kilifi while playing on the ground. The snake inflicted a protracted bite, and the child continued to bleed from the puncture wounds for several days (leukocytes = 17.1 × 10^9/L, hemoglobin 7.2 g/dL, hematocrit 22.5%, platelets 388 × 10^9/L). She received 5 units of blood and Sanofi-Pasteur Fav-Afrique antivenom that did not reverse the bleeding, but she ultimately recovered (Sanda Ashe, personal written communication with DAW, 2010).

4.1.1.7 Nigeria

Among 207 bites by identified snakes in northern Nigeria (1970–1975), seven were by proven non-front-fanged colubroid snakes, none resulting in significant symptoms: *Crotaphopeltis hotamboeia* (herald snake, red- or white-lipped snake; rooilipslang) (1), *Telescopus variegatus* (variegated tiger snake, West African cat snake) (2), *Psammophis sibilans* (olive grass or sand snake; olyfkleurige grasslang) (2), and *Lamprophis fuliginosus* (common African house snake, brown house snake; chakusa) (2) (Warrell, 1979).

4.1.1.8 Middle East

In Iraq and some other Middle Eastern countries, the black phase of the (European) whip snake, *Dolichophis (Coluber) jugularis* (Plate 4.70A and B), is greatly feared under the local names "arbid," "abrid," or "urbid" (Corkill, 1932; Thesiger, 1964). This reputation is based on its large size (up to 2.5 m in total length), aggressive display when cornered, and its resemblance to the black desert cobras (*Walterinnesia morgani* and *W. aegyptia*; Plate 4.71). There are no reliable reports of bites in the region, and the fatalities attributed to it by the local people are likely to have been caused by *Walterinnesia* spp. or by the blunt-nosed or Levantine viper (*Macrovipera lebetina*; Plate 4.72).

4.1.1.9 Guam: A Distinctive Set of Circumstances

Guam, the largest island in Micronesia, presents an unusual opportunity to assess the medical importance of a non-front-fanged colubroid species. Only two snake species are found on Guam. One is a fossorial member of the "primitive" superfamily

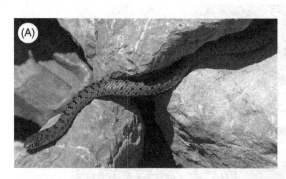
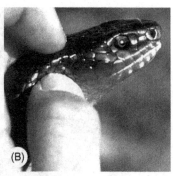

Plate 4.70 (A and B) European, green or large whip snake; fire snake; arbid, urbid
[*Dolichophis (Coluber) jugularis*], Greece. A former member of the formerly polyphyletic
genus *Coluber*, *D. jugularis* ranges throughout Cyprus, Turkey, Greece, and the Middle East.
It occurs at altitudes up to 1,400 m, and preys on rodents, lizards, and other snakes. It has a
bad reputation in Iraq and other Middle Eastern countries, based on its large size, aggressive
behavior, and similarity in appearance (particularly of the black phase of this species) to that of
the desert black cobra (*Walterinnesia aegyptia* and *W. morgani*; see Plate 4.71). Multiple field
observations have reported cannibalism among this species (Göçmen et al., 2008). The prey
preference (rats) of this colubrine species led to its use as an agricultural pest- (rat-) control
method in Cyprus (Göçmen and Yildiz, 2006). There are no well-documented cases of *D.
jugularis* bites, and anecdotal reports suggest only minor local effects from bites by this species.
(A) *Dolichophis jugularis*, Symi, Greece.
(B) *Dolichophis jugularis*, black phase, Kos, Greece.
Photos copyright to Matt Wilson.

Scolecophidia, the widespread Brahminy blindsnake (*Ramphotyphlops braminus*). It is
a very interesting ophidian species in that it is the only snake species proven to be par-
thenogenetic,[1] has been introduced all over the world, feeds almost exclusively on
insect larvae, and has notably reduced dentition. It does not figure in any snakebites
on Guam, or elsewhere.[2] However, the only other snake species found on Guam (also
introduced), the brown tree snake (*B. irregularis*), has inflicted a large number of bites
and has understandably attracted a great deal of concern regarding its medical importance. The distinctive factors surrounding this invasive and ecologically destructive
species are discussed in Section 4.4. A retrospective review of 446 *B. irregularis* bites
recorded at Guam Memorial Hospital, 1987–2004, identified several epidemiological

---

[1] Defined as the production of offspring by virgin females in the total absence of males, true parthenogene-
sis results in genetically identical clonal populations (Lampert and Schartl, 2010). Distinct from partheno-
genesis, some other ophidian species, such as the distinctive crotaline viperid, *Bothrops insularis* (golden
lancehead), occasionally have intersexual (females with hemipenes) individuals or populations. These
snakes are only found on Queimada Grande Island (coastal southeastern Brazil), and this partially intersexual population has been associated with declining fertility in this insular species (Duarte et al., 1995).
[2] However, Salomão et al. (2003) reviewed a series of purported bites inflicted by another Scolecophidian,
Liotyphlops spp. (an unspecified species of dawn blindsnake) that reportedly caused mild local effects in a
number of children (see Table 4.1).

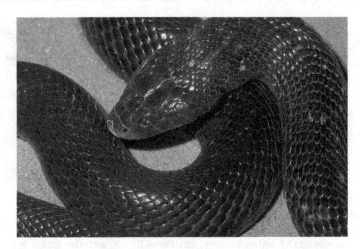

Plate 4.71 Desert black snake or cobra; Walter Innes' snake; iyah (*Walterinnesia aegyptia*), Saudi Arabia. An inhabitant of arid biotopes, *W. aegyptia* is a moderately large, usually glossy black elapid (often >1.0 m length) that resembles the nonvenomous *Dolicophis jugularis*. *Walterinnesia aegyptia* and its congener, *W. morgani*, are found in Israel, the lowlands of the Middle East, and range down into northeastern Egypt. Venom lethal potency is similar to some populations of the Asian cobra (*Naja naja*; average murine i.p. LD$_{50}$ is approximately 0.3 mg/kg), but yield is low (several specimens from Israel averaged around 2.5 mg; SAW, unpublished data). There are anecdotal reports of fatalities from envenomations by this species, but bites are rare, and well-documented cases are lacking. A bivalent antivenom effective for treatment of *W. aegyptia* envenomation is available.
Photo copyright to David A. Warrell.

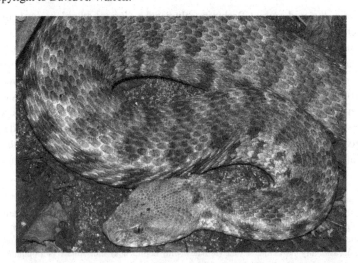

Plate 4.72 Blunt-nosed or Levantine viper (*Macrovipera lebetina lebetina*), Cyprus. A robustly large, Euro-Middle Eastern viperine viperid (up to 2 m in length) that is native to Cyprus, Lebanon, Syria, Iraq, Kuwait, Iran, Jordan, and Israel. It is a significant cause of snakebite, and envenomation can result in death. There is an effective antivenom for this species.
Photo copyright to David A. Warrell.

characteristics associated with these cases (Morocco et al., 2006). Bites most likely occurred during the rainy season in children (20% were infants younger than 1 year old), at night when the victim was sleeping, and were commonly inflicted on an extremity. This review included some of the cases detailed by Fritts et al. (1994), who reported risks and circumstances associated with 94 brown tree snakebites that occurred on Guam from 1989 to 1991. Similar to the data previously noted regarding reported peak incidence of bites from *P. olfersii* in Brazil and the three nonvenomous snake species surveyed in West Bengal, the highest frequency of *B. irregularis* bites in this series occurred during the early rainy season (May). The lowest incidence was noted in mid-dry season (January through March; Fritts et al., 1994). The mean number of bites during the rainy season (May–October) and the dry season (November–April) were 12.2 and 3.5, respectively (Fritts et al., 1994). The recorded increased frequency of bites during the rainy season correlates with the seasonal peaks in snakebite victims who present at the Guam Memorial Hospital emergency department (Fritts et al., 1990). However, in contrast with available data regarding *P. olfersii*, in cases ($n = 79$) of *B. irregularis* bite in which the victim's activity while bitten was documented, 63 (80%) were at home sleeping during the incident. Furthermore, of these, 33 (52%) were children younger than 5 years old (Fritts et al., 1994). Almost all of the bites inflicted on sleeping victims occurred between dusk and dawn, and 31 (49%) of the victims were bitten on the fingers or hand. The majority of victims had bites at various locations, including upper and lower extremities, back, and face. The majority of a small group of patients (13/17) with multiple bites were sleeping children younger than 16 years old (Fritts et al., 1994). Of the total number of cases, 71 included some data about the pre-senting symptoms/signs. Local pain was most common (56%), edema (49%), and "discoloration," probably mild ecchymoses (48%). In nine cases involving children, there were more extensive local effects (e.g., blistering, large hematomas at wound sites), and four were said to exhibit "respiratory difficulties and potential neurological impairment" (Fritts et al., 1994). The pediatric patients described were between 3 weeks and 4 months old. These cases are critically analyzed in Section 4.3. The studies by Fritts et al. (1990, 1994) identify children younger than 15 years old as having the highest risk of medically significant injury from *B. irregularis* bites on Guam.

4.1.2 Circumstances Associated with Species Capable of Inflicting Life-Threatening Envenoming

Although cases of life-threatening or fatal colubrid bites are rare, qualitative review of some well-documented histories provides a glimpse into some of the circumstances frequently associated with these cases. For example, consideration of a handful of thoroughly documented serious bites from *D. typus* or *Thelotornis* spp. (Table 4.1) reveals some victim characteristics and circumstances associated with these envenomings. These bites most commonly occur when a male victim (typically between 20 and 35 years old) is either attempting to capture a wild snake, or is handling a captive specimen. These victims are almost always bitten on the upper extremities, most often on the digits. Several reports describe children (primarily male, rarely female) receiving bites on the lower extremities while walking. The oldest victim in a well-documented fatal case was an 80-year-old prominent male herpetologist (Robert F.W. Mertens) who was bitten on the right thumb by a captive *T. kirtlandii* while offering the snake food (Table 4.1; Section 4.3). It is noteworthy that the victim had been bitten briefly ("quick release") by the same specimen some weeks earlier without any subsequent effects. Of 12 selected representative serious cases of *R. tigrinus* envenoming (see Table 4.1; Section 4.3), five (41%) were 6–14 years old (two, or 16%, were <10 years old); four (33%) were 49–57 years old, and the remaining two victims were 20 or 40 years old, respectively. All 12 victims were male, and at least eight (66%) of these were bitten while handling, attempting to collect, or otherwise intentionally interacting (e.g., attempting to photograph) with the culprit snake. All of the victims were bitten on the upper extremities, 10 (83%) were on the digits, the remainder on the wrist or dorsum of the hand. Interestingly, all of the victims in four cases of *R. subminiatus* envenoming were males between 20 and 25 years old, and all of these bites were inflicted on the digits of the upper extremities by captive snakes during intentional contact (e.g., during free handling; see Table 4.1 and Section 4.3).

Due to inconsistent documentation of circumstances (and victim characteristics) in many cases of serious envenoming by these species, there are too few well-detailed cases for significant statistical analysis. This emphasizes the need for careful, accurate, and detailed formal documentation of these fortunately uncommon cases.

There is a dearth of data on the risk of non-front-fanged colubroid bites in indigenous populations (see earlier for several countries) which are more likely to be accidental and associated with invasion of the snakes' arboreal domain. In coastal Kenya, for example, children are occasionally bitten by *D. typus* while raiding birds' nests or holes in trees (see earlier). In Cameroon, a man was bitten on the hand by a *D. typus* while climbing a palm tree (Knabe, 1939), and in South Africa, a farmer was bitten while picking bananas (Gerber and Adendorff, 1980), as well as a child bitten while walking through long grass (Aitchison, 1990). Snake charmers have also been bitten (Du Toit, 1980).

4.2 Some Representative Genera: Typical Features of Bites and an Overview of Their Natural History and Toxinology

4.2.1 Genus Boiga: Background and General Features of Documented Bites

Approximately 34 species of *Boiga* are currently recognized. Subspecies are recognized for several taxa with the mangrove or ringed cat snake, *B. dendrophila* (Plate 4.7A–D), having the most (nine) subspecies. Table 4.2 summarizes some of the dietary preferences, geographic ranges, and average adult sizes of representative *Boiga* spp. Documented cases of bites only involve about 10 species, and most of these are largely insignificant or limited to mild local effects [puncture wounds/lacerations, mild bleeding, minor

Table 4.2 Dietary Preferences, Average Adult Size and Range of Representative Non-Front-Fanged Colubroid Species

Species[a]	Family, Subfamily[b]	Average Adult Size (cm)	Dietary Preferences	Range	Remarks	Reference[c]
Boiga dendrophila	Colubridae, Colubrinae	180–213	Lizards, frogs, snakes, birds, small mammals	Malaysia, Indonesia, Philippine islands, southern Thailand	Primarily arboreal feeding behavior	Mehrtens (1987)
Boiga irregularis	Colubridae, Colubrinae	140–200	Birds, bird eggs, lizards, small mammals	Solomon islands, New Guinea, Australia (inadvertently introduced to Guam, Saipan, and other Western Pacific islands)	Unnatural range has occurred due to accidental widespread introductions	Cogger (1975)
Dispholidus typus	Colubridae, Colubrinae	120–155	Chameleons, frogs, small mammals, fledgling birds	Sub-Saharan Africa, extending down the east and south coast to Cape Town	Probably the widest ranging African tree snake. An active predator of the arboreal strata	Visser and Chapman (1978)
Hemorrhois ravergieri	Colubridae, Colubrinae	159 (max)	Lizards, birds, rodents	Northeastern Africa, Israel, Turkey, Afghanistan, Pakistan	Small prey swallowed live, large prey constricted	Latifi (1991)
Heterodon nasicus	Dipsadidae, Heterodontinae	35–45	Amphibians, reptiles, small mammals, birds, rarely lizards	Southwest Manitoba, south Alberta, southeast Saskatchewan, south to east and central Texas, New Mexico, and Zacatecas, Aguascalientes, San Luis Potosi Mexico. Occurs in isolated locales in Iowa, Illinois, Missouri, Wyoming	Common species kept by many amateur herpetologists	Ernst and Ernst (2003)

(Continued)

Table 4.2 (Continued)

Species[a]	Family, Subfamily[b]	Average Adult Size (cm)	Dietary Preferences	Range	Remarks	Reference[c]
Hierophis viridiflavus	Colubridae, Colubrinae	100–150	Lizards, small mammals, birds, snakes (including viperids)	France, Spain, Greece, Italy, Malta, Slovenia, Andorra, Croatia	Primarily saurophagous	Capula et al. (1997)
Hydrodynastes gigas	Dipsadidae, Xenodontinae	183–213	Primarily frogs, fish	East Bolivia, Paraguay, south Brazil, north Argentina	Reportedly utilizes both "venom" and constriction to subdue prey	Mehrtens (1987), Hill and Mackessy (2000)
Malpolon monspessulanus	Lamprophiidae, Psammophinae	152–183	Lizards, snakes, birds, small mammals	Western Morocco, Spain, Portugal, west to France, and northwestern Italy	Reportedly utilizes "venom" for lizards and constriction with rodents	Mehrtens (1987)
Philodryas olfersii	Dipsadidae, Xenodontinae	96–115	Frogs, birds, small mammals, lizards	West Brazil, east Peru, Bolivia, Paraguay, Uruguay, Argentina	Arboreal and terrestrial habitat use. Prey type varies with geographic range	Leite et al. (2009), Hartman and Marques (2005)
Platyceps najadum	Colubridae, Colubrinae	83–103	Lizards, small rodents	Bulgaria, Turkey	May range up to 1850 m elevation	Latifi (1991), Kumlutas et al. (2004)
Rhabdophis tigrinus	Natricidae	<100	Amphibians, small fish	Japan, China, Taiwan, Vietnam, eastern Russia, North and South Korea	Once sold in pet trade as nonvenomous	Gopalakrishnakione and Chou (1990)

Species	Family		Diet	Distribution		References
Thamnophis elegans vagrans	Natricidae	45–76	Small lizards, amphibians (including tadpoles), slugs, earthworms, leeches, and occasionally small mammals (mice)	Southwest Saskatchewan, south Alberta, south British Columbia;south Manitoba; South Dakota to western Washington, Oregon, and eastern central California (probably the widest ranging *Thamnophis elegans* subspecies)	Readily accepts small mammals in captivity. Has been observed at elevations up to 3200 m	Ernst and Ernst (2003), Kumlutas et al. (2004)
Thamnophis sirtalis sirtalis	Natricidae	45–66	Earthworms, small lizards, amphibians (including tadpoles), slugs, leeches, and occasionally nestling mice	Massachusetts and west New England westward through Ontario, and south through peninsular Florida and west to east Louisiana. Isolated occurrences in southeast Texas	Possibly, the snake most commonly maintained in captivity. Found farther north in Canada than any other snake species	Ernst and Ernst (2003), Kumlutas et al. (2004)
Thelotornis capensis	Colubridae, Colubrinae	60–80	Lizards (particularly chameleons), frogs, fledgling birds, snakes	East and South Africa	Prey is often swallowed while the snake suspends head downward	Visser and Chapman (1978)

[a]See Table 4.1 and text for common names.
[b]The listed taxonomic assignments are current to the date of publication of this book. These are susceptible to probable re-adjustment according to future taxonomic studies.
[c]Information is derived from these references, as well as personal observations of the authors.

pain, and edema etc.; see the seven species listed in Table 4.1, and there are also additional insignificant anecdotally reported bites by Forsten's cat snake, *B. forsteni* (Plate 4.8; Table 4.1), as well as the many-spotted or marble cat snake, *B. multimaculata*]. Most *Boiga* spp. attain an average adult length of 1.0–2.0 m, although some taxa (e.g., Blanding's tree snake, *B. blandingi* and the brown tree snake, *B. irregularis*) may exceed 3.5 m (Pitman, 1974; Fritts and McCoid, 1999; SAW personal observations).

Boiga (*Toxicodryas* Trape and Mané 2006) *blandingi* (Plate 4.5A and B) is subjectively viewed with suspicion by some authors (Groves, 1973; Levinson et al., 1976; Spawls, 1979; Goodman, 1985), although the few documented bites have featured only minor puncture wounds/lacerations, mild local pain, and slight bleeding (Table 4.1). Notably, around its range in the Kakamega Forest in western Kenya, this snake is feared by some of the local Luo people. The less spectacular, closely related, and sympatric *B.* (*Toxicodryas* LeGrand, 2002) *pulverulenta* (powdered or blotched tree snake) is not similarly perceived. Possibly, the large adult size and gaping mouth defensive display of *B. blandingi* (Plate 4.5B) adds to its somewhat fearsome reputation.

Despite several cases posted on the Internet that illustrate severe local swelling, bruising, and hemorrhagic blister formation following purported *B. dendrophila* bites (see Appendix A), the two published cases and several others from anecdotal accounts developed only mild symptoms (Table 4.1). This is concordant with the experiences of one of the authors (SAW), who received several insignificant bites (mild pain and brief bleeding) from *B. d. melanota* and *B. d. multicincta*. Although some observers have voiced concerns about the possible life-threatening risks of species such as *B. forsteni* in Sri Lanka, at this time there are no documented cases or other evidence that support these perceptions (De Silva, 1976a; Fritts and McCoid, 1999; Fritts et al., 1994). As noted earlier, the distinctive circumstances surrounding risks from *B. irregularis* are discussed in Section 4.4.

4.2.1.1 Overview of the Duvernoy's Gland and Associated Dentition of Boiga spp.

Although the presence of grooved, enlarged maxillary teeth is generally established for members of the genus, there are few data regarding the specific characteristics of the maxillary teeth present in various *Boiga* spp. Taylor (1922) reported that *Boiga* spp. found in the Philippines (including *B. dendrophila*) possessed "two or three" grooved posterior maxillary teeth. Fry et al. (2008) reported that *B. irregularis* had enlarged posterior maxillary teeth with deep grooves running their entire length. Plates 4.7C and D and 4.9E and F respectively show the enlarged, deeply grooved posterior maxillary teeth of *B. dendrophila* and *B. irregularis*. The teeth are gently recurved, notably larger than the preceding dentition, and the grooves span almost the entire length of the teeth.

In an extensive comparative histological study of colubrid oral glands, Taub (1967) assessed the morphology of Duvernoy's glands from several *Boiga* spp. He described the glands of *B. dendrophila*, *B. d. latifasciata*, and *B. blandingi* as having: capsules with "heavy" to "very heavy" thickness (that of *B. dendrophila* was slightly thicker than that of *B. blandingi* or *B. d. latifasciata*); noted vascularity; and numerous thin (*B. d. latifasciata*) or "heavily thick" trabeculae. The glands lacked mucous

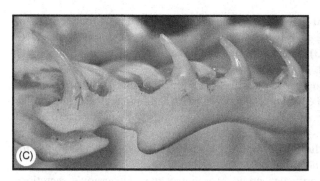
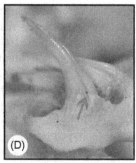

Plate 4.7 **(C) Lateral upright view of posterior maxilla of *Boiga dendrophila*.**
(D) Close-up of enlarged posterior maxillary teeth of *Boiga dendrophila*. The
posteriormost maxillary teeth are notably enlarged, recurved, and deeply grooved (arrows).
Plate 4.7C and D, AMNH specimen #R73608, photos copyright to Arie Lev.

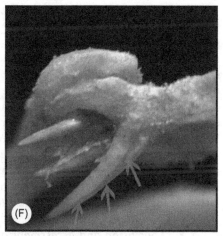
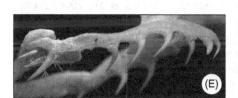

Plate 4.9 **(E and F) Close-up of enlarged maxillary teeth of *Boiga irregularis*.** The
posteriormost maxillary teeth are notably enlarged, recurved, and deeply grooved (arrows).
Plate 4.9E and F, AMNH specimen #114498, photos copyright to Scott A. Weinstein.

cells and were composed of columnar cells, but in *B. blandingi* there were mucous
cells associated with the glands. A lumen was noted in ≥90% of the tubules of the *B.
dendrophila* and *B. d. latifasciata* Duvernoy's glands, but in only 10% of the tubules
of the glands from *B. blandingi* (Taub, 1967).

4.2.1.2   Summary of the Toxinology and Properties of Duvernoy's Secretions from Boiga spp. (Excluding B. irregularis)

There is relatively limited information regarding yield and toxicity of Duvernoy's
secretions from these species (see Appendix B). Weinstein and Smith (1993) reported
a yield of 147.5 μL (1.6 mg solids) from *B. blandingi*. The protein content of secretion

from two specimens ranged between 75% and 100%. Intraperitoneal murine LD_{50} of *B. blandingi* secretion ranged between 2.85 and 4.88 mg/kg (Levinson et al., 1976; Weinstein and Smith, 1993). Standardization for protein content resulted in a lower LD_{50} (Weinstein and Smith, 1993).

Similarly, *B. d. melanota* yielded 127.5 µL, but with 8 mg solids, while *B. d. multicincta* yielded 87.5 µL with only 1 mg solids (Weinstein and Smith, 1993). The murine i.p. LD_{50} of *B. d. melanota* and *B. d. multicincta* secretions (protein standardized and weight/volume) were: 3.26–4.04 mg/kg and 3.91–7.17 mg/kg, respectively (Weinstein and Smith, 1993). An earlier study reported a murine i.v. LD_{50} of 4.85 mg/kg for *B. dendrophila* secretion (Sakai et al., 1984).

Proteolytic and/or hemorrhagic activity was detected in Duvernoy's secretions from *B. blandingi*, *B. d. melanota*, and *B. d. multicincta* (Hill and Mackessy, 2000; Sakai et al., 1984; Weinstein and Smith, 1993). Pulmonary and/or subendocardial hemorrhage has been noted in mice injected i.v. or i.p. with *Boiga dendrophila*, *B. d. melanota*, and *B. d. multicincta* secretions (Sakai et al., 1984; Weinstein and Smith, 1993). *Boiga dendrophila* secretion contained moderate levels of phospholipases A_2 (PLA_2; Hill and Mackessy, 2000). Phosphodiesterase was detected in *B. dendrophila* saliva, but not in Duvernoy's secretion (Hill and Mackessy, 2000).

Although postsynaptically active neurotoxins have been detected in Duvernoy's secretions from *B. blandingi*, *B. irregularis*, and *B. dendrophila*, as noted previously, these toxins ["denmotoxin," a monomeric 77 amino acid polypeptide containing five disulfide bridges from *B. dendrophila* Duvernoy's secretion, and "irditoxin," a heterodimeric polypeptide from *B. irregularis* Duvernoy's secretion (see Section 4.4)] have marked specificity for saurian or avian subjects (Pawlak et al., 2006, 2009). To date, there is no evidence of any clinical significance of these toxins. Similarly, although Sakai et al. (1984) reported *in vitro* coagulant activities of *B. dendrophila* Duvernoy's secretion, there are no documented cases of systemic effects in humans, including coagulopathy, resulting from bites inflicted by this species.

4.2.1.3 Conclusion and Assessment of Boiga spp.

The mild effects reported in the few documented cases of bites from these species, as well as the limited data regarding Duvernoy's secretion toxicity and yield from these snakes, suggest a very low medical risk to humans. However, a protracted bite inflicted by a large specimen might cause significant local effects.

Assessment of *Boiga* spp. (excluding *B. irregularis*) based on available evidence: Hazard Level 3/4 (typically only mild local effects such as puncture wounds/lacerations, erythema, edema, and insignificant bleeding, with potential for more pronounced local effects such as more extensive edema and pain).

4.2.2 Genus Philodryas spp.: Background and General Features of Documented Bites

Of the 18 species of South American racers, *Philodryas*, five (and one subspecies) have been reported to inflict medically significant bites (Table 4.1). These fast-moving, active snakes feed on a broad variety of prey and exhibit a wide range in South America (see Table 4.2 for examples). An uncommon characteristic of some Uruguayan populations of *P. patagoniensis* (Plate 4.41) is that they are known to participate in communal nesting (Vaz-Ferreira et al., 1970).[3] The biology, taxonomy, and perceived medical risks of this genus have been comprehensively reviewed by Campbell and Lamar (2004). Campbell and Lamar (2004) also described the habitats of various taxa and illustrated the recognized species. Of 16 genera included in a broad study of colubrid snakebite in Brazil, Salomão et al. (2003) ascribed 11 symptoms to *Philodryas* spp. bites as noted from records of Hospital Vital Brazil, Instituto Butantan—more than for any of the other species. Among these *Philodryas* spp. bites, the authors reported a 1.3% incidence of "gum hemorrhage" (Salomão et al., 2003), implying uncommon antihemostatic systemic effects from these bites and thereby suggesting "envenoming." In contrast, Ribeiro et al. (1999), who reviewed 43 cases of *P. olfersii* (Plate 4.39A and B) bites that presented to Instituto Butantan between 1982 and 1990, described only local effects. Whole blood clotting tests performed in 11 cases were unremarkable (Ribeiro et al., 1999). These authors also cited several unpublished cases characterized by mild-to-moderate local effects but lacking any systemic manifestations. Two pediatric cases were misdiagnosed as *Bothrops* spp. envenoming and treated with polyvalent anti-*Bothrops* antivenom (Ribeiro et al., 1999). Similarly, Nishioka and Silveira (1994) reported a case of mild local effects ("mild edema and warmth") in a 5-year-old patient bitten by *P. patagoniensis*. The patient was incorrectly diagnosed as having been envenomed by a *Bothrops* spp. and was given polyvalent anti-*Bothrops* antivenom. Salomão et al. (2003) reported the case of a 17-year-old male admitted to Hospital Vital Brazil with "all the symptoms of a *Bothrops* envenomation." The victim described the snake responsible as a "green snake with a brown head." When shown a specimen of *P. olfersii*, he immediately confirmed that it was the snake that had bitten him, and he was therefore not given antivenom (Salomão et al., 2003). These cases may suggest that misidentification of *Philodryas* spp. for crotaline species (e.g., some *Bothrops* spp.) could account for some reports of "bleeding gums" and other symptoms/signs reflecting systemic effects. As described earlier, antivenom may also be given inappropriately to patients with moderate local effects from a *Philodryas* spp. bite, as this may be wrongly ascribed to *Bothrops* spp. envenoming.

Misunderstanding of snakebite management and misinformation about differences between medical risks posed by front-fanged venomous snakes and "colubrids" contribute to the inappropriate treatment of bitten patients with clinically significant local effects. Ironically, this may assume greater importance in some hospitals admitting patients bitten by local species such as *Philodryas* spp. A patient bitten by a verified *P. olfersii* in Recife, Brazil, presented with local pain, moderate edema, erythema, and mild ecchymoses of the right hand, and was given eight ampoules of anti-*Bothrops*

---

[3] Communal nesting is well known among a number of Nearctic, Palearctic, and a few Australian snake taxa, but is quite rare among Neotropical species. The only South American species known to participate in this behavior are specific populations of *Dipsas oreas* (Ecuador snail eater; Cadle and Chuna, 1995), *Sibynomorphus mikanii* (Alburquerque and Ferrarezzi, 2004), *Psomophis obtusus* (wide ground snake), and *P. patagoniensis* (Vaz-Ferreira et al., 1970).

spp. (polyvalent) antivenom (Correia et al., 2010). Sometimes, the victim may be better informed than the medical team responsible for his or her care. For instance, a female technician maintaining an institutional venomous animal collection was bitten on the distal phalanx of her right fifth digit while handling a *P. olfersii* (De Araújo and dos Santos, 1997). Although there was no immediate pain or bleeding, edema involving the entire hand developed 15 min after the bite. She presented at an emergency department where all her vital signs and results of tests (unspecified) were reportedly within normal limits. However, the medical team recommended administration of anti-*Bothrops* spp. (polyvalent) antivenom, which the patient wisely declined. She was treated only with an "antihistaminic" injection (De Araújo and dos Santos, 1997).

The most frequently documented symptoms from *Philodryas* spp. include: lacerations/puncture wounds, mild local pain, edema, erythema, and ecchymoses (Table 4.1; Ribeiro et al., 1999; Salomão et al., 2003). A report of vertigo that developed several days after a bite from *P. o. latirostris* (Table 4.1) is considered in Section 4.4. A frequently cited fatal case attributed to a *P. olfersii* bite is discussed later. An anecdotal case mentioned by Means (2010) as communicated by Professor William Lamar described an alleged *P. viridissimus* (green palm snake or common green racer; Plate 4.42) bite inflicted on a pet shop worker in Virginia, USA. The victim suffered severe local effects and, ultimately, compartment syndrome was diagnosed. It was suggested that the severity of the "envenoming" may have been due to manual pressure exerted on the snake's head during attempts to extricate its jaws from the victim, leading to manual expression of gland contents into the wound (William Lamar, written personal communication with SAW, April 2010). However, the lack of any significant storage capacity in Duvernoy's glands of most species studied to date, including *Philodryas* spp., makes it more likely that stimulation of sustained glandular secretion contributed to the severity of this case. Acquired hypersensitivity to snake secretions or venom constituents must also be considered, especially in a person with a probable history of close contact with multiple ophidian species (see Section 4.6 and Table 4.1). Due to reportedly severe edema, fasciotomy was performed (Means, 2010; William Lamar, personal written communication with SAW, April 2010). Despite numerous attempts to review the hospital case notes, we have been unable to obtain full clinical documentation of this case. It is unclear whether specific compartmental pressures (e.g., by Wick catheter or Stryker intracompartmental pressure transducer) were obtained (see Table 4.2) in order to support surgical intervention. The victim also reportedly suffered considerable postfasciotomy disability. Fasciotomy has a known adverse effect profile and a history of inappropriate use in snakebite, resulting in long-term morbidity.[4] Therefore, without further data on the foregoing case, it is impossible to separate possible local venom-induced

---

[4] Unfamiliarity with the local effects of some snake bites may mislead medical professionals into considering fasciotomy. García-Gubern et al. (2010) reported a Puerto Rican racer or culebra corredora puertorriqueña, *Alsophis portoricensis*, bite in a pediatric patient that caused significant local edema. The patient was transferred for surgical consultation in consideration for a fasciotomy. As noted above, only objectively measured and markedly elevated intracompartmental pressures (typically well exceeding 30 mmHg) can justify consideration of surgical management of any snake bite. This is rarely needed, even in cases of bites from known medically important viperids and elapids.

morbidity from likely treatment-induced morbidity. This case emphasizes the essential need for adequate, objective, detailed documentation in cases of unusual and severe envenoming, including formal medical evaluation by a physician, preferably with experience in clinical toxinology (see Section 4.5). Publication of cases lacking sufficient clinical information must be discouraged, particularly when they report atypical serious effects of bites from species that are generally considered to have mildly toxic Duvernoy's secretions, or are "mildly venomous." Such anecdotal and unvalidated case reports can create false perceptions of the potential hazards associated with bites from particular colubroid species (Section 4.5).

Although well-documented case reports suggest that bites from these snakes can cause local medically significant bites resembling mild-to-moderate crotaline envenoming, as indicated previously, there are very few cases in which systemic envenoming could be inferred. An example of a patient bitten by a verified *P. olfersii* who developed systemic effects that were manifested by widespread ecchymoses is shown in Plate 4.40A and B. Therefore, large specimens of *Philodryas* spp. should not be carelessly handled in view of the known hemorrhagic, fibrinogenolytic, and possibly neurotoxic properties of their Duvernoy's secretions. The medical significance of bites from most species remains only partly characterized.

4.2.2.1 Overview of the Duvernoy's Gland and Associated Dentition of Philodryas *spp.*

The two *Philodryas* spp. that have received the most attention, *P. olfersii* and *P. patagoniensis*, have enlarged posterior, grooved maxillary teeth. The posterior maxillary teeth of *P. olfersii* have a deep groove occupying most of their length (Fry et al., 2008). *Philodryas baroni* has enlarged posterior maxillary teeth with deep grooves present on almost the entire length of the teeth (Plate 4.38C–E). Although there is limited information, it is likely that many, if not all, members of the genus exhibit similar dentition.

There is also little information regarding the ultrastructure and functional morphology of the Duvernoy's gland of this genus. However, Taub (1967) described the gland

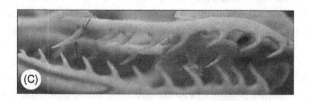

Plate 4.38 (C and D) Skull and enlarged maxillary teeth of *Philodryas baroni.* The teeth are recurved, and the posterior maxillary teeth are significantly enlarged (indicated by arrows). (E) Close-up of enlarged posterior maxillary teeth of *Philodryas baroni.* There is a prominent diastema between the anterior, and the notably enlarged, deeply grooved posterior maxillary teeth. The grooves extend along almost the entire length of the teeth (indicated by arrows). Plate 4.38A, photo copyright to Daniel E. Keyler; Plate 4.38B, photo copyright to Maik Dobiey; Plate 4.38C–E, AMNH #62831, photos copyright to Arie Lev.

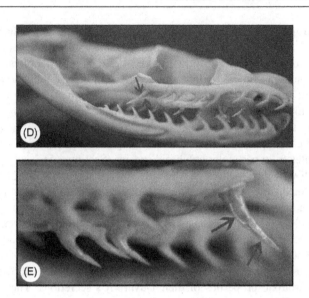

Plate 4.38 *(Continued)*

of *P. schotti* Boulenger, 1896 (*P. patagoniensis*, Hoge, 1964) as moderately vascular, with many thin trabeculae and an associated mucous-secreting supralabial gland. He also reported a thick capsule and an absence of intraglandular mucous-secreting cells (Taub, 1967). A morphological–histochemical study of Duvernoy's gland cytology of *P. patagoniensis* showed that acini of the gland were formed by seromucous cells containing neutrally staining mucosubstance and protein radicals (Lopes et al., 1982). Several calcium-binding proteins with molecular masses of 17, 28, and 67 kDa were detected in the Duvernoy's glands of *P. patagoniensis* (Goncalves et al., 1997).

4.2.2.2   Summary of the Toxinology and Properties of Duvernoy's Secretion from Philodryas *spp.*

The yield of Duvernoy's secretions from *Philodryas* spp. is unknown. In a study using pilocarpine stimulation to boost extracted yields (quantities were unreported), Duvernoy's secretions from specimens of *P. olfersii* and *P. patagoniensis* contained between 75% and 90% protein (da Rocha and de Furtado, 2007). These authors reported approximate murine i.v. LD_{50} of 3 mg/kg for both species. Assakura et al. (1992) reported a murine i.p. LD_{50} of 2.79 mg/kg for Duvernoy's secretion from *P. olfersii*, and a murine minimal hemorrhagic dose of 0.5 μg/mouse for Duvernoy's secretion from *P. olfersii*. Similarly, rapidly acting hemorrhagic activity and a minimum edematogenic dose of about 1 μg/mouse were reported for Duvernoy's secretion from *P. olfersii* and *P. patagoniensis* (da Rocha and de Furtado, 2007). Acosta de Pérez et al. (2003) reported a much higher murine minimal edematogenic dose (310 μg) for *P. olfersii* Duvernoy's secretion. Further, using the murine model, no defibrinating activity was detected in secretion from either *P. olfersii* or *P. patagoniensis* (da Rocha and de Furtado, 2007). In contrast, Peichoto et al. (2005) reported potent fibrinogenolytic activity in Duvernoy's secretion of *P. patagoniensis*. The activity was inhibited by several chelating agents, such as ethylenediaminetetraacetic acid (EDTA), benzamidine, and/or phenylmethylsulfonyl-flouride (PMSF). This suggested that the fibrinogenolytic activity was due to metalloproteases and serine proteases (Peichoto et al., 2005). This finding is supported by the previously reported fibrinogenolytic activity and subsequent characterization from *P. olfersii* Duvernoy's secretion of four acidic and one basic fibrinogenolytic proteases (one serine protease and four metalloproteases) ranging in molecular mass between 36 and 58 kDa (Assakura et al., 1992, 1994). One of the metalloproteases ("ProfibH") also exhibited hemorrhagic activity (Assakura et al., 1994). Similarly, an acidic 53.2-kDa α-fibrinogenolytic metalloprotease with hemorrhagic activity ("patagonfibrase") has been purified from Duvernoy's secretion of *P. patagoniensis* (Peichoto et al., 2007a,b). Fibrinogenolytic metalloproteases can directly cleave fibrinogen into fibrinopeptides A or B without producing a clot (Figure 4.1). This can potentially contribute to depletion of fibrinogen available for formation of a fibrin clot via thrombin action (Figure 4.1). Thus, the presence of these enzymes in *Philodryas* spp. Duvernoy's secretion could conceivably contribute to coagulopathy from a bite by some of these snakes. Documentation of hemostatic laboratory tests from verified cases of *Philodryas* bites is needed in order to confirm coagulopathic envenomations by members of this genus.

Some of these contrasting findings may be due to variability in Duvernoy's secretion components and/or ontogenetic variation, as has been demonstrated in secretion from *B. irregularis* (Mackessy et al., 2006; Weinstein et al., 1993; see Section 4.5). Conversely, experimental methods may lead to some incommensurability between laboratories.

Similar to the avian- and saurian-specific toxins characterized from Duvernoy's secretions of *B. dendrophila* and *B. irregularis* (see chapter 3), an avian-specific neurotoxin has been detected in Duvernoy's secretion from *P. olfersii* (Prado-Franceschi et al., 1996). In addition, an acidic, 182 amino acid myotoxin has been characterized from the Duvernoy's secretion of this species (Prado-Franceschi et al., 1998), and a 24.858 kDa CRISP with myotoxic activity ("patagonin") has been characterized from Duvernoy's secretion of *P. patagoniensis* (Peichoto et al., 2009).

Several of the aforementioned investigators frequently compared the documented edematogenic, hemorrhagic, proteolytic, and/or necrotic activities detected in *Philodryas* spp. Duvernoy's secretions to those of venoms from various *Bothrops* spp. (Acosta de Pérez et al., 2003; Assakura et al., 1992, 1994; Peichoto et al., 2005; de Perez et al., 2003). It is noteworthy that de Pérez et al. (2003) estimated the edematogenic activity of *P. olfersii* secretion from more than 3.5 to less than 10 times that of venoms from four taxa of *Bothrops* spp. [*B. alternatus* (urutu or half-moon viper), *B. jararaca* (jararaca), *B. jararacussu* (jararacussu), and *B. neuwiedi* (*sensu lato*; Neuwied's lance-headed viper); see Plates 4.73–4.75 for representative *Bothrops* spp.].

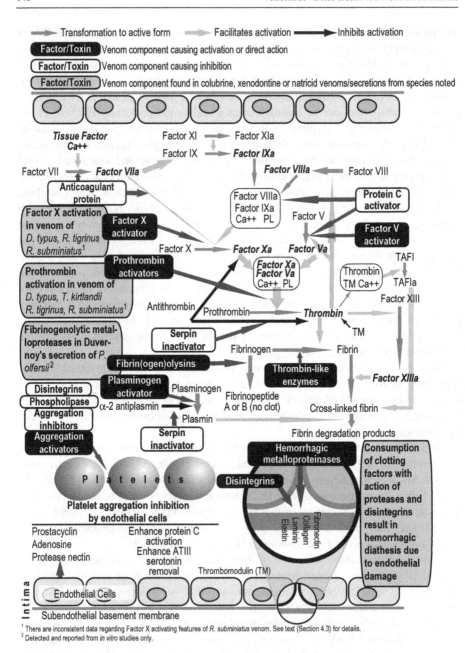

Figure 4.1 The effects of characterized toxins from non-front-fanged colubroids on hemostasis. Coagulation is accomplished through a complex cascade of proteolytically active clotting factors that act on successive factors and ultimately form a fibrin clot through the action of thrombin on fibrinogen. As a simplified summary, there are two classic pathways of activation: the intrinsic pathway and the extrinsic pathway. The intrinsic pathway is less significant than the extrinsic pathway to the maintenance of hemostasis under normal

(Continued)

◄ physiological conditions. It requires the action of Factors VIII, IX, X, XI, XII, and high molecular weight kininogen, prekallikrein, Ca^{2+} as well as platelet-derived phospholipids. The intrinsic pathway is initiated through exposure of several factors (prekallikrein, Factor XI, and Factor XII) to a negatively charged surface ("contact phase"). Exposure of these factors to phospholipids with a net negative charge (e.g., phosphatidylethanolamine) present on circulating lipids can initiate this pathway, and this partly accounts for the prothrombotic tendencies of hyperlipidemic states. The extrinsic pathway begins at the site of tissue (endothelial) injury, and the cascade is initiated by the release from the site of injury of Factor III ("tissue factor"). Factor III participates in the activated Factor V-activation of Factor X [forming activated Factor X (Factor Xa), the beginning of the common pathway that links the intrinsic and extrinsic cascades]. Factor Xa in turn proteolytically activates prothrombin to thrombin (Factor IIa), and this occurs on the surface of activated platelets. Factor IIa then proteolytically cleaves fibrinogen (which is comprised of three pairs of polypeptides that are covalently linked) to form fibrin through the aggregation of monomers produced via the digestion of the fibrinogen. The fibrin acts as a mesh-like lattice that stabilizes the forming platelet aggregate (fibrin clot). Factors VIII and V can be inactivated (regulated) by proteins C and S, and these regulatory components are activated by thrombin. Inhibition of several factors is accomplished by antithrombin.

As shown in the figure, hazard level 1 colubrid venom toxins may act on these clotting mechanisms by activating Factor X, thereby producing indirect activation of prothrombin, or by directly activating prothrombin. These toxins will thereby cause a coagulopathy that will rapidly consume the available clotting factors. As these venoms also contain proteolytic toxins that cause damage to blood vessel endothelium, massive hemorrhage may occur. In addition, the consumptive coagulopathy causes microthrombi that may lodge in the renal vasculature and result in mini-infarcts. The envenomated victim may hemorrhage extensively and develop hypovolemia, anemia, severe ecchymoses, hemorrhagic infarcts, and acute kidney injury. Bleeding may be brisk and life threatening. In addition, *P. olfersii* Duvernoy's secretion contains a fibrinogenolytic toxin that may prevent formation of a stable fibrin clot, and therefore could act as an anticoagulant. However, unlike the well-documented correlation between the pharmacology of hazard level 1 colubrid venom toxins and the pathophysiology of envenomation, there has been no clinically documented or confirmed coagulopathy from an envenomation by *P. olfersii*. Figure copyright to Julian White.

4.2.2.3   Summary of Experimental Pathophysiological Effects of Duvernoy's Secretion from P. patagoniensis

Peichoto et al. (2006) investigated the pathophysiological changes induced in rats by s.c, i.m., or i.v. administration of *P. patagoniensis* Duvernoy's secretions. Intravenously administered doses between 0.23 and 0.90 mg of secretion resulted in reported multifocal hemorrhage involving the cerebellum, cerebrum, and lungs. Noted also were renal peritubular capillary congestion and hepatic hydropic degeneration (Peichoto et al., 2006). The s.c. and i.m. routes exhibited similar effects aside from a lack of cerebellar and/or cerebral hemorrhage, while i.v. and s.c. administration were associated with elevated hepatic enzymes [aspartate aminotransferase (AST) and alanine aminotransferase (ALT); Peichoto et al., 2006]. The authors concluded that *P. patagoniensis* Duvernoy's secretion induced moderate histopathological changes in the vital organs of rats shortly after administration. They opined that the observed changes might be associated with functional abnormalities of the affected organs during envenoming (Peichoto et al., 2006).

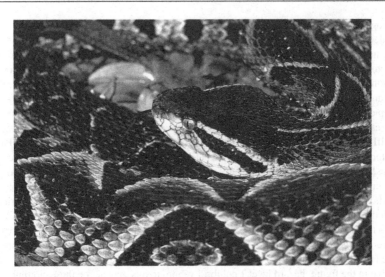

Plate 4.73 Jararacuçu (*Bothrops jararacussu*), Brazil. *Bothrops jararacussu* is a
medically important, large, heavy-bodied crotaline viperid that may attain a body length of
approximately 2.2 m. It is known by a multitude of common names (e.g., Cabeça de Sapo,
Jararacuçu, Jararaçucu Malha de Sapo). It is found in Brazil, Argentina, Bolivia, and Paraguay.
Bothrops jararacussu envenomation can feature coagulopathy, rhabdomyolysis, local necrosis,
and hypovolemic shock.
Photo copyright to David A. Warrell.

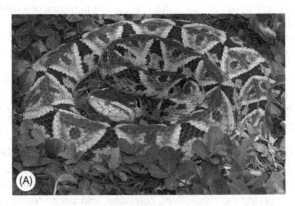

**Plate 4.74 (A and B) Terciopelo; barba amarilla; boquidorada; cachete de puinca;
tepoxo; many others (*Bothrops asper*).** One of the most important venomous snakes of Latin
America, this crotaline viperid has large volumes of toxic venom and sizeable, distensible
fangs ("solenoglyphous" dentition). Many indigenous people suffer long-term morbidity due
to bites from this species. Fatalities are common, and antivenom is often inaccessible in rural
communities where this snake is medically important.
(A) Terciopelo (*Bothrops asper*), Caucasia, Colombia.

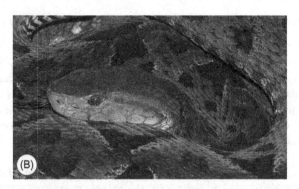

Plate 4.74 (*Continued*) **(B) Terciopelo (*Bothrops asper*), Mexico.**
Photos copyright to David A. Warrell.

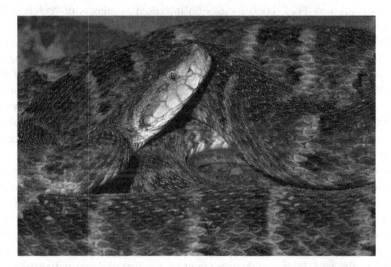

Plate 4.75 Common lancehead; barba amarilla; mapanare; caissaca; cuatro narices; many others. (*Bothrops atrox*), Morona, Santiago, Ecuador. Another medically important crotaline viperid of Latin America, this species is responsible for a large proportion of snakebite-related morbidity and mortality that occurs within its range. It has a reputation for an aggressive attitude when disturbed, and under some circumstances is quick to strike. Along with other *Bothrops* spp., this species may be incorrectly called, "fer-de-lance". The "true" fer-de-lance (*Bothrops lanceolatus*) is an insular species restricted to Martinique. Photo copyright to David A. Warrell.

4.2.2.4 Reported Fatal Outcome from a P. olfersii Bite: Rumor or Reality?

There is a single report of a purported fatality that resulted from a *P. olfersii* bite (Centro de Informações Toxicológicas do Rio Grande do Sul, 1996). This report has been frequently cited in the literature and is used to support a perception of lethal potential of this species. However, further scrutiny of this report fails to provide evidence supporting the reported fatality. The report is primarily an anecdotal account of *P. olfersii* ("Cobra verde, Cobra cipó") bites reportedly inflicted on two children, with one of them purportedly succumbing to the effects of the bite:

> In 1992, two children bitten by a Vine Snake were brought to the CITRS. Based on the childrens' relatives' testimonies, this animal showed itself very aggressive, wrapping around the arm of one of the children and biting it several times. One of the children from the Region sanitária de Cachoeira do Sul was killed
>
> **Centro de Informações Toxicológicas do Rio Grande do Sul (1996)**

Most of this very brief report focuses on increased awareness of "colubrids" and the *potential* "grave risks" in pediatric patients, including third spacing/massive edema and electrolyte disturbances. The authors do soundly recommend a 24-h observation period for any patient presenting with a medically significant *Philodryas* spp. bite. These warnings and recommendations do not include referenced examples of representative cases, but in relation to "rear-fanged colubrid snakes," the authors comment that "… the potential gravity of these accidents and the significant number of testimonies from the international literature … has set an alert for all of the doctors of all of the risks presented, especially in children" (Centro de Informações Toxicológicas do Rio Grande do Sul, 1996). Written 4 years after the cited incidents, the report contains no information about the specific identification of the reportedly culprit snake(s), the presentation, clinical features, or the specific cause of death. Also, as the cited reference (Centro de Informações Toxicológicas do Rio Grande do Sul, 1996) is very difficult to procure, some subsequent authors may have translated only a small section of available sections of the original paper, and these were likely taken out of context (e.g., descriptions for awareness of possible effects of a hypothetical bite incorrectly assigned to the very brief anecdotal account of the two children purportedly bitten by *P. olfersii*). It must be considered that the bite may have been inflicted by a crotaline because some—such as the two-striped forest pit viper, Amazonian pit viper or palm viper, *Bothrops* (*Bothriopsis* Campbell and Lamar, 2004) *bilineata* (Monzel and Wüster, 2008) (Plate 4.76)—are also known in some Brazilian communities as "Cobra verde." As the extralimital range of *B. bilineata* is north of the reported site of the two cases, this species is provided only as an example of how local names may be broadly applied to very different snakes. In fact, the alleged death itself is unproven as reported, and if it did occur may have resulted from causes unrelated to a *P. olfersii* bite (e.g., trauma from a motor vehicle accident on the way to a hospital), if it even occurred at all. In other words, due to a lack of any minimal standard of supporting data/information (see Section 4.5), the report must be classified as anecdote. As there are no specific clinical data, established linkage of the purported fatal outcome with the reported bite or detailed description of the victim's circumstances/cause of death, this case cannot be accepted as confirmed evidence of lethal potential of *P. olfersii*. Some of the

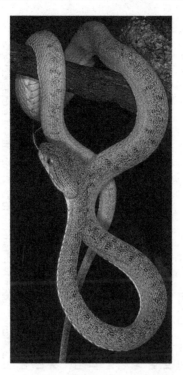

**Plate 4.76 Two-striped forest pit viper or Amazonian tree viper; surucucu de patioba
[*Bothrops (Bothriopsis) bilineata smaragdinus*], Napo, Ecuador.** This arboreal crotaline
viperid is sometimes locally named "cobra verde," a common name shared with several South
American racers, *Philodryas* spp. This could contribute to cases of mistaken identity, and may
lead to inappropriate management of *Philodryas* bites, or, conceivably, suboptimal treatment
of a *B. bilineata* envenomation.
Photo copyright to David A. Warrell.

deficiencies of this report have been noted previously by Ribeiro et al. (1999). Further,
as none of the cases of *P. olfersii* bites documented to date have been life threatening,
there are no patient-based data to support further citation of this case when assessing
the medical significance of this species.

4.2.2.5   Conclusion and Assessment of Philodryas spp.

The small number of well-documented cases of medically significant bites from
Philodryas spp. (primarily *P. olfersii*, *P. baroni*, and *P. patagoniensis*; Table
4.1) describe only mild-to-moderate local effects resulting from these incidents.
Uncommon cases that include systemic effects (widespread ecchymoses) have
occurred, but rarely documented. However, data characterizing several fibrinogenolytic enzymes and myotoxins suggest that large specimens of these species may
be capable of inflicting a bite resulting in significant systemic effects.

Assessment of *Philodryas* spp. based on available evidence: Hazard Level 3
(see Table 4.3).

Table 4.3 Summary of Management Recommendations and Assessment of Medical Risk of Some Selected "Colubrids"

Species	Hazard Index[a]	Management Recommendations[b]
Group I: Potential for fatal envenoming		
Boomslang, *D. typus*	1	ABC; i.v. access, preferably in two sites. Remove all constricting jewelry and scrutinize all recent dental work, piercing and/or tattoo sites as these may be subject to profuse bleeding.
		Consultation with a clinical toxinologist and a poison control center is strongly advised.
		ICU admission is strongly recommended. In the event of cardiac comorbidities, cardiology consultation is advisable.
		Minimize venipuncture; beware of placement of central lines due to probability of uncontrolled bleeding.
		Fluid resuscitation as indicated.
		Tetanus prophylaxis as indicated (delay administration until major coagulopathy with bleeding is resolved to avoid hematoma formation).
		Serial lab testing: CMP, CBC with differential and reticulocyte count, PT/INR/APTT, fibrinogen (measured, not calculated), fibrin(ogen) degradation products (d-dimer is sufficient), Proteins C and S, antithrombin III, CK.
Cape twig snake or African vine or bird snake, *T. capensis*	1	If available,[c] urgently obtain one to two ampoules of monospecific antivenom. *D. typus* antivenom does not provide any paraspecific protection. There is no available antivenom against *Thelotornis* spp. Anti-*R. tigrinus* antivenom may provide some neutralization capacity against *R. subminiatus* and should be used if available for *R. subminiatus* envenoming. Antivenom skin testing or pretreatment with steroids and/or antihistamines is not supported by current evidence and is not recommended (Weinstein et al., 2009).

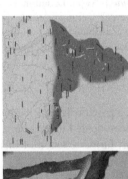
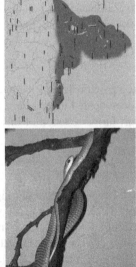
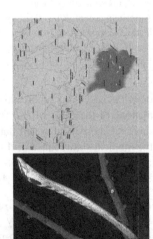

If indicated, give one ampoule of antivenom reconstituted with 10 mL saline in 100 mL of Ringer's lactate or saline. Infuse over 30 min and closely monitor for signs of anaphylaxis. Follow serial labs and provide a second ampoule if the coagulopathy is not reversed.

Treat pediatric patients with the same dose as adults. Treat pregnant women as indicated. In the USA, patients must be informed of the lack of FDA approval of these products.

Anaphylaxis protocol should be immediately available prior to provision of antivenom (see Section 4.6 for recommendations for managing envenoming in the sensitized patient).

In delayed presentations of serious *D. typus* envenoming, antivenom can be given up to 5–6 days following the bite. The delayed treatment of *R. tigrinus* or *R. subminiatus* envenoming is less established, but is likely to be similarly effective.

Replace PRBCs as indicated; strive to maintain a low normal hematocrit (remain aware of the potential for hemoglobinuric nephropathy; see Section 4.6).

Role of FFP is controversial; it is unlikely to provide benefit.

There are no data to support use of heparin or antifibrinolytics (e.g., ε-aminocaproic acid) and these are contraindicated. The use of synthetic protease inhibitor may be considered. It is unproven, but will likely not exacerbate bleeding.

Coagulation and renal function must be closely serially monitored. Diuretics have not been effective in re-establishing diuresis in cases featuring ARF. Dialysis may be necessary but may not confer clinical improvement of renal failure. In the event of ARF, nephrology consult is recommended.

(Continued)

Kirtland's twig snake or African vine or bird snake, *Thelotornis kirtlandii* (and other *Thelotornis* spp.)[d]

1

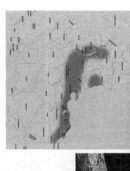
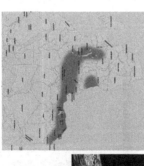

Tiger keel-back or yamakagashi, *Rhabdophis tigrinus*

1

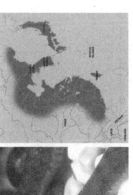
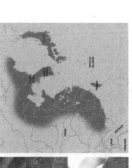

Table 4.3 (*Continued*)

Species	Hazard Index[a]	Management Recommendations[b]
Red-necked keel-back, *Rhabdophis subminiatus* 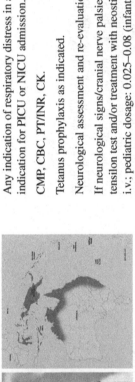	1	In cases featuring life-threatening DIC (especially with altered sensorium), consider CT without contrast of the head in order to exclude brain hemorrhage. Patients envenomed by these species often require extended admissions, careful monitoring, and renal/hematologic support. Extended admissions will require attentive nursing care. Until hemostasis is fully restored, protracted recumbent dependency may lead to serious ecchymoses. Renal function may slowly recover days-weeks after hemostasis is re-established. See Section 4.6 for further discussion of management.
Group II: Potential for significant effects/morbidity		
Brown tree snake, *Boiga irregularis* 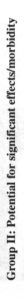 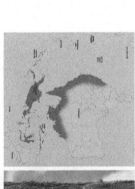	2/3	ABC, i.v. access Any indication of respiratory distress in a pediatric patient should be indication for PICU or NICU admission. CMP, CBC, PT/INR, CK. Tetanus prophylaxis as indicated. Neurological assessment and re-evaluation as indicated. If neurological signs/cranial nerve palsies are present, consider the tension test and/or treatment with neostigmine bromide (0.5–2.0 mg i.v.; pediatric dosage: 0.025–0.08 (infants) or 0.025–0.10 (children) mg/kg/dose). Pretreatment with atropine 0.6–1.2 mg i.v. (pediatric dosage 0.02 mg/kg/dose × 1) given several minutes prior to the provision of the neostigmine bromide is strongly recommended.

Montpellier snake, *Malpolon monspessulanus* 2/3

Meticulous wound management. Do not use antibiotics unless there is evidence of infection. Wounds in patients with comorbidities (i.e., Type 2 diabetes mellitus) should be closely monitored.

DO NOT GIVE ANTIVENOM OF ANY KIND. There are no antivenoms against these snakes and there are no data supporting any cross-neutralization from any poly- or monovalent antivenom. Due to this as well as the obvious high risk:low benefit profile, the use of antivenom is contraindicated for any of these snakes.

Close follow-up is advisable.

Careful verification of the identity of the snake and documentation of the case are integral.

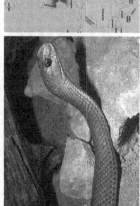
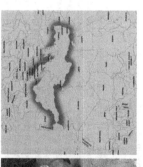
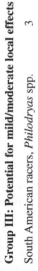

Group III: Potential for mild/moderate local effects

South American racers, *Philodryas* spp. 3

Local wound care as indicated. Wounds in patients with comorbidities (i.e., Type 2 diabetes mellitus) should be closely monitored.

Lab tests as indicated.

Antibiotics are indicated only with evidence of infection.

Tetanus prophylaxis as indicated.

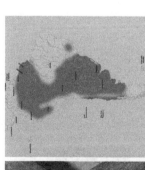
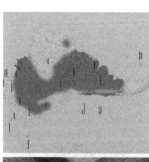

(Continued)

Table 4.3 (*Continued*)

Species	Hazard Index[a]	Management Recommendations[b]
Western hognose snake, *H. nasicus*	3	Observation as deemed clinically necessary in order to rule out any significant sequelae. This is important as although there are no data to support very serious sequelae from many genera (including *Philodryas* spp.), the possibility of such effects exists. Rare cases of widespread ecchymoses suggesting systemic effects have occurred following *P. olfersii* bites. Therefore, bites from larger specimens or protracted bites should be carefully reviewed. DO NOT GIVE ANTIVENOM OF ANY KIND. There are no antivenoms against these snakes and there are no data supporting any cross-neutralization from any poly- or monovalent antivenom. Due to this as well as the obvious high risk:low benefit profile, the use of antivenom is contraindicated for any of these snakes. Close follow-up as indicated.
Several other assorted taxa [*Alsophis* (*Borikenophis*) *portoricensis, Platyceps rhodorachis,* etc; see Table 4.1]	3	Careful verification of the identity of the snake and documentation of the case are integral.

Abbreviations: ABC, airway, breathing, circulation, and associated emergency measures; ARF, acute renal failure; APTT, partial thromboplastin time; CBC, complete blood count; CK, creatine phosphokinase; CMP, complete metabolic panel; CT, CAT scan; DIC, disseminated intravascular coagulation; FFP, fresh-frozen plasma or cryoprecipitate; ICU, intensive care unit; INR, international normalized ratio; NICU, neonatal intensive care unit; PICU, pediatric intensive care unit; PRBCs, packed red blood cells; PT, prothrombin.

[a]Hazard Index is defined following a modification of the criteria of Weinstein et al. (2009): Level 1—serious and potentially fatal envenoming is possible; Level 2—systemic envenoming is possible, but uncommon; Level 3—usually mild-to-mildly moderate local effects and often related to protracted bite.

[b]The representative species and recommendations for management listed here were selected due to the availability of data sufficient to assess the potential medical significance of bites inflicted by each taxa. Due to the limited number of documented cases involving most of these and the majority of "colubrid" species, this assessment and management recommendations can only be considered a preliminary guide and should not be considered a fully inclusive list.

[c]Antivenom: Anti–*D. typus* antivenom is only available from the South African Vaccine Producers (SAVP; 1 Modderfontein Road, Sandringham, Johannesburg, South Africa, Tel.: + 27 11 882 9940; fax: + 27 11 882 0812; E-mail: savpunit@global.co.za / savpqual@global.co.za, web site: www.savp.co.za). Anti-*Thelotornis* spp. antivenom is not available. Anti-*R. tigrinus* antivenom is only available from the Japan Snake Institute, Yabuzuka-honmachi Nittagun, Gunma Prefecture 379-2301, Japan, Tel.: + 81 277 78 5193; fax: + 81 277 78 5520; E-mail: snake-a@sunfield.or.jp. In any case of serious envenoming by these species, it is strongly advised to contact any available antivenom index center (in the USA, call 800-222-1222), Poison Control Center and an experienced clinical toxinologist.

[d]The photo depicts *Thelotornis mossambicanus*, while the map illustrates the range of *T. kirtlandii*. In addition to *T. capensis* and *T. kirtlandii*, other members of the genus such as *T. mossambicanus* should be considered as probable hazard level 1 species.

4.2.3 Genus Thamnophis spp.: Background and General Features of Documented Bites

North American natricids such as the garter and ribbon snakes (*Thamnophis* spp.; approximately 27 species) are the best-known members of the tribe, Thamnophini (about 31 taxa), and among the most popular snakes maintained (often by children) in captivity. They are medium-sized (most species average between 40 and 80cm in total length), and prey on a wide variety of small vertebrates and invertebrates (Table 4.2). Rossman et al. (1996) thoroughly reviewed the biology and evolution of the genus. Although *Thamnophis* spp. are abundant and among the most studied North American snakes, their phylogenetic relationships have received relatively limited scrutiny (de Quieroz et al., 2002). The phylogeography of *Thamnophis* spp. may have resulted from at least one invasion of northern North America from Mexico (Alfaro and Arnold, 2001). Several cases of bites from a couple of these species that caused mild local effects (e.g., puncture wounds/lacerations, edema, and, uncommonly, ecchymoses) have been well documented (Table 4.1). As these snakes have long been popularly viewed as totally "harmless," some authors have assigned acquired hypersensitivity as a likely factor contributing to these effects (Ernst and Barbour, 1989), while others have rejected this possibility on the basis of absent "urticaria" after bites from *T. s. similis* (Plate 4.53; blue-striped garter snake; Nichols, 1986). As discussed later in Section 4.6, Type 1 hypersensitivity manifests quite variably and urticaria, while often present, does not develop inevitably in all cases. Misinterpretation of clinical signs/symptoms features prominently in these reports (see Section 4.5), and commonly obfuscates or complicates analysis of real versus perceived risks posed by many of these species. Several documented cases suggest that two *Thamnophis* taxa [*T. e. terrestris* (western terrestrial garter snake), Plate 4.52A, and *T. e. vagrans* (wandering garter snake), Plate 4.52D] are capable of inflicting mild local effects, and that two others [*T. s. similis* and some populations and/or large adults of nominate *T. sirtalis* (common garter snake, Plate 4.54A, D–J)] may also have this potential (Table 4.1). As noted previously, these effects may cause greater surprise and concern because of the preconceived perception of complete "harmlessness" of these snakes. Also, medical personnel confronted by the unfamiliar scenario of a snakebite may be similarly predisposed to "expect the worst." This may be more likely in the case of a species of unknown medical importance or when a culprit specimen is misidentified and/or confused with a known medically important crotaline or elapid species (see previous section regarding *Philodryas* spp. and Section 4.5).

4.2.3.1 Overview of the Duvernoy's Gland and Associated Dentition of Thamnophis spp.

Some of the members of the genus have slightly enlarged, ungrooved posterior maxillary teeth. Ruthven (1908) noted that members of the genus *Thamnophis* exhibited maxillary teeth that were "rather abruptly longer near the posterior end of the maxillary bone than anteriorly." However, in citing Cope (1892), Ruthven (1908) added that "the excess in the length of the posterior teeth is so small in many specimens ...

that it is impossible to distinguish them from apparently isodont specimens of these forms...." Similarly, Rossman (1961) noted that *T. sauritus* (eastern ribbon snake) and *T. proximus* (western ribbon snake) had the greatest number of maxillary teeth among the genus. He also reported that these taxa exhibit maxillary teeth that increase in size only slightly posteriorly, but the posteriormost two or three teeth abruptly increase in size. Fry et al. (2008) described the maxillary teeth of *T. elegans* as smooth (without grooves).

Gross examination of the maxillary teeth of eight live specimens of *T. sirtalis sirtalis* and three live specimens each of *T. proximus* and *T. marcianus* (checkered garter snake or Marcy's garter snake) suggested nearly imperceptible differences in maxillary tooth size among the specimens examined (SAW, personal observations). Close examination of a *T. sirtalis* skull showed no size differences among the maxillary dentition. The maxillary teeth are recurved, equal in size, and ungrooved (Plate 4.54B). The maxillary dentition appears very similar to that of a typical non-front-fanged colubroid without any specialized dentition [e.g., Taiwan beauty snake, *Orthriophis (Elaphe taeniura friesi* Tiedemann and Grillitsch, 1999) *taeniurus* Cope, 1861; see Plate 4.54C; in addition, this species lacks a Duvernoy's gland]. Two young adult live specimens of *T. e. vagrans* exhibited two or three slightly but perceptibly enlarged posteriormost maxillary teeth (SAW, personal observations). These observations were concordant with those from examination of the maxilla of a *T. e. vagrans* specimen (Plates 4.54B and 4.77). The posteriormost maxillary teeth are slightly enlarged, smooth, and without perceptible grooves (Plates 4.54B and 4.77).

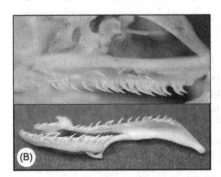 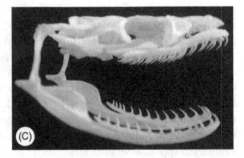

Plate 4.54 (B) Comparison of maxillae of *Thamnophis sirtalis sirtalis* and *Thamnophis elegans vagrans*. The posterior maxillary teeth of *T. s. sirtalis* have no gross enlargement or grooves (main panel), while several of the most posterior maxillary teeth of *T. e. vagrans* (inset panel) are slightly enlarged but also lack grooves.
(C) Skull and maxilla of the Taiwan beauty snake (*Orthriophis taeniurus*). Formerly synonymized with the genus *Elaphe* (rat snakes), these colubrine snakes lack any significantly specialized dentition as well as Duvernoy's glands. Several subspecies of *O. taeniurus* are popular in private collections. Plate 4.54B, *T. sirtalis sirtalis*, AMNH #70096; *T. e. vagrans*, AMNH #R148051, photos copyright to Arie Lev; Plate 4.54C, photo copyright to Javier José Carrasco Araújo.

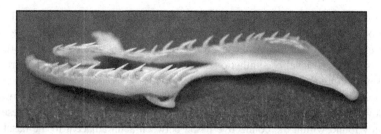

**Plate 4.77 Maxilla of the wandering garter snake (*Thamnophis elegans vagrans*),
Sandoval, New Mexico, USA.** Several slightly enlarged, ungrooved posterior maxillary teeth
are present. Bites by this species have uncommonly produced mild-to-moderate edema, pain,
and hemorrhagic blistering (see text). AMNH #R148051, photo copyright to Arie Lev.

In a detailed morphological comparison of Duvernoy's glands of three *Thamnophis*
taxa, Taub (1967) reported that *T. sirtalis* had a thin gland capsule and a moderate number of thin-walled trabeculae, while the glands of *T. elegans* and *T. cyrtopsis* (black-
necked garter snake) exhibited heavy-to-thick capsules and many moderately thick
trabeculae. Other significant differences among these glands were noted. The glands of
T. elegans and *T. cyrtopsis* were composed of columnar cells, but there were pyrami-
dal cells in the *T. sirtalis* gland (Taub, 1967). About 10% of the tubules in the *T. sirtalis* gland were lumenate, in comparison to 50% and 90% of the tubules present in the
glands of *T. elegans* and *T. cyrtopsis*, respectively. The glands of *T. sirtalis* and *T. cyrtopsis* were moderately vascular, whereas that of *T. elegans* was highly vascular (Taub,
1967). The *T. elegans* gland contained a mixture of serous and mucous cells; that of
T. cyrtopsis had mucous cells common throughout; and the *T. sirtalis* gland lacked
mucous cells. None of these taxa had a mucous supralabial gland associated with the
serous Duvernoy's gland (Taub, 1967). Fry et al. (2008) reported that the *T. elegans*
gland contained isolated mucoid cells or patches and a relatively large ovoid duct.

Kardong and Luchtel (1986) performed a gross and ultrastructural study of the
Duvernoy's gland of *T. elegans vagrans* and reported that the gland was encased by
a thin coat of collagenous connective tissue. The gland was multilobulated, and these
consisted of numerous acini (= secretory units containing serous cells). These authors
reported absence of any significant secretion storage volume, although there were variably sized lumenae defined by the acini (Kardong and Luchtel, 1986). A main duct
contained the only mucous cells found within the gland and, along with scattered
serous cells, comprised the simple columnar epithelium lining the duct. The duct ultimately emptied into the buccal cavity near the posterior maxillary teeth. The study
demonstrated that the ultrastructure of the *T. e. vagrans* Duvernoy's gland closely compared with that of another natricid, the medically important *R. tigrinus*. The glands
of both taxa exhibit serous and myoepithelial cells, but lack mitochondrial-rich cells;
secretory granules of the serous cells are abundant and homogenously dense (Kardong
and Luchtel, 1986; Yoshie et al., 1982; see the subsection on *R. tigrinus* in Section 4.3).
Unlike in *R. tigrinus*, the serous cells of *T. e. vagrans* have endoplasmic reticulum and
Golgi complexes that lack extensive cisternae (Kardong and Luchtel, 1986; Yoshie
et al., 1982). Similar to *D. typus* and *N. tessellata*, the serous cells of *T. e. vagrans*

exhibit extensive intracellular distribution of secretory granules (Kardong and Luchtel, 1986; Kochva, 1978). Interestingly, the secretory granules of *D. typus* and *N. tessellata* appear less electron-dense than those of *T. e. vagrans*. It is unclear whether this difference is related to level of synthetic activity, taxa-specific variation, or experimental methods (Kardong and Luchtel, 1986; Kochva, 1978).

Kardong and Luchtel (1986) found rich unmyelinated innervations in the *T. e. vagrans* Duvernoy's gland, with bundled nerves encased in folds of Schwann cells. These were commonly found within the connective tissue between acini adjacent to the basal laminae. The authors attributed the flow of secretions to release of secretory granules into the luminae, thereby creating secretory pressure that forces secretion through the glandular channels (Kardong and Luchtel, 1986). Contraction of local bulging striated muscles may augment secretory pressure (Kardong and Luchtel, 1986), as has been suggested from study of *T. sirtalis* Duvernoy's gland secretion (Jansen and Foehring, 1983).

4.2.3.2   Summary of the Toxinology, Properties and Pathophysiology of Duvernoy's Secretion from Thamnophis spp.

There is very limited information regarding the toxinology of *Thamnophis* spp. Duvernoy's secretions. In a relatively early study, Vest (1981b) used aspiration as well as micropipette extraction (see Weinstein and Kardong, 1994, for a review of these methods) in order to obtain secretions from *T. e. vagrans*. He reported a yield of $0.71\,\mu L$ containing $0.057\,mg$ solids. The secretion protein content was 46% (Vest, 1981b). Collection of Duvernoy's secretion from many non-front-fanged colubroids (especially the smaller fossorial taxa) presents technical difficulties that can result in contamination of Duvernoy's secretions with other buccal secretions and vice versa (Hill and Mackessy, 2000; Weinstein and Kardong, 1994). Therefore, it is not clear if Vest (1981b) assayed material primarily from Duvernoy's glands or, more likely, a sample of mixed buccal secretions.

Other investigators have increased the yield of *Thamnophis* spp. secretions by using parasympathomimetic agents, such as pilocarpine in sedated specimens (Fry et al., 2003; Hill and Mackessy, 1997, 2000; Rosenberg et al., 1985). Using this method, Rosenberg et al. (1985) obtained from *T. s. parietalis* an average yield of $3\,\mu L$ secretion containing $3.8\,mg/mL$ of protein. With a similar method, Hill and Mackessy (2000) obtained from *T. e. vagrans* a mean yield of $23\,\mu L$ secretion containing $0.39\,mg$ of protein (51.6% protein).

To date, lethal potency studies have demonstrated low toxicities for Duvernoy's secretions of *Thamnophis* spp. Vest (1981b) reported a murine i.p. LD_{50} of $13.85\,mg/kg$ for *T. e. vagrans* secretions, while Rosenberg et al. (1985) reported an i.p. LD_{50} of $33.0\,mg/kg$ for *T. s. parietalis* secretions.

There are few data regarding the pathophysiological effects of *T. e. vagrans* Duvernoy's secretion in mice. Intravenous injection of *T. e. vagrans* secretion reportedly caused "massive pulmonary hemorrhage" (Vest, 1981b). Additional hemorrhagic effects in other organs appeared to be dose dependent. Administration of mixed buccal secretions devoid of significant amounts of Duvernoy's secretions resulted in minor, diffuse local hemorrhage (Vest, 1981b). Myonecrosis has been reported in mice injected with Duvernoy's secretion of *T. e. vagrans* (Jansen, 1987). Confirmation of these reported pathophysiological effects is needed.

From field observations, Finley et al. (1994) suggested that the buccal secretions of *T. e. vagrans* may have a digestive function. These authors based their hypothesis on the observed partial depilation of a vole (*Microtus mexicanus*) while the animal was being grasped and swallowed by a 68-cm *T. e. vagrans*. In addition, Jansen (1987) reported that buccal secretions of *T. e. vagrans* exhibited antibacterial properties as has been described for venoms from several species of elapids and viperids.[5]

4.2.3.3 Conclusion and Assessment of Thamnophis spp.

Most bites inflicted by *Thamnophis* spp. are insignificant. However, bites from these taxa can cause puncture wounds/lacerations, mild edema, erythema, and, occasionally, ecchymosis. The very low yields of Duvernoy's secretions, as well as the sparse lethal potency data indicating very low toxicity, underscore the lack of any significant medical risk from these snakes.

Assessment of *Thamnophis* spp. based on available evidence: Hazard Level 4 (typically only mild lacerations, reactive erythema and edema, and rarely mild ecchymoses).

4.2.4 Genus Heterodon spp.: Background and General Features of Documented Bites

Concerns about the potential toxicity of bites by hognose snakes (*Heterodon* spp.; four species; for photos of three of these species (see Plates 4.24A–C, 4.25A–D, and 4.78A and B) have been expressed at least since the late nineteenth century (Blatchley, 1891; Schneck, 1878). Recently assigned to the family Dipsadidae, subfamily Heterodontinae, most of these snakes are anuran (frogs and particularly toads) specialists, while *H. nasicus* (western hognose, Plate 4.24A–C; see also Plate 4.91B–F later Section 4.5.1.1) in particular will prey opportunistically on a wider variety of animals (Table 4.2). Another genus popular in private collections, hognose snakes (most commonly, *H. nasicus*; Table 4.1) can inflict bites that produce mild-to-moderate local effects (Table 4.1; see Plate 4.24D–J). Almost all of these cases involved protracted bites sustained during feeding of captive snakes. It is noteworthy that several of these cases featured local effects (edema, blistering, ecchymoses, joint stiffness, or other joint dysfunction) that lasted for weeks to months (Weinstein and Keyler, 2009). To date there are no reports of systemic effects from bites by any *Heterodon* spp. (Weinstein and Keyler, 2009; Table 4.1).

---

[5] Antimicrobial components identified in and/or purified from some elapid and viperid venoms have included well-known enzymes such as L-amino oxidases (Stiles et al., 1991) as well as novel peptides (Gomes et al., 2005; Nair et al., 2007). As noted when considering the relative paucity of information about numerous specific components of Duvernoy's secretions and venoms of most non-front-fanged colubroids, the lack of idenitifed antimicrobial activities of these secretions may reflect the comparatively limited research of these, rather than absence of these substances from these secretions/venoms.

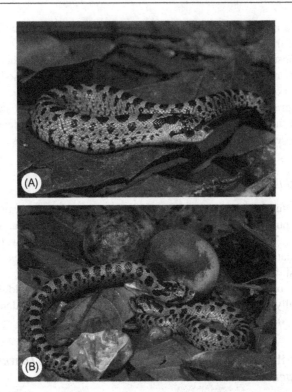

Plate 4.78 (A and B) Hatchling specimens of the Southern hognose snake (*Heterodon simus*). This secretive and lesser-known *Heterodon* species feeds exclusively on anuran amphibians. There are no documented bites by this species.
Photos copyright to Mark O' Shea.

4.2.4.1 Overview of the Duvernoy's Gland and Associated Dentition of Heterodon spp.

The genus *Heterodon* is named for their heterologous dentition (= heterodont). Hay (1892) reported that the enlarged posterior maxillary teeth of *Heterodon* spp. lacked canals and grooves. Similarly, Ditmars (1896) noted that "… the posterior maxillary tooth is considerably larger than those in front, but not grooved …." However, Ditmars (1912) later reported that when examined with light microscopy, the posterior maxillary teeth had faint anterior grooves. Kapus (1964) agreed with the earlier assertion of Ditmars (1896), as he did not find any grooves during examination of 15 skulls of *H. nasicus*, *Heterodon platirhinos* (eastern hognose), or *Heterodon simus* (southern hognose). Similarly, Kroll (1976) reported that *H. nasicus* and *H. platirhinos* possessed ungrooved enlarged posterior maxillary teeth. The teeth probably rotate to a 45° orientation on the maxilla, thereby penetrating grasped prey (Kroll, 1976). Taub (1967) hypothesized that the mobility of the maxilla might aid infliction of a wound amenable to inflow of Duvernoy's secretion. *Heterodon platirhinos* possesses a row of recurved maxillary teeth, unequal in length and separated by a diastema from two enlarged, slightly curved posterior teeth that are almost three times the length of the anterior teeth and are angled 30° to the maxilla (McAlister, 1963). Fry et al. (2008) described the maxillary teeth of *H. nasicus* and *H. platirhinos* as having smooth surfaces and lacking an "enclosed venom canal." These investigators also reported that the "venom" duct opened directly into the oral cavity rather than into the "lumen of the fang sheath" and the surface of the "fang" (Fry et al., 2008). The notably enlarged, smooth posterior maxillary teeth of *H. platirhinos*, *H. simus*, and *H. nasicus kennerlyi* are shown in Plate 4.79A–E.

The enlarged posterior maxillary teeth of *Heterodon* spp. have been popularly perceived to perform prey manipulation and "deflation" functions. The deflation function, specifically, puncturing a grasped toad with the enlarged maxillary teeth during deglutition, was considered to be a response to the toads' (*Bufo* spp.—a favored prey item of *Heterodon* spp.) antipredator defense mechanism of inflating themselves with air (Edgren, 1955; McAlister, 1963; Pope, 1947). However, these teeth have been considered too short to effectively perform this function (Kroll, 1976). An opposing view opines that the enlarged maxillary teeth probably only reinforce the grip on prey (Ditmars, 1896; Kroll, 1976), as well as possibly facilitate entry of Duvernoy's secretion into the resulting wounds (Averill-Murray, 2006; Weinstein and Kardong, 1994). Although the latter hypothesis is probably correct, close examination of the markedly enlarged, ungrooved, posterior maxillary teeth suggests that these could support such a prey-handling function (toad "deflation") if approximately two-thirds of the length of the respective teeth protrude from the buccal mucosa during deglutition (see Plate 4.79A–E). This interesting question deserves further formal study, as it may clarify *Heterodon* prey-handling strategies as well as add some clues about Duvernoy's secretion function(s).

The source of toxic oral secretions of *Heterodon* spp. has been long debated. Hay (1892) indicated that the enlarged posterior maxillary teeth were "… not connected with any source of poison …." Similarly, McAlister (1963) reported that the "superior labial gland" lacked posterior enlargement. He concluded that the enlarged posterior maxillary teeth were not primarily associated with facilitating penetration of "saliva" into prey. Kapus (1964) reported the presence of a "parotid" gland in *H. nasicus*, *H. n. kennerlyi*, and *H. simus*, and that the gland of *H. nasicus* was notably larger than that of *H. simus*. Some authors hypothesized that local effects of *Heterodon* spp. bites in humans were possibly due to residual toxic skin secretions from anuran prey left in the snake's buccal cavity (Anderson, 1965). Smith and Brodie (1982) considered that *Heterodon* spp. may have a generalized salivary toxicity: "… the fangs do not deliver a venom, although the saliva is believed to be toxic."

However, several authors favored probable toxic secretions produced in a specific oral gland (Bragg, 1960; Morris, 1985). This was demonstrated by Kroll (1976), who identified in *H. nasicus* and *H. platirhinos* a "seromucous venom gland" (Duvernoy's gland) associated with the enlarged posterior maxillary teeth. This gland is readily found in dissected specimens of *H. nasicus* and *H. platirhinos* and clearly produces a secretion with variable toxicity and probable specificity for anuran amphibians (McAlister, 1963; Young, 1992). Taub (1967) found that the Duvernoy's glands of *H. nasicus* and *H. platirhinos* had moderately thick-"heavy" thick capsules and moderate numbers of moderately thick trabeculae. Ninety percent of the intraglandular

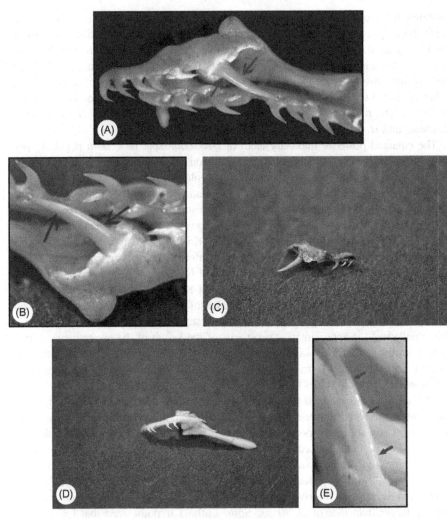

Plate 4.79 (A–E) Posterior maxillae of the hognose snakes (*Heterodon* spp.). Some
authors have speculated, without confirmative evidence, that the enlarged posterior maxillary
teeth of these heterodontine dipsadids are used to deflate air from toads (*Bufo* spp.), as these
amphibians use inflation as an antipredator mechanism. These teeth are probably too short for
this theoretical function, but this speculation is worthy of further study. These enlarged teeth
are without grooves, but may facilitate entry of Duvernoy's secretion into inflicted wounds.
**(A and B) Enlarged posterior maxillary teeth of the Mexican hognose snake (*H. nasicus
kennerlyi*).** Note the markedly enlarged, ungrooved, smooth posterior maxillary tooth (arrows;
AMNH #58234).
(C) Enlarged posterior maxillary teeth of *H. simus*, South Carolina, USA. As in other
Heterodon spp., there is a diastema between the notably enlarged, ungrooved posterior
maxillary teeth, and the smaller recurved anterior teeth (AMNH #38165).
**(D and E) Enlarged posterior maxillary teeth of the Eastern hognose snake (*H.
platirhinos*).** Note the diastema between the recurved, smaller anterior maxillary teeth, and the
enlarged, ungrooved maxillary teeth (arrows; AMNH #63590).
Photos copyright to Arie Lev.

tubules had a lumen and the gland substance was comprised of columnar cells. The *H. nasicus* gland was highly vascular and had serous as well as mucous cells, while that of *H. platirhinos* was moderately vascular and lacked mucous cells. Neither species possessed mucous supralabial glands associated with their Duvernoy's glands (Taub, 1967). In comparison, Fry et al. (2008) reported that both species exhibited glandular epithelium with mucous cells or patches and a "venom duct" that opened only into the oral cavity, not into the vicinity of any specific dentition. The diameter of the duct appeared reduced and surrounded by circular connective tissue (Fry et al., 2008).

4.2.4.2 Summary of the Toxinology and Duvernoy's Secretion Properties of Heterodon *spp.*

The scarce data regarding yield of Duvernoy's secretion from *Heterodon* spp. indicate limited average volumes from a small series of specimens. Mean liquid yields from two specimens each of *H. nasicus nasicus* and *H. n. kennerlyi* (Mexican hognose, *H. kennerlyi*; Smith et al., 2003) were 24 and 15 µL, respectively (Hill and Mackessy, 2000).

There are few data regarding components of Duvernoy's secretions from *Heterodon* spp. Hill and Mackessy (2000) found low phosphodiesterase, moderate-to-high proteolytic activity, but no PLA_2 activity in *H. nasicus* Duvernoy's secretion. They found that enzymatic constituents of *Heterodon* spp. saliva and Duvernoy's secretions differed. Saliva from the nominate form, *H. n. nasicus*, lacked proteolytic activity and exhibited high levels of PLA_2 (Hill and Mackessy, 2000). None of the *Heterodon* spp. secretions studied contained detectable thrombin-like, hyaluronidase, or kallikrein-like activities (Hill and Mackessy, 2000).

As noted with *Boiga* spp., the *in vitro* detection of postsynaptically active neurotoxins present in Duvernoy's secretions from *H. platirhinos* (Young, 1992) appears to be irrelevant to elucidating the basis for the observed clinical effects of bites from this species. Young (1992) reported induction of acetylcholinesterase-like neuromuscular blockade by *H. platirhinos* Duvernoy's secretion in the frog sciatic nerve-gastrocnemius preparation, as well as antagonism of acetylcholine and histamine responses of isolated rat duodenum. It is likely that many of these toxins are prey (anuran amphibians) specific, following preferences of these snakes, although *H. nasicus* readily preys upon small mammals.

4.2.4.3 Conclusion and Assessment of Heterodon *spp.*

Well-documented bites from *Heterodon* spp. (almost all from *H. nasicus*) feature mild-to-moderate local effects including puncture wounds/lacerations, mild-moderate edema, blistering, ecchymoses and, uncommonly, mild lymphadenopathy (Table 4.1). Several reports describe extended convalescence (weeks to months) of patients after protracted bites from these snakes. However, as with *Thamnophis* spp., despite the many thousands of these snakes kept in captivity, bites and local "envenomations" are exceedingly rare. This genus does not deserve to be considered venomous or dangerous (Weinstein and Keyler, 2009).[6] They should not be subject to regulation or restriction. Captive specimens should be handled with care, particularly during feeding or after handling potential prey items.

Assessment of *Heterodon* spp. based on available evidence: Hazard Level 3 (see Table 4.3)

4.2.5 Genera Hemorrhois *spp.*, Platyceps *spp.*, Hierophis *spp.*, and Coluber *spp.*: Background and General Features of Documented Bites

The colubrine genera *Coluber* (North American racers, approximately 23 species; see Plate 4.80A and B), *Platyceps* (Old World whipsnakes or racers, eight species; see Plates 4.13A–C and 4.14), *Hierophis* (Old World whipsnakes, three species; see Plates 4.16A–D and 4.81), and *Hemorrhois* (Asian racers, four species; see Plate 4.23A–C) occupy a wide variety of biotopes that reflect their geographic distribution and opportunistic/nonfastidious diet (see Table 4.2 for examples). Medically significant bites consisting of only mild local effects, such as lacerations/puncture wounds, mild edema, erythema, and, occasionally, blistering, have been reported for several taxa (Table 4.1). Among *Platyceps* spp., case reports have included *P. najadum* (Dahl's whipsnake; Plate 4.13A–C) and *P. rhodorachis* (Jan's desert or wadi racer; Plate 4.14; Table 4.1). A very unusual case involving a presumed *P. najadum* bite is discussed in Section 4.4. Several authors have published data describing mild local effects resulting from *P. rhodorachis* bites (Table 4.1), and Malik (1995) reported leukocytosis and elevated creatine phosphokinase (CK) among three patients bitten by this species, although no specific systemic effects were documented.

Similarly, several cases of bites from *Hemorrhois nummifer* (coin snake; Plate 4.23D–F) and *H. ravergieri* (mountain racer or leopard snake) featured mild local effects, although one case of *H. ravergieri* bite reported by Mamonov (1977) suggested moderately severe edema (Table 4.1). This is similar to the pediatric case reported involving *Boiruna maculata* (mussurana, Santos-Costa et al., 2000; Table 4.1) and may be a result of individual human inflammatory responses to minor trauma.

As the previous genera were re-assigned from the genus *Coluber*, it is not surprising that some reports would involve members of this genus. This genus has been extensively revised and is still under taxonomic review. A bite reported here from *C. rubriceps* (red-headed whipsnake) produced only mild, transient insignificant effects (Table 4.1; Plate 4.15). Numerous bites inflicted by several taxa of *Coluber* spp. [e.g., *C. constrictor* (eastern racer, including several of the approximately 10 subspecies), *C. mormon* (western racer), *C. elegantissimus* (elegant racer or most beautiful

---

[6]As noted previously, the term "venomous" should not be used simply due to the presence of oral secretions with laboratory-determined toxicity for experimental animals (typically, mice). "Venomous" implies verified use in prey capture and/or subjugation functions. These functions have not been verified in *Heterodon* spp., and these snakes commonly swallow their prey alive (SAW, personal observations). Therefore, the term should be carefully applied as it confers specific biological (and, secondarily, clinical) significance.

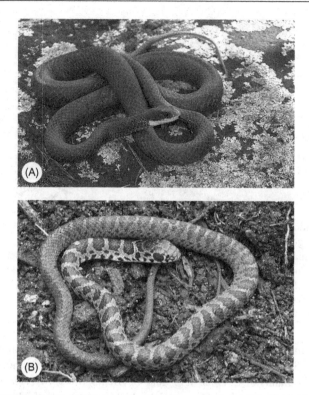

Plate 4.80 (A and B) Common black racer (*Coluber constrictor*), Virginia, USA. Fast, alert, and often quick to bite when caught, these diurnal colubrine snakes typically inflict medically insignificant bites (see text).

(A) *Coluber constrictor*, adult.

(B) *Coluber constrictor*, juvenile. Juvenile specimens of *C. constrictor* may be mistaken for juvenile *Crotalus* spp. or *Agkistrodon* spp., especially as these snakes often beat or vibrate their tails in dead leaves when approached, and this can contribute to their misidentification. Photos copyright to John White.

whip snake)], either personally experienced or observed by some of the authors, consisted of insignificant puncture wounds, lacerations, brief bleeding, and slight pain/erythema.

In contrast, a *Hierophis viridiflavus* (green whipsnake; Plate 4.16A–D) bite resulted in an ICU admission that was probably attributable to the patient's alcoholic intoxication (Table 4.1). This case is briefly considered in Section 4.4.

4.2.5.1   Overview of the Duvernoy's Gland and Associated Dentition of Hemorrhois *spp.*, Platyceps *spp.*, Hierophis *spp., and* Coluber *spp.*

In several anesthetized living specimens of *Coluber* spp. [*C. constrictor* ($n = 4$), *C. rubriceps* ($n = 2$), and *C. mormon* ($n = 2$)] there were no grooves in the posterior

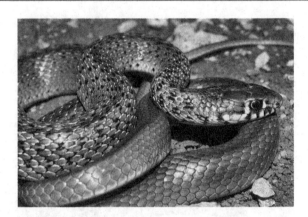

Plate 4.81 Balkan whip snake or Balkan racer (*Hierophis gemonensis*). Another former member of the genus *Coluber*, this fast-moving, active colubrine species ranges from Croatia, Slovenia, Bosnia-Herzegovina, Albania, Montenegro, and into southern Greece. It is reportedly a threatened species due to habitat loss. There are no documented medically significant bites by this species.
Photo copyright to Daniel Jablonski.

maxillary teeth, nor gross enlargement of these teeth (SAW, personal observations). Fry et al. (2008) reported that the dentition of *C. constrictor* had a smooth surface.

Duvernoy's glands of *C. constrictor* and *C. (Hemorrhois) ravergieri* were similar in size. Although the gland of *C. constrictor* had a moderately thick capsule, that of *C. ravergieri* was thin, but both species had moderate numbers of thin trabeculae and a lumen was noted in about 50% of tubules in the gland (Taub, 1967). Both species lacked mucous cells in the glands, but had a supralabial mucous gland associated with their Duvernoy's glands. The Duvernoy's glands were moderately vascular and comprised of columnar cells (Taub, 1967). Fry et al. (2008) reported that the "venom glands" (Duvernoy's glands) of *C. constrictor* had a relatively large ovate duct, contained isolated mucous cells/patches and possessed a "venom duct" that opened only into the oral cavity. As discussed later (see pp. 150-153, section 4.4.7, and the Summary and Conclusions section), it is essential to avoid inappropriate and premature use of terminology (e.g. "venom glands", "venom duct") implying unproven biological function of oral secretions from species such as *C. constrictor*. As noted, this also popularly and incorrectly may be mis-interpreted as as suggesting potential medical significance. To date, there is no detailed information about dentition or specific morphology of Duvernoy's glands of *Hierophis* spp. or *Platyceps* spp.

4.2.5.2   *Summary of the Toxinology and Duvernoy's Secretion Properties of* Hemorrhois *spp.,* Platyceps *spp.,* Hierophis *spp., and* Coluber *spp.*

The yield, toxicity, and components of Duvernoy's secretions from these species are unknown. Bites by these taxa typically feature mild effects without any significant sequelae.

4.2.5.3 Conclusion and Assessment of Hemorrhois spp., Platyceps spp., Hierophis spp., and Coluber spp.

Little information is available about properties of Duvernoy's secretions from these taxa, and the few documented bites have featured only mild effects. Two aberrant cases involving *Hierophis viridiflavus* and *P. najadum* reported in the literature were serious or fatal, but these consequences are most unlikely to have been related to "envenomation" by either of these snakes, and identification of the snake responsible is questionable in at least one of these cases (see Section 4.4). Therefore, available evidence supports only mild, local effects resulting from bites by these taxa. Large specimens of *P. najadum* and *P. rhodorachis* might produce more significant local pathology.

Assessment of *Coluber* spp., *Hemorrhois* spp., *Hierophis viridiflavus*, *Platyceps* spp. based on available evidence: Hazard Level 3/4 (see Table 4.3).

4.2.6 Genus Alsophis spp.: Background and General Features of Documented Bites

The genus *Alsophis* (West Indian, Caribbean or Central American, South American, and Galapagos racers) belongs to the family Dipsadidae, subfamily Xenodontinae, tribe Alsophiini, and contains approximately 14 species. Some taxa have multiple subspecies with the Cuban racer or jubo, *A. cantherigerus*, probably having largest number of subspecies (approximately eight). Most taxonomic studies have supported monophyly of the West Indian species (Hass et al., 2001; Vidal et al., 2000; Zaher, 1999) that are probably derived from a South American stock origin. This group has also been subjected to ongoing systematics investigations, and the tribe Alsophiini has recently been reorganized with reclassification of the alsophiines into 10 genera (seven previously named, and three new; Hedges et al., 2009). This included recommendation for reassignment of *A. portoricensis* (Puerto Rican racer; culebra corredora puertorriqueña; Plate 4.2A–F) and *A. cantherigerus* to the new genera, *Borikenophis* and *Cubophis*, respectively (Hedges et al., 2009). This is especially relevant due to the occasional reports of medically significant bites by these species (Table 4.1). For purposes of the present discussion, the previous taxonomic designations will be used as, to date, these terms are used exclusively in the body of limited literature about bites by these snakes. Most *Alsophis* spp. attain an average total body length of about 0.8–1 m (although some specimens may be significantly longer), are fast moving, and are found in a diverse range of tropical habitats including sparsely vegetated scrub, arid sandy coastal tussock, moist meadow/grasslands, cultivated fields, and rainforest as well as rocky terrain. Although most species feed on a wide range of prey, including small mammals, and occasionally bats or nestling birds, many species exhibit preference for amphibians [especially hylid frogs (treefrogs such as *Osteopilus* spp.)], lizards (e.g., anoles, *Anolis* spp., gekkonids, and other taxa), and other snakes [e.g., *Tropidophis* spp. (dwarf boas or wood snakes; family Tropidophidae)]. Schwartz and Henderson (1991) reported that gekkonids [e.g., *Sphaerodactylus* (reef or dwarf geckos)] and the hylids, peeping, chirping, or robber rainfrogs (*Eleutherodactylus* spp.) comprised a large proportion of the diet of *A. cantherigerus*. *Alsophis* spp. (e.g., Plate 4.3A–E) are active diurnal foragers that will ascend low-lying bushes, shrubs, trees, and occasionally man-made structures in search of prey. Juvenile *A. portoricensis* utilize caudal luring as a foraging strategy, but this behavior has not been confirmed in adults (Leal and Thomas, 1994). Although mostly terrestrial, *A. portoricensis* has been observed in water (Barun et al., 2007).

There are only a few documented cases of bites by *Alsophis* spp., and almost all of these are by *A. portoricensis* (Table 4.1). The signs/symptoms consisted of local pain, edema (in a few cases this has been progressive, and reportedly involved the entire affected upper extremity), mild ecchymoses, and occasionally minor blistering (Tables 4.1 and 4.4). It is noteworthy that one pediatric victim exhibited progressive edema significant enough to prompt a surgical consultation (Table 4.1), although as noted previously, local effects of snakebites may be notoriously misinterpreted. The "impaired coagulation" reported anecdotally by Rodriguez-Robles and Thomas (1992) requires clinical confirmation by appropriate formal medical review, and laboratory investigations [prothrombin time, international normalized ratio (PT/INR), activated partial thromboplastin time (aPTT), see Section 4.6]. Until and if proven otherwise, this must be considered a misinterpretation of brisk bleeding from puncture wounds. Such descriptions smack of the pitfalls discussed in Section 4.5. To date, there is absolutely no evidence of systemic effects from bites of any *Alsophis* spp.

A communicated case (Kevel Lindsay, written communication with SAW, February 2011) occurred on Mosquito Island, British Virgin Islands (September 2007). An 870mm (total body length), 51.7g female *A. portoricensis* was encountered in the vicinity of an abandoned building, and grabbed by the victim. The snake bit the victim on the distal and proximal phalanges, second digit of the left hand. The snake "... moved its head ..." in a "slow side-ways" ... and "downward motion" for a few seconds, and "bit down" twice. The snake remained attached for about 1 min, and the bite was not immediately painful. The victim indicated that he did not immediately remove the snake due to his concerns of damaging it as well as wishing to prevent its escape. Within minutes, the victim noted "tingling" and "numbness" at the wound site as well as minor swelling. In less than 1 h (Plate 4.4), the bitten finger and immediate metacarpal region were swollen, tingling, with increased "numbness" as well as mild "stiffness." Several hours later, noted were: progressive edema reaching the upper forearm, accompanied by "throbbing"; increased "numbness" at the wound site; and mild ecchymoses. The bitten finger was mildly-to-moderately painful. By morning, the victim noted pain, edema, and throbbing involving the entire forearm, and mild ecchymoses of the hand. The victim was eventually examined by a physician (within 36h of the bite) and was prescribed two different medications (specifics are unavailable; probably an antihistamine and an antibiotic). The edema almost fully resolved within 48h, and the victim noted a dull ache that lasted for about 2 days. The victim also reported occasional "tingling" and an episodic rash on the left shoulder and arm. The only significant sequelae (2 weeks duration postbite) consisted of soreness in the joints, including the left elbow and shoulder. The victim was fully recovered 2 weeks after the bite. It is noteworthy that the victim had been bitten previously by a *A. portoricensis*, but the bite was negligible (K. Lindsay, personal written communication with SAW, February 2011).

Table 4.4 Overview of Reported Serious Evidence-Supported Symptoms and Signs Associated with Documented "Colubrid" Bites[a]

Symptom/Sign[b]	Species[c]	Comments
Blistering/Blebs	*Alsophis (Borikenophis) portoricensis*, *Heterodon nasicus*, *Platyceps rhodorachis*, *Madagascarophis meridonalis*, *Oxybelis* spp., *Philodryas chamissonis*, *Thamnophis elegans vagrans*	The bites of some species produced relatively transient blistering (e.g., *T. e. vagrans*), while the bites of others (e.g., *H. nasicus*) have occasionally produced a more protracted blistering disease (see Plate 4.24D–J).
Ecchymoses[d]	*Boiga irregularis*, *Boiga nigriceps*, *Boiruna maculata*, *Dispholidus typus*, *Erythrolamprus bizona*, *Helicops angulatus*, *Ithycyphus miniatus*, *Liophis poecilogyrus sublineatus*, *Philodryas baroni*, *Philodryas olfersii*, *Rhabdophis subminiatus*, *R. tigrinus*, *Thamnodynastes pallidus*	*P. olfersii* has produced widespread ecchymoses, suggesting systemic envenoming, in at least one documented case (see text and Plate 4.40A and B). The ecchymoses caused by envenoming from Hazard Level 1 species may encompass large areas of dependent sites on the victim (posterior thighs, flanks; see Plate 4.20M–O and 4.46C).
Edema[d]	*Alsophis (Borikenophis) portoricensis*, *Boiga irregularis*, *Boiga nigriceps*, *D. typus*, *Hemorrhois ravergieri*, *H. nasicus*, *Hydrodynastes gigas*, *Ithycyphus miniatus*, *Philodryas olfersii*, *P. patagoniensis*, *P. viridissimus*, *Psychophis flavovirgatus*, *Rhabdophis subminiatus*, *R. tigrinus*, *Symphimus* spp., *Thamnodynastes pallidus*, *Thelotornis capensis*, *Thrasops flavigularis*	The cases included contain relatively well-documented expanding or persistent edema. For examples of local edema from some of the listed species, see Plates 4.24I and J, 4.26E, and 4.44B and C. Excluded are cases without supportive documentation, or with descriptions suggestive of limited edematous effects. Those with clinically less significant edema are included in Table 4.1.
Lymphadenopathy	*Platyceps rhodorachis*, *H. nasicus*, *Malpolon monspessulanus*, *P. olfersii*, *R. tigrinus*	Additional published cases have described isolated instances of more transient lymphadenopathy (see Table 4.1 and Plate 4.24D–J).
Cranial nerve palsies	*Malpolon monspessulanus*	Several reports with one well-documented, verified case demonstrating the medically significant neurotoxic properties of Duvernoy's secretions from this species.
Coagulopathy[e]	*Dispholidus typus*, *R. subminiatus*, *R. tigrinus*, *T. capensis*, *T. kirtlandii*	May be delayed, asymptomatic, and, occasionally, initially undetected without laboratory investigations. However, often severe and accompanied by hemorrhage and profuse bleeding.
Systemic hemorrhage/DIC	*D. typus*, *R. subminiatus*, *R. tigrinus*, *T. capensis*, *T. kirtlandii*	All of the well-documented bites from *R. subminiatus* occurred while handling captive specimens.
Death	*D. typus*, *R. tigrinus*, *T. capensis*, *T. kirtlandii*	There are no reported deaths from *R. subminiatus* bites. There are probably a number of unrecorded deaths among agricultural workers bitten (and other regions) by *D. typus* in Kenya.

[a]Included are only summarized serious signs/symptoms that were reported after qualified medical review, and caused prolonged distress and/or serious injury to the victim.

[b]This table omits reported cases of "respiratory difficulty" or ptosis linked to pediatric patients bitten by *Boiga irregularis* on Guam, as well as alleged systemic effects attributed in a single case to a bite from a *Hydrodynastes gigas*. Further confirmation of the etiology of the observed effects in these cases is desirable (see Section 4.4).

[c]For common names, see Table 4.1 and relevant text.

[d]Only cases that contain descriptions of clinically extensive or significantly progressive ecchymoses or edema are included. Therefore, this summarized list does not include all of the cases listed in Table 4.1.

[e]There is a single documented report of "mild coagulopathy" after a *P. patagoniensis* bite, as has been made regarding a bite from *Sibynomorphus mikanii*. There are also several anecdotally referenced reports of hemostatic disturbances after *P. olfersii* bites without any supporting clinical documentation. Confirmation is desirable of these alleged systemic effects from bites of these species.

4.2.6.1 Overview of the Duvernoy's Gland and Associated Dentition of A. portoricensis

Alsophis cantherigerus have two posterior enlarged, ungrooved maxillary teeth separated from the anterior teeth by a diastema (Kardong, personal verbal and written communication with SAW, June–July 2009). There are few data about the presence or absence of grooves in other *Alsophis* spp., and available information supports a lack of any grooves or other significant dentitional modifications. Further study of a large number of specimens would clarify the specific characteristics of dentition among alsophiines. Kardong (1980b) detailed the jaw musculature and associated innervation of *Alsophis cantherigerus brooksi* (*Cubophis cantherigerus schwartzi* Hedges et al., 2009).

The Duvernoy's glands of two *A. portoricensis* specimens (AMNH #1332 and #28126) both had gland capsules with "heavy thickness" and a mucous supralabial gland associated with the serous Duvernoy's gland. However, the Duvernoy's glands of these two specimens did have some subtle differences in: number of trabeculae (#1332 < #28126); presence of lumen in tubules (50% in #1332, 90% in #28126); degree of vascularity ("very high" in #1332, "moderate" in #28126); and #28126 had very limited storage space, while #1332 had none (Taub, 1967). A specimen of *A.* (*Cubophis* Hedges et al., 2009) *vudii* (Bahaman racer; AMNH #34178) had a Duvernoy's gland with: a heavy, thick capsule; moderate number of trabeculae; absent lumena in tubules; no storage space; a mucous supralabial gland associated with Duvernoy's gland; and no appreciable gland vascularity (Taub, 1967). The Duvernoy's glands of all three of the *Alsophis* specimens examined by Taub (1967) had columnar cells, as well as an absence of mucous cells within the glands. Weldon and Mackessy (2010) compared the organization of the "venom gland" (Duvernoy's gland) of *A. portoricensis* to that of *B. irregularis*. They noted a series of lobular subunits arranged into secretory tubules lined by serous secretory cells. These secretory cells were distinguished from those of the supralabial salivary gland by differential staining with hematoxylin/eosin or periodic acid-Schiff. They also noted an absence of any storage capacity and a lack of any "venom" (Duvernoy's secretion) in most of the secretory tubules (Weldon and Mackessy, 2010).

4.2.6.2 Summary of Duvernoy's Secretion Properties and Toxinology of Alsophis spp.

Although there is very limited information about the toxinology of the tribe Alsophiini, there has been some investigation of the Duvernoy's secretions of *A. portoricensis* that shed light on several of its properties and components. In an early investigation, Hegeman (1961) described hemolytic and proteolytic activities of *A. portoricensis* Duvernoy's secretion, as well as a low level of cholinesterase. An unpublished screening of direct hemolytic activities in Duvernoy's secretions of several non-front-fanged colubroids, including *A. vudii*, did not detect any significant activity (Weinstein and Bernheimer, 1986, unpublished observations). In the most thorough study to date of *A. portoricensis* Duvernoy's secretion, Weldon and Mackessy (2010) found that the secretion had a protein content of about 89%, high metalloproteinase and gelatinase activities, and low levels of acetylcholinesterase and phosphodiesterase. They also detected the rapid hydrolysis of the α-subunit of human fibrinogen by the whole "venom" (secretion). Polyacrylamide gel electrophoresis revealed about 22 bands with most molecular masses ranging between 25 and 62 kDa, but mass spectroscopy resolved a complex group of proteins in the 1.5–13 kDa range, and low intensity signals in the 6.2–8.8 kDa range may have represented the presence of three-finger-fold toxins (Weldon and Mackessy, 2010). A 25-kDa peptide was found to have sequence homology with tigrin, the CRISP from venom of *R. tigrinus*. The "venom" had higher lethal potency for mice (2.1 μg/g) than for the American or green anole, *Anolis carolinensis* (3.8 μg/g; Weldon and Mackessy, 2010). Intradermal injection of 1.0 μg or 5.0 μg of crude secretion caused hemorrhage in mice, and a dose-related magnitude of induced hemorrhage was noted. Mice and anoles included in the lethal potency determinations reportedly exhibited extensive pulmonary hemorrhage (Weldon and Mackessy, 2010). These investigators speculated that the *in vitro* fibrinogenase activity may account for reports of prolonged bleeding ("… by disrupting the blood clot cascade and inducing hypofibrinogenemia …") in cases of bites from these and other non-front-fanged colubroids (e.g., *Philodryas* spp.). They also hypothesized a role for the multiple proteinases/hemorrhagins present in this secretion in the local effects of bites from this species (Weldon and Mackessy, 2010).

4.2.6.3 Should Alsophis portoricensis *Duvernoy's Secretion Be Called "Venom"?*

Unlike most other species of non-front-fanged colubroids, the possible biological functions of *A. portoricensis* Duvernoy's secretions have been investigated by both laboratory study and field observations. Several investigators have described the preferential engagement of the enlarged posterior maxillary teeth in response to struggling movements of seized anoline prey (Rodriguez-Robles, 1992; Rodriguez-Robles and Thomas, 1992; Thomas and Prieto-Hernandez, 1985). Rodriguez-Robles (1992) described the specific response of *A. portoricensis* specimens to anoles attempting to escape the snake's grasp. He reported that anoles were always held following successful strikes, and if the grasped lizard struggled after capture, the snakes "chewed" in order to embed the posterior maxillary teeth. Vigorously struggling prey was held firmly, and forceful "chewing" ensued until the lizard was still. The jaw movements did not seem to facilitate swallowing as the snake did not reposition the grasped prey, and therefore were considered to be a possible means to introduce "venom" into the prey (Rodriguez-Robles, 1992). This suggests active use of these secretions in either prey subjugation or tranquilization. Interestingly, Rodriguez-Robles (1992) also reported personal and communicated observations of *A. portoricensis* accomplishing prey [laboratory mice and a teiid lizard, *Ameiva exsul* (Puerto Rican ground lizard)] capture/restraint with constriction alone. As noted by Rodriguez-Robles (1992), prey subjugation strategies using constriction or oral secretions are not mutually exclusive and have precedent in some Australian elapids [e.g., the apparently preferential use of venom by some tiger snakes (*Notechis* spp.) and brown snakes (*Pseudonaja* spp.) in capture of mammalian prey versus the use of constriction by these snakes when capturing lizards and frogs; Shine and Schwaner, 1985]. Shine and Schwaner (1985) even noted that frequency of prey constriction among some Australian elapids was statistically identical to that of some nonvenomous snakes. Therefore, the selective use of venom may be an indicator of a prey-specific capture strategy possibly applied to reduce the likelihood of reprisal from a more physically imposing prey item, while constriction may be used to subdue prey that is more resistant to the subjugating effects of a given venom.

In a rare study addressing the possible digestive function of Duvernoy's secretions of a non-front-fanged colubroid, Rodriguez-Robles and Thomas (1992) assessed the extent of digestion by *A. portoricensis* of a natural prey item, *Anolis cristatellus* (Puerto Rican crested anole) by comparing lizards recovered from the snakes' gastrointestinal (GI) tract 6 h after natural capture/deglutition, force-feeding of intact lizards, or those with experimentally administered puncture wounds (by puncturing the lizards with sterilized sewing needles). The force-feeding was conducted by shielding the snakes' teeth in order to prevent accidental introduction of oral secretions, and the artificially punctured anoles served to assess the possible role of puncture wounds facilitating digestion by providing a pathway for the entrance of digestive enzymes into the body cavity (Rodriguez-Robles and Thomas, 1992). The anoles were recovered from the snakes' GI tract 6 h after natural deglutition or force-feeding, and a qualitative scoring system was used to estimate the degree of digestion by examination of the condition of several body structures ("body wall," forelimbs, etc.), and visceral organs (liver, lungs, etc.). The results were statistically analyzed, and the authors reported that the general digestion of "envenomated" anoles was faster than those of "nonenvenomated" anoles. In addition, digestive rates for several structures and visceral organs were faster in "envenomated" lizards in comparison with the "nonenvenomated" group (Rodriguez-Robles and Thomas, 1992). The study had several flaws that modify interpretation of the results. For example, the scoring system was notably (but understandably) subjective; the induced artificial puncture wounds were probably poor facsimiles of actual tooth-inflicted wounds, and as the experimental groups of lizards were force-fed to the snakes, the possible role of cephalic-natural olfactory stimulation of a prey item was probably absent. The last process could conceivably play an important independent factor in the speed of digestion. However, in a similarly uncommon study of nutrient signals that potentially stimulate digestion in a henophidian, the Burmese python (*Python molurus*), Secor et al. (2002) reported that neither cephalic, gastric, or intestinal (physical) signals, nor the luminal presence of bile, lipids, or glucose, induced an intestinal response. Rather, a combination of nutrients, especially amino acids and peptides (also, provision of a homogenized rat mixture) induced an intestinal response resembling that after ingestion of intact rodent prey (Secor et al., 2002). Secor et al. (2002) emphasized the carnivorous diet per ingestion of large whole prey items by *Python molurus*, thus the natural gastric response to a rich proteinaceous bolus. Therefore, the experiments of Rodriguez-Robles and Thomas (1992) may have produced a digestive response, as they did introduce a natural prey item to the snakes' digestive tracts. The relatively high proteolytic activities of *A. portoricensis* Duvernoy's secretion (Weldon and Mackessy, 2010) could be viewed from the standpoint of both a potential digestive role, and as potential, but unverified, contributors to the local effects in some victims bitten by this species. McCue (2005) commented on the higher levels of proteolytic activities of venoms from the more recently derived crotalines, and this could suggest that the evolution of these venoms may be influenced by their digestive function. Although some research has provided evidence of a digestive function for venom of *Crotalus atrox* (Thomas and Pough, 1979), other investigations have not demonstrated any significant contribution of venom to the digestive process of *C. atrox* (McCue, 2007). This may reflect individual venom properties of snakes included in specific studies, as well as differences in experimental methods and the complexities of studying a dynamic, multifactorial physiological process. *Crotalus atrox* venoms have notably marked individual, population/geographic, and ontogenetic variability (Minton and Weinstein, 1986). However, it must be noted that studies such as those briefly outlined earlier are crucial to the clarification of potential fundamental biological roles of venoms and other ophidian oral secretions.

Considering that there are accumulating field and laboratory observations that support active use of *A. portoricensis* Duvernoy's secretions in subjugation, and possibly digestion, of prey, as well as demonstrated toxicity to favored prey species, the criteria for the formal term "venom" have been met. Therefore, the Duvernoy's secretions of *A. portoricensis* offer an uncommon example of oral secretions of a non-front-fanged colubroid species that have been studied from a functional biological perspective. This research provides sufficient evidence to consider this secretion as venom, or, prey-specific venom, as suggested elsewhere in this book. The putative medical effects from bites by this species remain of unknown etiology, and, as noted previously and later, should not in any case influence the biological–functional definition of venom.

4.2.6.4 Conclusion and Assessment of Alsophis spp.

There are only a handful of formally documented cases of bites by alsophiine snakes. The very limited toxinological information about most species in this group further complicates objective risk assessment. However, *A. portoricensis* has inflicted several medically significant bites that consisted of mild-to-moderate local effects. To date, there is no evidence of systemic "envenomation" by any of these snakes. Due to the identification of fibrinogenases and high levels of other proteases in *A. portoricensis* venom, handling of these snakes is discouraged, and large specimens may be capable of inflicting a more clinically significant bite. Field and laboratory observations/findings support the recognition of *A. portoricensis* Duvernoy's secretions as venom, independent of any medical risks. There is no evidence supporting any medical significance for the vast majority of alsophiines, but aside from *A. portoricensis*, the scant biomedical information about most species in this taxonomically unsettled group is insufficient for a thorough risk analysis.

Assessment of *Alsophis* (*Borikenophis*) *portoricensis*, *A.* (*Cubophis*) *cantherigerus*, and *Alsophis* spp. based on available evidence: Hazard Level 3 [*A.* (*Borikenophis*) *portoricensis*] and 3/4 [*A.* (*Cubophis*) *cantherigerus* and *Alsophis* spp.].

4.3   Life-Threatening and Fatal Cases: "Venomous Colubrids" and Assessment of Evidence-Based Risk

4.3.1   Dispholidus typus, Thelotornis capensis, and Thelotornis kirtlandii: Background and General Features of Documented Bites

The African non-front-fanged colubroids, *D. typus* (Plate 4.20A–F), *T. capensis* (Plate 4.56A–C), and *T. kirtlandii* have inflicted multiple well-documented fatal and life-threatening envenomations (Table 4.1). It is likely that the two additional species of *Thelotornis*, *T. usambaricus* (Usambara vine or twig snake) and *T. mossamibicanus* (Mozambique twig, vine or bird snake; Plate 4.56D–G) have similar potential, but no cases have yet been reported. The several subspecies of *D. typus* (*D. t. typus*, *D. t. punctatus*, and *D. t. kivuensis*) are uncommonly identified with specificity in the reporting of envenoming cases. Similarly, the subspecies status is usually not documented for *Thelotornis* spp. (e.g., *T. capensis capensis*, *T. c. oatesii*, and, possibly, *T. c. shilisi*) involved in envenomation. However, a prolonged bite by *T. c. oatesii* (Oates' twig, bird, or vine snake; Oate's savannah twig snake; Plate 4.56B) resulted in bleeding complications, defibrination, prolonged prothrombin, and partial thromboplastin times lasting 3 days, but without renal complications (Saddler and Paul, 1988). The recently described and closely related Uluguru dagger-tooth vine snake, *Xyelodontophis uluguruensis* (Broadley and Wallach, 2002), is very rare and has not been involved in any reported bites. This poorly known species exhibits unique, ungrooved, multiple-ridged dentition, and an ecological niche similar to *Dispholidus* and *Thelotornis*. This species and other remaining members (*Thrasops* spp., African tree snakes; three species, and *Rhamnophis* spp., African large-eyed tree snakes; two species) of the tribe, Dispholidini, are of unknown medical importance. However, there is a single documented case that occurred in 2004 of a medically significant bite from a *Thrasops* spp. The victim, a 40-year-old female, without any reported pre-existing significant medical history, presented to a medical facility after she was bitten on the thumb (side and specific site unspecified) by an adult *T. flavigularis* (yellow-throated tree snake) while cleaning the glass of the snake's terrarium (Ineich et al., 2006; Table 4.1). The authors suggested that the victim's hand movements performed during the cage cleaning provoked the bite. The snake grasped the victim's thumb and advanced its jaws ("chewed") for about 1 min. It is noteworthy that the victim did not "actively react to the bite, since this species is commonly accepted as harmless" (Ineich et al., 2006; see Section 4.5.2). The authors noted that a sustained grip with continuous "chewing action" probably allowed penetration of "venom" into the wound (Ineich et al., 2006). Within minutes after the bite, the victim experienced a "strong burning feeling" involving the whole thumb, and rapid swelling. Approximately 20 min later, movement of the thumb was restricted, and the edema involved the entire hand. The edema progressed, reached the forearm 2 h after the bite, and the hand was reportedly "double" in size (Ineich et al., 2006). Similar to some cases reporting blisters or hemorrhagic blebs appearing distant from the bite site (e.g., after a medically significant bite from the western hognose snake, *H. nasicus*; Weinstein and Keyler, 2009; Plate 4.24D–J; Table 4.1), a hematoma appeared along the arm between the elbow and the axilla, as well as at the bite site (Ineich et al., 2006). The patient was observed in an emergency room for 12 h and treated with an i.v. antihistamine. There were no laboratory results included in this report, and no other symptoms or signs were mentioned. There were no signs of neurotoxicity, and no significant bleeding was reported (Ineich et al., 2006). The patient's edema persisted for 5–6 days; mild residual pain in the affected thumb remained for several additional days. The hematoma on the arm remained visible for almost 1 week, and slowly diminishing pain in the "arm lymphatic tract" was reported (Ineich et al., 2006). Some of these effects could be interpreted as lymphatic spread of introduced Duvernoy's secretion, or lymphatic drainage related to regional hypersensitivity (see Section 4.6).

As with *B. dendrophila*, anecdotal reports posted on the Internet (Appendix A) describe prolonged bleeding and/or edema following protracted bites from captive specimens of *Thrasops jacksoni* (western black tree snake, Jackson's black tree snake or isilukanga; there are other names as well). However, as these were not formally medically reviewed, risk assessment and clinical evaluation of this taxon are not feasible using the information in these cases of unconfirmed provenance (see later and Section 4.5). Similarly, there are no data available about possible risks by bites of the third species, *T. occidentalis* (also often referred to as the western black tree snake).

Although some authors are eager to ascribe perceived significant risk to some ophidian species of little-known importance (i.e., *Boiga (Toxicodryas) blandingi*), others have underestimated the lethal potential of some of the Dispholidini. Sweeney (1971) stated that bites from *Thelotornis* spp. caused edema, pain, and fever, but did not cause "true hemophilia." Although the lethal potential of *D. typus* was clearly identified as early as 1909 (FitzSimons, 1909), Cansdale (1955) questioned the documented hazard posed by *D. typus* and opined that *Thelotornis* spp. was "almost harmless." These mixed and incorrect popular perceptions of the danger of these snakes may have contributed to the deaths of Robert Mertens, Karl Schmidt, and probably others as well.

Envenomation by these snakes often features severe consumptive coagulopathy with disseminated intravascular coagulation (DIC) causing spontaneous systemic bleeding that can pose a clinical management challenge for the attending physician. In cases of *D. typus* envenomation, symptoms may appear very soon after the bite or be delayed for 12–48 h, resulting in premature discharge from the hospital (Lakier and Fritz, 1969; Nicolson et al., 1974; Reitz, 1989). Persistent bleeding from the "fang" or maxillary teeth puncture marks is often the first symptom. Dizziness, syncope, shock, and seizures within the first 15 min after the bite have been described. Within a few hours, nausea, vomiting, colicky abdominal pain and severe, often occipital, headache may develop (Broadley, 1960). There may be bleeding from old and recent wounds such as venepunctures and scratches, as well as spontaneous systemic bleeding from gums, nose, conjunctivae, and external auditory meatus. Numerous documented cases have included: hematemesis, hemoptysis, rectal bleeding, hematochezia or melena, subarachnoid and intracranial hemorrhages, hematuria, and extensive superficial ecchymoses as well as hematomas (Plate 4.20J–L). In fatal cases, widespread petechial hemorrhages are seen at autopsy in serosal cavities, heart, walls of the great vessels, and elsewhere with obvious sites of severe bleeding in the stomach and bladder (Spies et al., 1962). Histopathological appearances included diffuse fibrin microthrombi in brain, liver, and lungs, and hemoglobin casts in the renal tubules (Lakier and Fritz, 1969; Spies et al., 1962). Both intravascular and microangiopathic hemolysis leading to hyperbilirubinemia and hemoglobinuria have been described (Lakier and Fritz, 1969; see Section 4.6). The misleading term "hemolytic uremic syndrome" is sometimes applied (Du Toit, 1980). Most fatalities occurred within a few days of the bite but some, attributable to acute tubular necrosis, were delayed for many days. Local envenomation is usually trivial apart from some pain, but several patients developed local swelling; one had swelling of the entire bitten arm, with sloughing of necrotic skin at the bite site on his hand

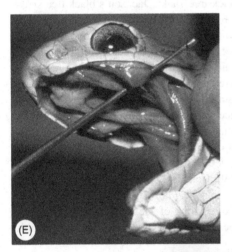
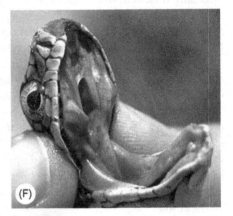
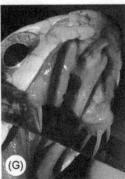

Plate 4.20 (E) *Dispholidus typus*, view of the enlarged posterior maxillary teeth. (F and G) Additional views of the enlarged posterior maxillary teeth of *Dispholidus typus*. Plate 4.20F **Male, Ghana;** Plate 4.20G **Kenya** (see also Plate 2.13).

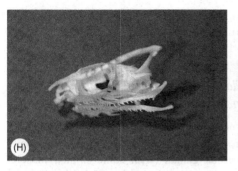
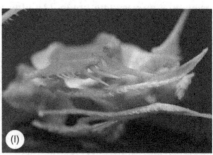
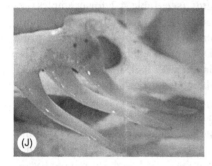
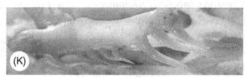

Plate 4.20 (*Continued*)
(H–K) *Dispholidus typus*, **osteological specimen.** Note the multiple enlarged posterior maxillary teeth with prominent lateral sharp ridges, and deep grooves running about 65% of the length of the respective teeth. These adaptations, and a potentially wide buccal gape, probably influence the lethal potential of bites by this species.
Plate 4.20E, photo copyright to Dave Ball; Plate 4.20F and G, photos copyright to David A. Warrell; Plate 4.20H–K, AMNH #75722, photos copyright to Scott A. Weinstein.

which took 5 weeks to heal (Knabe, 1939), and another had massive swelling with blood-filled bullae (Spies et al., 1962). Local tender lymphadenopathy may develop. Laboratory investigations confirm incoagulable blood, defibrinogenation, elevated fibrin(ogen) degradation products, severe thrombocytopenia, anemia, and complement depletion via the alternative pathway (Nicolson et al., 1974; see also Table 4.1).

As there is no commercial antivenom for *Thelotornis* envenomations, a cascade of symptoms often ensues. Patients may present with local edema, uncontrolled bleeding from the gums, and healing pre-existing wounds (Broadley, 1959; Muguti and Dube, 1998), extensive ecchymoses, hematuria, coagulopathy, raised fibrin(ogen)-related degradation products, thrombocytopenia, intravascular hemolysis, multiple organ hemorrhage, and acute kidney injury [AKI; often manifested as acute renal failure (ARF) characterized by acute tubular necrosis, probably primarily from hemoglobinuric nephropathy; see Section 4.6] that is unresponsive to diuretics or dialysis, such as occurred after Robert Mertens was bitten by a *T. kirtlandii* that resulted in death 18 days later (Table 4.1). Patients may also develop signs of envenomation very late (up to 24 h after the bite), present with substantial delay after a bite from one of these species, and exhibit coagulopathy without any outwardly concerning signs on examination.

4.3.1.1   Overview of the Duvernoy's Gland and Associated Dentition of D. typus and Thelotornis spp.

The medical risks from these snakes are associated with their notably enlarged and relatively numerous posterior, deeply grooved maxillary teeth (Plates 2.15, Plate 4.20D–J, and 4.56C, H–K), markedly serous glands (with some limited muscle attachment), and highly toxic venoms. Consistent with the arboreal habits of these snakes, their prey often includes lizards and birds (see Table 4.2 for examples). A Fischer's chameleon (*Chameleo fischeri*) seized by a *T. usambaricus* in northern Tanzania succumbed within a few minutes, turning a deep black color just prior to death (SAW, personal observations). The Duvernoy's glands of this tribe display size variability that may have some correlation with their medical importance. *Thrasops* spp. and *Rhamnophis* spp. possess relatively small glands. The gland size is increased in *Thelotornis* spp. and *Xyelodontophis* and reaches an apex in *D. typus* (Broadley and Wallach, 2002). In his histological study of oral glands of approximately 180 colubrid species, Taub (1967) emphasized the distinctive character of the *D. typus* Duvernoy's gland as these glands were readily distinguished from all other non-front-fanged colubroid glands that were examined. Although he reported variability in the thickness of the gland capsule (one specimen, CM #6340, had a thin capsule; the other, AMT No. 5, had a "very heavy, thick" capsule), he observed several features that highlighted the active secretory function of the *D. typus* Duvernoy's gland. The glands had: "very many" trabeculae of variable thickness; >90% of tubules had lumenae; mucous cells and mucous supralabial glands were absent; also, high vascularity was noted. The gland substance was composed of either columnar or cuboidal cells (Taub, 1967). He similarly described the Duvernoy's gland of *T. kirtlandii* as having: a "heavy thick" capsule; with many thick trabeculae; >90% of tubules with a lumen; intraglandular mucous cells as well as a supralabial mucous gland were absent (Taub, 1967). The highly tubuloacinous gland of *D. typus* exhibits extensive folding. This provides some limited space for venom storage, thus constituting a minimal cisternae (Broadley and Wallach, 2002; Weinstein et al., 2010). Taub (1967) noted the lobular evaginations and invaginations of the *D. typus* gland that contributed to the substantial secretory and storage space, and compared these to the "folding" (rugae) present in the mammalian gall bladder.

The multiple, enlarged posterior maxillary teeth of *D. typus* possess a deep groove that is restricted to between approximately 50% and 65% of the tooth length (see Plate 4.20H–J), while those of *T. capensis* have a deep groove that runs most of the tooths' length (Jackson and Fritts, 1995; Fry et al., 2008). The multiple enlarged posterior maxillary teeth of *T. kirtlandii* have similar deep grooves that run almost the entire length of the teeth (Plate 4.56H–K). Meier (1981) described blade-like modifications of the surface of these teeth. This modified surface presumably facilitates the introduction of venom through the integument of prey or human victim. *Thelotornis*

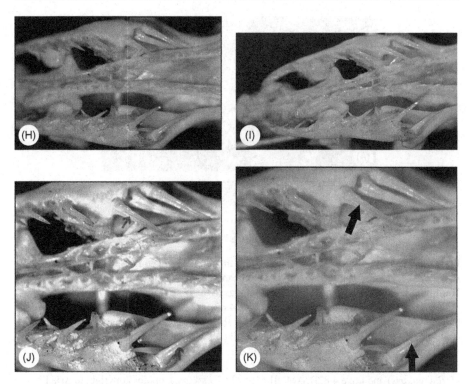

Plate 4.56 (H–K) Maxilla and enlarged posterior maxillary teeth of *T. kirtlandii*. Note the multiple enlarged, deeply grooved posterior maxillary teeth (arrows). Chameleons (*Chameleo* spp.) are favored prey, and these lizards succumb rapidly when grasped by a *T. kirtlandii*. Plate 4.56H–K, AMNH #75091, photos copyright to Scott A. Weinstein.

spp. and *D. typus* retain this prominent ridge on the anterior surface of the teeth, and the ridge arises within the groove in *Thelotornis* spp., thus dividing the "venom canal" (= groove) (Broadley and Wallach, 2002). The division formed by this modification terminates well before the tip of the respective posterior maxillary teeth (Broadley and Wallach, 2002). This is particularly significant, as Broadley (1968) noted that *D. typus* can strike with the enlarged maxillary teeth in a forward orientation thereby increasing contact with the intended target. The jaw kinetics of this species probably adds an additional dimension to this capability, as these snakes exhibit a wide gaping capacity (to about 170°; Marais, 1985) that increases the likelihood of greater biting contact and bitten surface area. However, with the posterior venom-delivery apparatus, some bites will fail to result in envenoming. Cooper and Reid (1976) discussed several asymptomatic and insignificant *D. typus* bites reported by Ionides. Therefore, although rapid envenoming (i.e., strike and release) by "opisthoglyphous" and "aglyphous" snakes certainly occur (Warrell, 2004), "dry" bites are likely common, as they are with some viperids.

Little information is available about the specific dentitional characteristics of *Thrasops* and *Rhamnophis*. The three posteriormost maxillary teeth of *T. flavigularis*

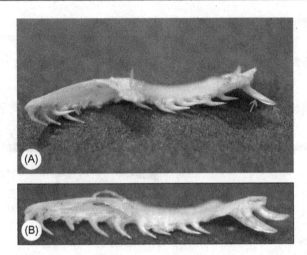

Plate 4.82 (A) Maxillae of the African yellow-throated-big-eyed tree snake (*Thrasops flavigularis*), French Cameroon and (B) Jackson's tree snake (*Thrasops jacksoni*), Kampala, Uganda. The genus, *Thrasops*, belongs to the tribe Dispholidini. *Thrasops flavigularis* (Plate 4.82A) and *T. jacksoni* (Plate 4.82B) are active arboreal species that feed on lizards and birds. Relatively little is known of their natural history. The markedly enlarged, blade-like posterior maxillary teeth have a leaf-like morphology and are ungrooved (Plate 4.82A, arrows). There is a single documented case of a bite by *T. flavigularis* that caused moderate local effects including edema and pain. Plate 4.82A, AMNH #R50573 (*T. flavigularis*) and Plate 4.82B, AMNH #50572 (*T. jacksoni*), photos copyright to Arie Lev.

are enlarged and separated from the anterior teeth by a diastema (Broadley and Wallach, 2002). They taper from base to tip and have slight anterior and posterior ridges, but are ungrooved (Broadley and Wallach, 2002; Chippaux, 1999). Plate 4.82A and B show the respective blade-like, markedly enlarged, ungrooved posterior maxillary teeth in specimens of *T. flavigularis* and *T. jacksoni*. The same teeth in *R. aethiopissa ituriensis* (Ituri large-eyed green tree snake or nataymankeema; see Plate 4.83A and B) and *R. batesi* (Bates' tree snake) are slightly enlarged, curved, and possess sharp anterior and posterior ridges. However, these adaptations are less developed than those of *X. uluguruensis*, in which the leaf-shaped (narrowed at the dentary base) posteriormost maxillary teeth exhibit ridges that are broadest midway along their length (Broadley and Wallach, 2002).

4.3.1.2 Overview of the Properties, Toxinology, and Pharmacology of Venoms of D. typus and Thelotornis spp.

The life-threatening pathology observed after some of the bites from these snakes exhibits some correlation with lethal potency studies. Reported *D. typus* venom i.v. LD_{50} have ranged between 0.060 and 0.10 mg/kg and i.p. LD_{50} have ranged between 1.32 and 1.80 mg/kg (Christensen, 1968; Minton, 1974; Minton and Minton, 1980; Weinstein and Smith, 1993). The reported LD_{50} for *T. kirtlandii* and *T. capensis* venoms were 0.25–1.24 mg/kg (i.v.) and 0.50 mg/kg (i.p.), respectively (Christensen, 1968; Kornalik et al., 1978; Weinstein and Smith, 1993; see Appendix B).

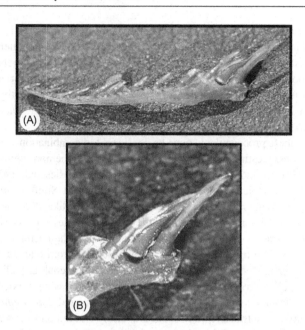

Plate 4.83 (A and B) Maxilla of the African (Congolese) large-eyed green tree snake or nataymankeema (*Rhamnophis aethiopissa ituriensis*), Niapu, Belgian Congo. Another little-known member of the Dispholidini, *R. a. ituriensis* has enlarged posterior maxillary teeth that are recurved, and the posteriormost tooth is notably larger than the anterior preceding teeth (Plate 4.83A, arrows). The suggestion of a groove in the second to last posterior maxillary tooth in this specimen is likely an artifact/defect of age. AMNH #12500, photos copyright to Arie Lev.

Although effects of most bites by non-front-fanged colubroid snakes cannot easily be explained by the toxins known to be present in their secretions, there is clear correlation between the pharmacology of toxins of Dispholidini studied to date and the pathophysiological effects observed in envenomated patients. Kornalik and Taborska (1978) described the similarity between hemorrhage in mice injected with *T. kirtlandii* venom and that caused by venom of *Bothrops jararaca* (jararaca). Similarly, Weinstein and Smith (1993) compared hemorrhagic effects in mice succumbing to i.p. injections of either *D. typus* or *T. capensis* venoms with those resulting from injection of *C. atrox* (western diamondback rattlesnake) venom.

Several investigators have described the prothrombin-activating activity of venoms from *D. typus* (Bradlow et al., 1980; Guillin et al., 1978) and *T. kirtlandii* (Kornalik and Taborska, 1978; Kornalik et al., 1978). Bradlow et al. (1980) also reported that *D. typus* venom could activate Factor X and possibly Factor IX. The prothrombin-activator was identified as a 58-kDa species that generated fragments 1, 2, and α-thrombin in the absence of Ca^{2+} and phospholipid. The mechanism involved the intermediate formation of meizothrombin in the presence of hirudin and therefore functioned similarly to that of ecarin from venom of the Indian saw-scaled viper, *Echis carinatus* (Gullin et al., 1978). *Thelotornis kirtlandii* venom exhibited strong *in vivo* defibrinating activity. Fibrinogen was undetectable within 10min after i.v. injection of a gland extract into rats (Kornalik and Taborska, 1978). The afibrinogenemia persisted for 24h with restored fibrinogen levels noted after about 72h. *In vivo* hemolytic activity was also reported (Kornalik and Taborska, 1978). Figure 4.1 summarizes the essential features of human coagulation, and the mechanisms of coagulopathy induced by toxins currently known from venoms of the dispholidines, *D. typus, Thelotornis* spp., and the natricids, *R. tigrinus* and *R. subminiatus* (see later).

The action of these procoagulants must be considered in combination with strong proteolytic activities (suggesting the presence of possible rhexic hemorrhagins) detected in these venoms (Grasset and Schaafsma, 1940; Hiestand and Hiestand, 1979; Kamiguti et al., 2000; Robertson and Delpierre, 1969; Weinstein and Smith, 1993). Some of these, such as the metalloproteases that exhibit disintegrin-like domains (likely that of P-III/P-IV metalloproteases) as noted in the 65-kDa species characterized from *D. typus* venom by Kamiguti et al. (2000), in combination with the Factor II and X activators, likely account for most of the life-threatening sequelae from bites of these snakes. Section 4.6 considers the possibility of direct and indirect intrarenal[7] as well as procoagulant-related prerenal[8] pathology contributing to the concerning nephrotoxicity associated with envenoming from the medically important Dispholidini and *Rhabdophis* spp.

A recent study of the transcriptomes and Duvernoy's gland and venom gland morphology of representative colubroid genera included *T. jacksoni* (Fry et al., 2008). This study reported that the transcriptome of *T. jacksoni* contained toxin transcripts (particularly, P-III-type metalloproteases and a disintegrin-metalloprotease) closely similar to those of *D. typus*. On this basis, the authors warned of a possible medical risk from this species (Fry et al., 2008).

4.3.1.3 Dispholidus typus: A Colubrid Important in Veterinary Medicine

There are very few data regarding the veterinary importance of non-front-fanged colubroid species. *Boiga irregularis* is known to actively prey on domestic animals (see Section 4.4.1), but there is little information regarding specific cases of dogs or cats bitten by this species. However, there are several well-documented cases of serious *D. typus* envenoming in dogs (Hoole and Goddard, 2007; Leisewitz et al., 2004; Vaughan and Lobetti, 1995), and a case of persistent bleeding (from the presumed bite wound) in a dog after it was bitten by a *T. capensis* (Otto and Blaylock, 2003). Dogs with clinically significant *D. typus* envenomation exhibit consumptive coagulopathy, often with profuse hemorrhage (Hoole and Goddard, 2007; Vaughan and Lobetti, 1995). Animals seriously envenomated by *D. typus* respond rapidly to monospecific *D. typus* antivenom. As reported in humans treated with this antivenom (Section 4.6), dogs treated with monospecific anti-*D. typus* antivenom may develop early anaphylaxis that is responsive to i.v. cortisone (we recommend epinephrine)

---

[7] This refers to toxin effects within the kidney.

[8] Any process or substance that reduces blood flow to the kidney has prerenal effects. This may include toxins, nonsteroidal anti-inflammatory medications (NSAIDS), loss of blood volume (hypovolemia), and many others.

and symptomatic management (Hoole and Goddard, 2007). Although the effects of *D. typus* envenomation in dogs and humans appear very similar, there are differences in management of envenomated dogs compared with that of humans, as discussed by Leisewitz et al. (2004). Pet owners living within the range of *D. typus* or *Thelotornis* spp. should be aware of the possible threat posed by these snakes, and should take appropriate precautions to protect their pets from envenomation.

4.3.1.4 Conclusion and Assessment of D. typus and Thelotornis spp.

As with the vast majority of bites from snakes in the artificial colubrid assemblage, the most publicized bites are inflicted by these snakes while being handled by herpetologists and amateur snake collectors. However, in some parts of Africa (e.g., the Kenyan coast), local agricultural workers are occasionally bitten by *D. typus*. Many documented bites from *D. typus* and *Thelotornis* spp. have produced life-threatening clinical effects and fatalities typified by consumptive coagulopathy/DIC and hemorrhagic diathesis. The morphological adaptations outlined earlier combined with high venom toxicity for humans endow these snakes with notable lethal potential. Aside from a single documented case of moderate local effects from a *T. flavigularis* bite, the clinical importance of other Dispholidini (*Rhamnophis* and *Thrasops*) is unknown. Partial characterization of the transcriptome of *T. jacksoni* suggests an array of toxins similar to those of *D. typus*. Therefore, other members of this tribe should be approached with caution. Any bites from these snakes should be assessed by a physician, and serial blood coagulation assays should be included in the assessment of a patient bitten by any of these species.

Assessment of *D. typus*, *T. capensis*, and *T. kirtlandii* based on available evidence: Hazard Level 1 (see Table 4.3).

4.3.2 Rhabdophis subminiatus and Rhabdophis tigrinus: Background and General Features of Documented Bites

The Asian natricid genus, *Rhabdophis* (the Asian keel-backs), consists of 18 species. Of these, only *R. subminiatus* and *R. tigrinus* (Plates 4.45A–C and 4.46A and B, respectively) have caused medically significant bites. These include several thoroughly documented fatal and life-threatening envenomations consisting of consumptive coagulopathy, DIC, hemorrhagic diathesis, anemia, AKI, and severe ecchymoses (see Plate 4.46C; Table 4.1). For example, a 25-year-old Thai man was bitten five times while feeding his pet *R. subminiatus helleri* in Ranong. He went to the local hospital with bleeding gums and was inappropriately given 10 ampoules of Malayan pit viper antivenom together with 6 units of fresh frozen plasma (FFP). On the second day, his hand was swollen and, after 5 days, he was referred to Chulalongkorn Hospital in Bangkok with incoagulable blood (PT > 100, PTT > 100 s). He was treated with a further 14 units of FFP, 13 units of packed red blood cells (PRBCs), 10 units of cryoprecipitate, and, again inappropriately, with 24 ampoules of green pit viper (*Cryptelytrops albolabris*) antivenom. After a further 5 days, the bleeding stopped (Kijjirak et al., 1998). This was the first reported case of *R. subminiatus* envenomation in South East Asia. A second South East Asian case was published by Seow et al. from Singapore in 2000.

Rhabdophis tigrinus (tiger keel-back or yamakagashi) has three subspecies (tigrinus, formosanus, and lateralis), while two subspecies (subminiatus and helleri) of R. subminiatus (red-necked keel-back) are currently recognized. The dietary preferences of Rhabdophis spp., summarized in Table 4.2, are similar to many other natricids. Careful review of documented envenomations inflicted by these two species suggests that they are among the most dangerous members of the former artificial colubrid assemblage. This threat results from the marked toxicity of their venoms to humans, and their occasional entry into the pet trade due to mistaken identity [they may be confused with several species of other keel-backs or, as they are popularly known, Asian garter snakes, Amphiesma spp. (e.g., A. stolata; Plate 4.84A–E)]. Although this circumstance has occurred occasionally with Dispholidus and Thelotornis spp., mistaken identity involving these species is now uncommon. The potential misidentification of R. tigrinus or R. subminiatus with Amphiesma spp. (compare Plates 4.45A and B and 4.46A and B with Plate 4.84A–E) has resulted in a periodically renewed concern among medical professionals and amateur collectors. A life-threatening case of R. subminiatus envenoming in 1981 resulted in the banning of private ownership of this species in Los Angeles (New York Times, September 13, 1981).[9] Conversely, in 1990, the New York City Health Department issued a citywide alarm due to concerns that Rhabdophis spp. had entered the retail pet trade. The alarm was issued after a self-taught amateur collector informed the health department that the snakes being sold as "garter snakes" were actually a species of Rhabdophis spp. Until correctly identified as Amphiesma spp., the initial misinterpretation resulted in the removal of several dozen Amphiesma spp. from the stock of a large New York pet store chain (New York Times, October 17, 1990). Some hobbyist periodicals highlighted the potential confusion (Walls, 1991) as collectors expressed concerns regarding the perceived danger of a potentially fatal misidentification.

4.3.2.1 Overview of the Duvernoy's Gland and Associated Dentition of R. subminiatus and R. tigrinus

Rhabdophis subminiatus and R. tigrinus possess enlarged, ungrooved posterior maxillary teeth (Plates 4.45C and 4.46E–G, respectively). These teeth have a sharp posterior edge and are notably recurved (Plate 4.46E–G). They are separated from the anterior teeth by a prominent diastema and, in R. tigrinus, are 2.25 times longer than the teeth immediately anterior to them (Mittleman and Goris, 1974; see Plate 4.46E and F). Although there are a number of documented "dry bites" from these species suggesting that protracted bites are more likely to result in serious envenoming (Viravan et al., 1992; Table 4.1), some cases have only involved brief biting/contact with the snake. In one life-threatening case, the R. tigrinus specimen was 55 cm long and had enlarged posterior maxillary teeth measuring 2.3 mm from tip

[9] See Appendix D for a critical opinionated essay regarding legal issues relevant to private ownership of dangerously venomous colubroid snakes.

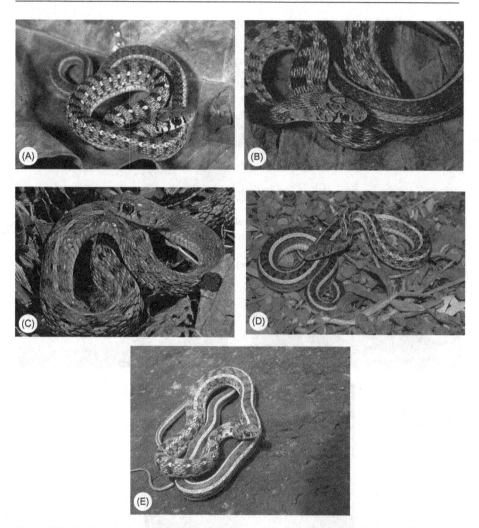

Plate 4.84 (A–E) Asian keel-backs, flower snakes, or garter snakes (*Amphiesma* spp.).
There are about 41 species of *Amphiesma*, and some of these Asian natricids are commonly
seen in the commercial snake trade. Due to pattern variability and appearance that may be
similar to some members of the genus *Rhabdophis*, some *Amphiesma* (particularly *A. stolata*)
have occasionally been mistaken for the hazard level 1 species, *R. tigrinus* and *R. subminiatus*
(see Section 4.3; compare with Plates 4.45A–C and 4.46A and B). There are no documented
medically significant bites by *Amphiesma* spp.
(A) Striped keel-back, flower snake, yellow-banded or yellow-necked water snake,
Amphiesma stolata, **Habarana, Sri Lanka.**
(B) *Amphiesma stolata*, **Nikaweratiya, Sri Lanka.**
(C) *Amphiesma stolata*, **South Asia.**
(D) *Amphiesma stolata*, **Sisaket, Thailand.**
(E) *Amphiesma stolata*, **Pune, India,** Plate 4.84A–C, photos copyright to Mark O'Shea;
Plate 4.84D, photo copyright to Wolfgang Wüster; Plate 4.84E, photo copyright to Shukla
Chaitanya.

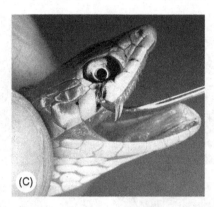

Plate 4.45C. Enlarged posterior maxillary teeth of the red-necked keel-back (*Rhabdophis subminiatus*). Note the markedly enlarged, ungrooved posterior maxillary teeth (also see Plates 4.46E-G).
Plate 4.45C, photo copyright to David A. Warrell.

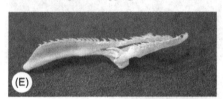

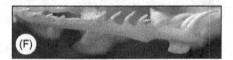

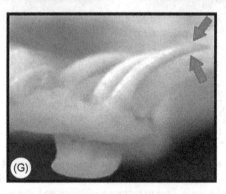

Plate 4.46 (E–G) Maxilla and posterior enlarged maxillary teeth of *R. tigrinus lateralis*, Korea. The posterior maxillary teeth are enlarged, but, unlike other hazard level 1 species (*Dispholidus* and *Thelotornis*), lack grooves or any other dentitional modifications (see Plate 4.46G, arrows). "Quick release" bites by these snakes occasionally may not be medically significant, but some brief bites have caused life-threatening envenomations.
Plate 4.46E–G, AMNH #R148038, photos copyright to Arie Lev.

to alveolar insertion. The brief bite from this snake produced a severe consumptive coagulopathy with DIC in a 57-year-old, 82-kg male (Mittleman and Goris, 1974).

In some non-front-fanged colubroids, selection for increased oral glandular size may have occurred in snakes whose mid- or posteriorly positioned maxillary teeth were already enlarged (Kardong, 1979; Weinstein and Kardong, 1994). Malnate

(1960) found that in natricines (now, provisionally natricids) there was a direct correlation between glandular development and increasing occurrence of specialized dentition, a selective adaptation that was reported to reach its zenith in *Balanophis* (*Rhabdophis*, Wall, 1921) *ceylonensis*. *Balanophis ceylonensis* has grooved, enlarged posterior maxillary teeth and well-developed Duvernoy's glands (Malnate, 1960). In the single documented case of a bite from this species, there were only minor local effects and nonspecific headache (De Silva and Aloysius, 1983; Table 4.1). However, this species should be treated with caution in view of its morphological adaptations and relationship to *R. tigrinus* and *R. subminiatus*.

The Duvernoy's glands of *R. subminiatus* and *R. tigrinus* are tubuloacinous, well developed, and comprise at least half of the total supralabial glandular structure (Mittleman and Goris, 1974). Yoshie et al. (1982) conducted an electron microscopic study of Duvernoy's glands of *R. tigrinus*. Secretory units of the gland consisted of columnar secretory and myoepithelial cells. There were well-developed organelles and homogenous, dense secretory granules accumulated in the apical cytoplasm for exocytotic release into the lumen (Yoshie et al., 1982). The duct epithelium was composed of mucous-secreting cells that contained cytoplasmic secretory globules. The myoepithelial cells encompassed the secretory units and had numerous autonomic innervations via the basement membrane (Yoshie et al., 1982). Histochemical study indicated that these nerve terminals were enriched with acetylcholinesterase-reactive and peptide histidine-isoleucine-like immunoreactive fibers (Yoshie et al., 1988). As many of the neuronal terminals contained small, clear vesicles as well as dense core granules, were devoid of Schwann cell coverage on the capillary side, and entered the pericapillary space, the authors hypothesized intravascular release of neurosecretions (Yoshie et al., 1982, 1988).

4.3.2.2 The Unusual Nuchal Gland of R. tigrinus

Rhabdophis tigrinus also possesses a nuchal (sometimes referred to as "cervical") gland that produces several novel polyhydroxylated steroid toxins, the bufadienolides (Azuma et al., 1986; Hutchinson et al., 2007). This can be considered analogous to the biosynthetic pathway for the batrachotoxins from a few genera of dendrobatid "poison dart" frogs (e.g., *Dendrobates* and *Phyllobates*), as the toxins present in this gland are probably derived from dietary sources (i.e., toads; Hutchinson et al., 2007; Mori and Burghardt, 2000). Some data suggest that the gland serves an antipredator function (Hutchinson et al., 2007; Mori and Burghardt, 2008). Although this gland and its secretion play no role in snakebite envenomation in humans, there have been documented cases of ophthalmia (resembling toxic chemosis) resulting from accidental ocular exposure to the secretion (Kawamoto and Kumada, 1989). The combined presence of Duvernoy's glands containing toxic venom and the poison-containing nuchal gland endows this snake with both venomous and poisonous properties.[10]

---

[10] As noted earlier, "venomous" implies introduction by biting or stinging (e.g., injection; introduction into or through the integument of prey or foe) per a specialized apparatus of a toxic mixture utilized for prey capture or defense. "Poisonous" implies the presence of a toxic substance that exerts its effects after ingestion or absorption.

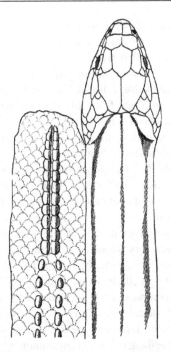

Figure 4.2 The dorsal-nuchal glands of the green keel-back (*Macropisthodon plumbicolor*). The well-known physician-herpetologist, Malcolm Smith (see also Plate 4.31C), drew this rendering of the unusual glands of *M. plumbicolor*. These appear similar to those of the hazard level 1 colubrid, the tiger keel-back or yamakagashi (*R. tigrinus*). The *R. tigrinus* nuchal glands produce several novel polyhydroxylated steroid toxins, the bufadienolides. Unlike the toxins present in Duvernoy's glands, these toxins are formed from dietary precursors. Although the *R. tigrinus* glands seem to provide an antipredator armamentarium, the function and components of the *M. plumbicolor* glands remain unknown. After Smith, 1938.

Similarly located glands have been described by Smith (1938) in the Asian green keel-back, *Macropisthodon plumbicolor* (Plate 4.14A; Figure 4.2). Neither their function or biochemical properties of their secretion(s) have been investigated.

4.3.2.3 Overview of the Properties, Toxinology, and Pharmacology of Venoms of R. subminiatus and R. tigrinus

There are few data regarding venom yield from these snakes. Using micropipette extraction, Ferlan et al. (1983) obtained 10–15 μL of secretion from *R. subminiatus*. Although solid yield was not reported, they detected 14.34 mg protein/mL secretion (Ferlan et al., 1983). Excision, maceration, and extraction of Duvernoy's glands from *R. tigrinus* yielded 8.5–20.5 mg solids (Sakai et al., 1983).

As noted with *Dispholidus* and *Thelotornis* (see previous section), significant envenomation from either *R. tigrinus* or *R. subminiatus* often presents the physician with a challenging case of a severely ill patient exhibiting varying degrees of consumptive coagulopathy/DIC, hemorrhagic diathesis, AKI, and anemia (Table 4.1). All of the *R. tigrinus* envenomations documented to date have occurred in Japan except for one case in the Russian literature (Orlov et al., 1990) of a 50-year-old man who developed bleeding from the bite wound, thrombocytopenia, increased PT, and hypofibrinogenemia. Only a few *R. subminiatus* envenomations have been described, mainly in amateur snake collectors in Western countries. Essentially all serious envenoming from these species resulted from handling of the snakes and frequently involved protracted bites (Table 4.1). However, as highlighted earlier, briefly administered bites from small specimens have resulted in life-threatening envenoming (Table 4.1; Mittleman and Goris, 1974). Predictably, Sakai et al. (1983) reported that i.m. or s.c. injection of *R. tigrinus* venom into mice resulted in widespread s.c. hemorrhage in the injected animals.

Although *R. tigrinus* and *R. subminiatus* have inflicted several life-threatening or fatal envenomations (to date, *R. subminiatus* has not caused a fatal envenoming), there are relatively few studies of the lethal potency of their venoms. Sakai et al. (1983) reported murine i.v., i.m., and s.c. LD_{50} of 2.65, 7.35, and 9.20 mg/kg, respectively, for Duvernoy's secretion (venom) from *R. tigrinus*. Sakai et al. (1990) reported an identical murine i.v. LD_{50}, 2.65 mg/kg, for *R. tigrinus* Duvernoy's secretion. Lethal potency determinations of *R. subminiatus* venom have indicated that venom from this species is probably twice the toxicity of *R. tigrinus* venom. Sakai et al. (1984) obtained a murine i.v. LD_{50} of 0.125 mg/kg for *R. subminiatus* venom, while Ferlan et al. (1983) reported an i.v. LD_{50} of 0.129 mg/kg for this species (see Appendix B).

The medical significance of these natricids and the lethal potency of their venoms correlate with their powerful procoagulant toxins. Nahas et al. (1976) reported that *R. tigrinus* venom activated Factor X in the presence of phospholipid and Factor V, while Sakai et al. (1983) found that *R. tigrinus* venom activated prothrombin in human plasma. The *in vivo* hemorrhagic effects of this venom were viewed as a result of the coagulopathy due to the procoagulant toxin-induced hypofibrinogenemia (Sawai et al., 1985). Spontaneous systemic hemorrhage implies the presence of vascular endothelium damaging hemorrhagins such as metalloproteinases, as coagulopathy alone does not cause hemorrhage unless there is vessel wall damage as well (Figure 4.1). Therefore, the *in vivo* actions of proteolytic enzymes that hydrolyze intrinsic proteins of blood vessels combined with the coagulopathy probably cause the hemorrhagic diathesis.

The prothrombin-activator present in *R. tigrinus* venom acts like ecarin. Cleavage of the zymogen occurs at the Arg 320-Ile 321 bond. This results in formation of meizothrombin, an intermediate that is autocatalytically cleaved to α-thrombin (Morita et al., 1988). This is very similar to the reported pharmacology of a 58-kDa prothrombin-activator partially characterized from *D. typus* venom (see previous section, pg. 187; Guillin et al., 1978). Kornalik et al. (1978) similarly reported that *T. kirtlandii* Duvernoy's gland extract contained powerful Ca^{2+} independent procoagulant activity mediated by direct conversion of prothrombin to thrombin. Their extract also showed potent defibrinating action. Kornalik and Taborska (1978) described *T. kirtlandii* venom as an activator of prothrombin and Factor X (see previous section). Thus, both *Thelotornis* and *Dispholidus* venoms have properties similar to those of *R. tigrinus* and *R. subminiatus* (see Figure 4.1), and the resulting pathophysiology from venoms of all of these species correlates closely with clinical manifestations in the envenomated patient.

Other studies have revealed different venom activities. For instance, Theakston et al. (1979) reported that *R. subminiatus* venom functioned as a Ca^{2+} independent, potent Factor X activator and a mild prothrombin-activator. In contrast, Zotz et al. (1991) described a potent prothrombin-activator present in gland extract from *R. subminiatus*. The thrombin thus generated was not inhibited by antithrombin III or by antithrombin III–heparin complex. Unlike Theakston et al. (1979), Zotz et al. (1991) found no direct Factor X activation. Several investigators have reported powerful Ca^{2+} independent Factor X activation in *R. subminiatus* or *R. tigrinus* venom or Duvernoy's gland extract (Nahas et al., 1976; Theakston et al., 1979), while others have emphasized prothrombin activation (Sakai et al., 1983; Zotz et al., 1991). All of these studies have reported potent defibrinating action of venoms from both species; none reported thrombin-like activity (Weinstein and Kardong, 1994).

Several investigators have detected proteolytic activity in venoms of *R. subminiatus* and *R. tigrinus* (Ferlan et al., 1983; Komori et al., 2006). Phospholipases A activity in *R. subminiatus* venom was reported by Ferlan et al. (1983). A recent study of hemorrhagic toxins in venom of *R. t. tigrinus* discovered and characterized a novel metalloprotease that may be regulated by the cysteine-switch mechanism (Komori et al., 2006). The authors considered that this protease was likely to be a matrix metalloprotease, rather than a snake venom metalloprotease (Komori et al., 2006). As previously discussed, proteases, related rhexic hemorrhagins, and, possibly, disintegrins, combined with the powerful defibrinating activity of potent procoagulant toxins are likely to contribute to the severe hemorrhagic diathesis/DIC observed in serious envenoming from these natricids, as well as the medically important Dispholidini, *Thelotornis* spp., and *D. typus* (Figure 4.1).

4.3.2.4 Summary of Experimental Pathophysiological Effects of Duvernoy's Secretion from R. tigrinus tigrinus

Pathophysiological studies of *R. tigrinus* venom in rats and mice have offered a glimpse into some of the potential pathology that might be induced by this venom in a mammalian system. Injected mice exhibited systemic hemorrhage, including subendocardial and pulmonary foci and alveolar as well as glomerular microthrombi (Sakai et al., 1983). The magnitude of pathological effects were correlated with dose as rats injected with either 300 μg or 1.5 mg of Duvernoy's gland extract developed consumption coagulopathy, while those injected with the lower dose recovered fibrinogen, platelets, and erythrocyte levels more rapidly than those receiving the higher dose. Animals injected with 1.5 mg developed marked pulmonary edema, hemorrhage and hyaline droplet degeneration, and renal casts. Glomerular deposition of fibrin thrombi and renal tubular necrosis were observed. They were especially marked in a rat succumbing 34 h postinjection.[11] Thymus hemorrhage and involution were also observed (Sakai et al., 1990). Within 1 h of i.m. injection of *R. t. tigrinus* venom into rats, fibrinogen was undetectable, PT was prolonged, and fibrin degradation products (FDP) increased (Sakai and Hatsuse, 1995). DIC, hemoglobinuria, anemia, and thrombocytopenia also developed. The authors suggested that fibrin thrombus formation accounted for most of the hemostatic abnormalities. Necropsy detected local and pulmonary hemorrhage/edema and renal tubule necrosis (Sakai and Hatsuse, 1995). Many of these pathophysiological changes have occurred in humans envenomated by these species.

4.3.2.5   Conclusion and Assessment of R. subminiatus and R. tigrinus

Both *R. subminiatus* and *R. tigrinus* have inflicted well-documented, carefully reported life-threatening, and/or fatal bites. Almost all of these have occurred as a consequence of handling captive specimens. Confusion of these snakes with harmless natricids, such as some species of *Amphiesma*, has resulted in recurrent concerns (most often unfounded) regarding the possible accidental presence of either species in the retail pet trade. Although the posterior maxillary teeth do not show the same extent of adaptation as in the medically important Dispholidini, the potent venom and potentially fatal consequences of bites inflicted by these species emphasize their medical importance.

Assessment of *R. subminiatus* and *R. tigrinus* based on available evidence: Hazard Level 1 (see Table 4.3).

4.3.3   Comparison of Major Features of Hazard Level 1 Colubrids (Figure 4.3) (Dispholidus typus, Thelotornis capensis, Thelotornis kirtlandii, Rhabdophis tigrinus, and Rhabdophis subminiatus)

- Serous Duvernoy's glands associated with markedly enlarged noncanaliculated posterior maxillary teeth. Although these are grooved in *D. typus* (deep grooves that extend over approximately 50–65% of the tooth surface) and *Thelotornis* spp. (deep grooves that traverse almost the entire tooth surface), *R. tigrinus* and *R. subminiatus* have ungrooved teeth. Figure 4.3 compares head and dentition profiles of *D. typus*, *T. kirtlandii*, and *R. tigrinus*.
- All produce potent procoagulant toxins that activate prothrombin, and Factor X, but some pharmacological studies suggest variability of these activities among different populations and/or individual snakes. The role of these toxins in the natural history of these taxa remains unclear and/or unverified.
- Clinical manifestations of envenoming by any of these snakes results in consumptive coagulopathy, DIC, bleeding, anemia, thrombocytopenia, and other serious hemostatic disturbances. Severe cases may result in AKI (see Section 4.6) and death.
- There are well-documented fatalities from envenomations by *D. typus*, *T. capensis*, *T. kirtlandii*, and *R. tigrinus*, but to date there are no documented fatalities from *R. subminiatus* bites.

---

[11] It is possible that due to some of the delayed effects (e.g., progressive renal tubular necrosis, possible microthrombi deposition in the splanchnic vasculature, and other evolving pathophysiology) the experimental lethal potencies of these species have been underestimated due to approximations from murine lethal potency studies conducted with 24-h observation limits.

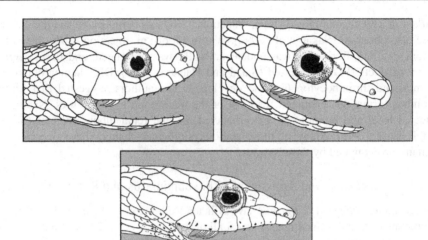

Figure 4.3 Profiles of three hazard level 1 colubrids. Depicted in the figure are head and
dentition profiles of the tiger keel-back, *R. tigrinus* (upper left panel), boomslang, *D. typus*
(upper right panel), and Kirtland's twig, vine, or bird snake, *T. kirtlandii* (bottom panel). All
three hazard level 1 colubrid species have inflicted well-documented life-threatening and/or
fatal envenomations. All have serous Duvernoy's glands associated with markedly enlarged
noncanaliculated posterior maxillary teeth. Although these are grooved in *D. typus* (deep
grooves that extend over approximately 50–65% of the tooth surface; some of these grooves
may be located on the medial-posterior surface of the teeth, and thus are not visible in this
profile; upper right panel; see also Plate 4.20E–K) and *Thelotornis* spp. (deep grooves that
traverse almost the entire tooth surface, bottom panel; see also Plate 4.56C, H–K), *R. tigrinus*
and *R. subminiatus* have ungrooved teeth (upper left panel; see also Plates 4.45C and 4.46D–
G). All produce potent procoagulant toxins that activate prothrombin, and Factor X, but some
pharmacological studies suggest variability of these activities among different populations
and/or individual snakes. The role of these toxins in the natural history of these taxa remains
unclear and/or unverified, but observations of wild and captive specimens indicate that these
species use their venoms in the capture and/or subjugation of prey. Clinical manifestations
of envenoming by any of these snakes results in consumptive coagulopathy, DIC, bleeding,
anemia, thrombocytopenia, and other serious hemostatic disturbances (see Plate 4.20L–O).
Severe cases may result in acute kidney injury (see Sections 4.3 and 4.6, and Figure 4.4) and
death. Figure copyright to Kevin M. McAllister.

4.3.4 *Proven Guilty Without a Trial: Three Additional Unsupported Reports of Fatal Outcomes after Bites by* Tachymenis peruviana, Oligodon arnensis, *and* Xenodon severus

4.3.4.1 Tachymenis peruviana: *An Undeserved Reputation of Lethal Potential?*

Of the six species in the dipsadid genus *Tachymenis* (slender snakes), only *T. peruviana* (Peruvian slender snake; Plate 4.49A and B) has acquired a reputation for lethal
potential. This species has enlarged, recurved posterior maxillary teeth that contain a

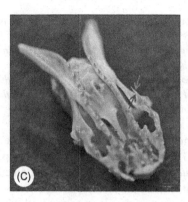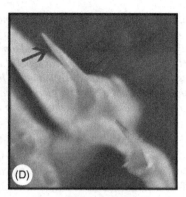

Plate 4.49 (C and D) Enlarged posterior maxillary teeth of *Tachymenis peruviana*. The most posterior (the last two teeth in the maxilla) enlarged maxillary teeth are gently recurved and contain a shallow groove that extends over almost the entire length of the tooth. Plate 4.49C and D, AMNH #5256, photo copyright to Arie Lev.

shallow groove present on approximately two-thirds of their length (Plate 4.49C and D). There are no well-documented cases of medically significant bites from this species; anecdotal reports suggest only mild-to-moderate local effects (Warrell, 2004).

One published paper frequently cited in support of a fatal envenomation by this species (Vellard, 1955) mentions no human fatality. Rather, the paper describes the effects of *T. peruviana* secretion on experimental animals (Vellard, 1955). There is, therefore, no evidence whatsoever of serious envenomation in humans from a *T. peruviana* bite. The report by Vellard (1955) should only be cited in relation to experimentally induced effects of *T. peruviana* secretion in animals. It must not be propagated in the literature as evidence of a "fatal bite" that in fact did not occur.

4.3.4.2 Oligodon arnensis: *Deadly Fear Without a Cause?*

The colubrine genus *Oligodon* (kukri snakes; Plate 4.67A and B) consists of approximately 68 species that feed on a variety of small vertebrates and invertebrates including nestling birds and their eggs, lizards and their eggs, frogs, and occasionally large insects (diet varies according to species). *Oligodon* spp. have a wide range in northern to western Asia, Southeast Asia, and the Indian subcontinent, and most average ≤89 cm in length (Cox, 1991; Smith, 1943; Wall, 1921; www.toxinology.com). There are no well-documented cases of medically significant bites from these snakes (Viravan et al., 1992). However, a case described by Wall (1921) has been cited as possible evidence of a fatal envenomation from a bite by the common, russet, or banded kukri snake, *O. arnensis*, near Bannu, Khyber-Pakhtunkhwa Province, Pakistan. The victim was described as having received a bite on the buttocks after lying down on his bed on the ground:

> *"He jumped up immediately rubbing his buttock, and declared that something had bitten him there. His companions searched his bedding, and there found a snake which they killed. They examined him, but could see no signs of a bite, and tried to persuade*

him, though without success, that he had not been bitten. The next morning he did not get up, and his companions could not rouse him. The hospital assistant was sent for and found him comatose ... he expired along the way. Captain Sumner here examined the body, and could find no local signs of the bite, and was much perplexed as to the cause of death. The snake was put into a bottle ... To my surprise I found the author of the mischief was a common kukri snake, 1 foot 71/2 inches long. It seems to me that the man must have died of fright, believing himself bitten"

(Wall, 1921, p. 233). Thus, Wall (1921) noted his own doubt regarding the actual disposition of this unfortunate case. Wall (1913) provides other examples of patients dying unaccountably after bites by *X. piscator* and *L. aulicus*. Deeply ingrained communal fear of a particular animal can result in dramatic symptoms after bites, in the absence of any evidence that the animal is in any way venomous. In the Turkana region of northern Kenya, bites by Ruppell's agama lizard (*Agama ruppelli orientalis*) are feared even more than bites by saw-scaled vipers (*Echis pyramidum*). Bitten patients may appear extremely ill or even comatose (MacCabe, 2009). Around Freeport, West Papua, the blue-tongued skink (*Tiliqua gigas*) is feared more than the death adder (*Acanthophis* spp.; DAW, personal communication; see also pp. 77; section 4.5.2 and 4.4.7). These cases further illustrate the power of psyche in the generation of symptomatology.

An alternative explanation is that the snake found in the man's bedclothes was not responsible for the bite which, given circumstances, was far more likely to have been a krait (*Bungarus* spp., Plate 4.64). There are no grounds for supposing that *O. arnensis* has venom or venom apparatus capable of causing fatal envenomation in humans.

4.3.4.3 A Fatal Bite by Xenodon severus?

There is a single obscure report (Orcés, 1948) of an alleged fatality from a bite by *X. severus* (Amazon false-Fer-de-Lance; Plate 4.59C; see also Plate 4.59A and B). To date, we have been unable to obtain a complete copy of the original report, and further efforts are underway to fully evaluate this case. In addition, the website for Instituto de Investigación Biológica de las Cordilleras Orientales[12] states the following:

The Yacu-jergon, Xenodon severus, is possibly extremely toxic: there are hospital records of bitings contributed to this very aggressive and somewhat common snake which showed severe effects-campesinos mention that this snake kills persons (sic).

Therefore, the very limited information about the toxic potential of this species is purely unsubstantiated anecdote and rumor without verifiable provenance. There is currently insufficient evidence for critical evaluation of any possible risk associated with this species. The single recorded case briefly described uncomplicated, minor, local effects (Quelch, 1893; Table 4.1).

---

[12] http://www.inibico.org/AreasInvestigaci%c3%b3n/Herpetolog%c3%ada/INIBICOUsers/ ReptilesandAmphibiansofSanMartin/tabid/57/Default.aspx

4.4 Aberrant Cases and Representative Cases Without Clear Etiology: A Critical Assessment of Risk

Things seen are mightier than things heard.

Lord Alfred Tennyson (1864)

4.4.1 Boiga irregularis

4.4.1.1 Background, History, and Aberrant Features of Bites

Boiga irregularis (Plate 4.9A–D) presents a unique and unusual opportunity to assess the medical importance of a non-front-fanged colubroid species. This is due to the relatively large number of medically reviewed snakebite incidents associated with this species, as well as the atypical circumstances surrounding its clinical importance.

Introduced to Guam (probably from Papua New Guinea) during the extensive ordinance transport operations in the Pacific Theater of World War II, *B. irregularis* rapidly established growing populations partly due to a lack of any natural predators. The burgeoning numbers of snakes had a severe impact on some of the native wildlife, especially birds (some species, including the endemic Guam rail, *Gallirallus owstoni*, and the Micronesian kingfisher, *Halcyon cinnamomina*, were extirpated), fruit bats (e.g., the Marianas fruit bat, *Pteropus mariannus*), and probably a number of scincid and gekkonid lizard populations [e.g., the scincid, *Emoia caeruleocauda* (Pacific blue-tailed skink) the gekkonid, *Gehyra mutilata* (four-clawed gecko or stump-toed gecko), and others; www.mesc.usgs.gov/resources/education/bts/impacts]. The decrease and disappearance of bird populations in the 1970s was the first worrying sign of the devastating ecological impact that this snake would cause in the coming decades on Guam, Saipan, Marianas, and other islands. In recent years, *B. irregularis* populations on Guam have often reached densities exceeding 50 snakes/hectare (http://www.anstaskforce.gov/Species%20plans/Brown%20Tree%20Snake%20Mgt%20Plan.pdf). *Boiga irregularis* is the only ophidian species ever to be targeted for control measures by an act of the United States Congress (e.g., Brown Tree Snake Control and Eradication Act of 2003, H.R. 3479, November 7, 2003).

In addition to its impact on native wildlife, *B. irregularis* rapidly affected the human inhabitants on Guam. This species has a predilection for frequent copulatory behavior, and predation on nestlings or scavenging birds electrocuted on power lines (Fritts and McCoid, 1999; see Plate 4.85A and B). From 1978 to 1994, this behavior resulted in numerous electrocutions of these snakes that caused approximately 1,200 power outages ("brownouts") on Guam (Fritts and McCoid, 1999). These incidents cumulatively resulted in a significant economic impact on the island's economy (Fritts and McCoid, 1999; Fritts et al., 1990, 1994). These snakes also actively preyed on domestic animals and, occasionally, ingested pet food left for dogs or cats (Fritts et al., 1994, 1999).

The medical importance of *B. irregularis* on Guam became evident during the mid-1980s to the late 1990s, when approximately 50 emergency visits per annum (about 1/1,200 emergency-room visits) were due to bites from *B. irregularis*

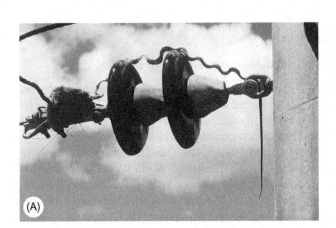
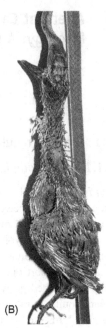

Plate 4.85 (A and B) A brown tree snake (*Boiga irregularis*) preying on birds nested (A) or electrocuted (B) on high power lines, Guam. The predilection of *B. irregularis* for mating and searching for avian prey on high power lines has resulted in repetitive "brown outs" on Guam due to the occasional electrocution of these snakes. This has caused significant economic loss on the island.
Photos copyright to Gordon Rodda.

(www.mesc.usgs.gov). As an example, from 1989 to 1994, 206 well-documented cases were recorded. In this series, 82% of the victims were bitten while sleeping, and 52% of these victims were younger than 5 years old (www.mesc.usgs.gov/resources/education/bts). This is reminiscent of some common features of krait (*Bungarus* spp.) envenoming in India and Sri Lanka (Warrell, 1995a). A published series of cases included three pediatric patients (mean age = 2.9 months) that reportedly exhibited ptosis, respiratory failure, and spasticity (Fritts and McCoid, 1994). Retrospective medical expert review of these presumed neurotoxic effects was equivocal (SA Minton, personal verbal communication with SAW, June 1995).

The majority of patients included in a retrospective review of 446 *B. irregularis* bites recorded at Guam Memorial Hospital, 1987–2004, were asymptomatic or exhibited mild local effects (Morocco et al., 2006). Several patients (most commonly children) developed more extensive local effects including bleb (blister) formation. These authors identified "systemic toxicity" ("generalized weakness," respiratory difficulty, and ptosis) in several victims, all younger than 1 year old (Morocco et al., 2006). The more severe effects in infants were ascribed to the introduction of larger "doses of venom" due to protracted bites/chewing inflicted on victims unable to disengage the snake (Morocco et al., 2006). A survey conducted from January 2008 to November 2008 yielded 11 documented cases of emergency-room review of *B. irregularis* bites on Guam (this study; Table 4.1). Of these, 10 consisted of minor lacerations, erythema, and slight bleeding. One 2-week-old male reportedly exhibited respiratory distress, thrombocytosis,[13] and required a 3-day neonatal intensive care unit (NICU) admission (Table 4.1).

However, as indicated in Table 4.1, the major presenting symptoms in the vast majority of victims are puncture wounds/lacerations, minor bleeding, mild edema, ecchymoses, and mild pain. As noted above, the few cases ($n = 4$) that suggest systemic signs and symptoms all involved infants. The paucity of cases from New Guinea and Australia (only one documented case) is likely due to far less frequent contact between humans and these snakes in their natural range. Interestingly, in part of the natural range of *B. irregularis*, some Aboriginal clans in the Arnhemland, Northern Territory, Australia, view *B. irregularis* as particularly dangerous to menstruating women and those with infants (Oscar Whitehead, personal verbal communication with SAW, April 1999, and SAW personal observations). The attraction of *B. irregularis* to human menstrual blood under laboratory conditions (David Chiszar, personal written and verbal communication with SAW, June 1993) adds some information that supports concerns regarding the unusual allure of certain human populations to these snakes.

4.4.1.2   Overview of the Duvernoy's Gland and Associated Dentition of B. irregularis

Boiga irregularis has enlarged, gently recurved posterior maxillary teeth containing deep grooves that run along almost their entire length and are separated from the anterior teeth by a diastema (Plate 4.9E and F). The enlarged posterior maxillary teeth are associated with a lobular Duvernoy's gland located in the temporal region, posterior to the maxilla (Weinstein and Kardong, 1994; Zalisko and Kardong, 1992). The gland features lobular and common lobular ducts, a minimal central cistern (of no appreciable secretion storage capacity), and an additional main duct (Zalisko and Kardong, 1992).

4.4.1.3   Summary of the Properties, Toxinology, and Variability of B. irregularis Duvernoy's Secretion

Several investigators have reported yields of Duvernoy's secretions from *B. irregularis*. Weinstein et al. (1991) reported an average liquid yield of 80.2 μL containing 6.7 mg solids with 100% protein content. Using two groups of *B. irregularis* classed by body length, Vest et al. (1991) reported that snakes <100 cm produced an average liquid yield of 9.63 μL with 0.642 mg solids, while specimens >100 cm yielded a liquid average 126 μL with 6.88 mg solids that contained only 22.8% protein. These

---

[13] This pediatric patient's platelet count and hemoglobin/hematocrit with normal ranges in parentheses: 493,000↑ (150,000–350,000), 13.4/37.8 (13.3–21 g/dL/31–69%).

marked differences are clearly related to size of the specimens studied. Further characterization of this body size–yield volume relationship was reported by Chiszar et al. (1992), who studied *B. irregularis* Duvernoy's secretion yields from several weight classes of *B. irregularis*. Specimens <300 gm body weight produced 40 μL of secretion with 2.3 mg solid, while those >900 gm yielded an average of 139 μL with 10.8 mg solids (Chiszar et al., 1992). Weight classes between these lower and upper limits produced intermediate volumes. The yield volume statistically correlated with the size classes of snakes (Chiszar et al., 1992). Similar findings were recorded by Mackessy et al. (2006), who reported a varied yield according to size and an average yield (collected with parasympathomimetic stimulation) of 500 μL with 19.2 mg solids (90% protein) from large specimens of *B. irregularis*.

Similarly, a further study of *B. irregularis* Duvernoy's secretion protein content found that different size classes of *B. irregularis* produced Duvernoy's secretions with protein content ranging between 66% and 100%, with smaller snakes having higher protein content (Weinstein et al., 1993).

Studies of the lethal potency of secretion from *B. irregularis* similarly reflect differences related to body size, rather than ontogeny, *sensu stricto* (Weinstein and Kardong, 1994). Vest et al. (1991) reported an i.v. LD_{50} of 80 mg/kg for secretion from smaller-intermediate-sized specimens, while Weinstein et al. (1991) reported an i.p. LD_{50} of 10.33 mg/kg for secretion from larger specimens (see Appendix B). This size-related difference was further investigated by Weinstein et al. (1993), who reported i.p. LD_{50} for *B. irregularis* secretion that ranged between 10.5 mg/kg (large snakes) to 34.13 mg/kg (small snakes). The size-related differences in *B. irregularis* Duvernoy's secretion yield, toxicity, and protein content are reflected in the secretion toxin content. Weinstein et al. (1993) reported that acetylcholine receptor-binding (AchRB) activity of the secretion was higher in smaller snakes. Duvernoy's secretion from larger snakes had little, if any, AchRB activity (Weinstein et al., 1993). These observations were further expanded by Mackessy et al. (2006), who reported that an azocaseinolytic metalloprotease and acetylcholinesterase increased in activity with size/age of the *B. irregularis* specimens studied, while toxicity, highest in neonate snakes, decreased. These investigators described prey specificity (saurian and avian) of the toxic activities detected in these secretions (Mackessy et al., 2006). Secretions from either juveniles or adults lack hemorrhagic activity (Vest et al., 1991; Weinstein et al., 1991).

Fast protein chromatographic fractionation of Duvernoy's secretion from large-size *B. irregularis* resulted in two lethal fractions (Weinstein et al., 1991). The major fraction contained three proteins with molecular masses 12.5–52 kDa and had an i.p. murine LD_{50} of 7.3 mg/kg. The second fraction exhibited proteolytic and myotoxic activities and consisted of two proteins with molecular masses of 14.5–17 kDa. It had an i.p. murine LD_{50} of 3.7 mg/kg and caused myoglobinuria in mice injected with lethal doses of the fraction (Weinstein et al., 1991).

Recently, a unique, heterodimeric, covalently linked three-finger-fold neurotoxin ("irditoxin," as noted earlier) from Duvernoy's secretion of *B. irregularis* was characterized and structurally analyzed (Pawlak et al., 2009). This distinctive 17,112-Da three-finger-postsynaptic neurotoxin exhibited specificity for birds and lizards and was nontoxic to mice. This specificity was noted also in nerve-muscle preparations in which the toxin produced potent neuromuscular blockade at the avian neuromuscular junction, but was three orders of magnitude less effective in blocking the mammalian neuromuscular junction (Pawlak et al., 2009). Thus, this toxin may account for the prey-specificity shifts reported for this snake (e.g., juveniles favor lizard prey; Greene, 1989) as well as the decreasing level of neurotoxin with increasing size and age (Mackessy et al., 2006; Weinstein et al., 1993).

4.4.1.4 What Is the Etiology of the Medical Effects of B. irregularis Bites?

The distinctive circumstances involving medical risks from *B. irregularis* on Guam (and other islands) present a rare opportunity to scrutinize the source of risks from bites of a given non-front-fanged colubroid species. There is a relatively large series (*n* > 450) of well-documented emergency-room presentations after bites from *B. irregularis*. Also, as these occurred in an insular environment, factors influencing variability in snakes, victims, and medical facilities were likely to be relatively restricted. The vast majority of these cases featured puncture wounds, lacerations, mild edema/ecchymoses, and bleeding (Table 4.1). Only five cases, all involving infants younger than 6 months old, reportedly contained clinical signs that suggested systemic effects ("ptosis," "respiratory distress" or "respiratory difficulty," "spasticity"; Table 4.1). However, the size-related/ontogenetic variability in *B. irregularis* Duvernoy's secretion properties and the predatory behavior of these snakes complicate interpretation of these limited cases that suggest systemic effects, including neurotoxicity. For example, *B. irregularis* swallows smaller prey directly while large prey is actively constricted (Rochelle and Kardong, 1993), and "envenomed" rodents retain in their integument almost 50% of the secretion introduced during predation (Hayes et al., 1993). As noted previously, the secretion of this species exhibits low lethal potency, contains a postsynaptic neurotoxin that is avian/saurian-specific, and is in significantly higher concentrations in secretions from smaller/younger snakes (Mackessy et al., 2006; Pawlak et al., 2009; Weinstein et al., 1993). Also, metalloprotease and acetylcholinesterase activities increase with size and age, along with the variable increase in lethal potency (Mackessy et al., 2006). Aside from *B. irregularis*, only specimens or populations of the crotaline viperids, *Lachesis muta stenophrys* (Central American bushmaster, *L. stenophrys*; McDiarmid et al., 1999; see Plate 4.86), and the jararaca (*Bothrops jararaca*) exhibit an ontogenetic increase in venom toxicity, respectively (Gutiérrez et al., 1990; Antunes et al., 2010). All other ophidian species studied to date that have detectable ontogenetic change in venom properties typically exhibit ontogenetically decreased lethal potency and increased proteolytic activity (Chippaux et al., 1991; Mackessy, 1988; Minton and Weinstein, 1986).

Therefore, the potential basis for systemic effects after *B. irregularis* bites in this small group of pediatric patients is unclear and contrasts with available biomedical data regarding the biology of this species. The following points are considered: some larger snakes (>1.4 m) produce a secretion that exhibits a higher murine toxicity and has very low postsynaptic neurotoxin content; all of the concerning bites inflicted on humans (principally, four of the five pediatric cases mentioned earlier; Table 4.1) were from large snakes (average length about 1.17 m); juvenile/smaller snakes have a lower murine toxicity and higher postsynaptic neurotoxin content; larger prey are actively

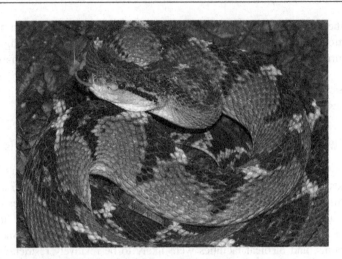

Plate 4.86 Bushmaster; surucucu; cuaima; culebra sibucano; mapepire z'ananna; others (*Lachesis muta*), Peru. The largest species of crotaline viperid, although average adult specimens attain total body lengths of approximately 1.60 m, exceptional specimens can reach 3.5 m or more. The lighter-colored Central American species, *L. stenophrys*, is one of only two front-fanged colubroids (the other is the jararaca, *Bothrops jararaca*) with populations and/or individuals known to have increasing venom toxicity with age. The non-front-fanged colubroid, the brown tree snake (*B. irregularis*), is the only other ophidian known to show increased oral secretion (Duvernoy's secretion) toxicity associated with ontogeny. Photo copyright to David A. Warrell.

constricted; and bites delivered during prey handling sequester large volumes of low toxicity secretion in the integument and, to date, the only neurotoxin characterized from *B. irregularis* secretion is a distinctive, heterodimeric species that has marked prey specificity for avians and saurians with very low toxicity for mammals.

Therefore, although *B. irregularis* clearly presents a medical risk on Guam, particularly to infants, the precise etiology of the medical sequelae remains elusive. There may be uncharacterized postsynaptic neurotoxins in *B. irregularis* secretion that could be active at the mammalian AchR. However, the evidence for neurotoxicity in humans is equivocal. Spasticity is not usually observed concomitantly with hypotonicity in neurologically affected pediatric patients (David Kaufman, personal verbal communication with SAW, August 2010). Thus, clinical interpretation of the reported signs is not straightforward and without alternative explanation. Some of the concerning symptoms observed in the five infants bitten by *B. irregularis* may have resulted from trauma (i.e., constriction involving the head, neck, and/or thoracic region, causing airway compromise, as well as repetitive biting that may or may not have included repeated introduction of Duvernoy's secretion). A well-documented, efficacious clinical response after provision of an acetylcholinesterase inhibitor such as neostigmine could clarify whether postsynaptic neurotoxicity contributes to the syndrome observed in infants bitten by *B. irregularis* (see Table 4.3). Also, proteolytic activity detected in *B. irregularis* secretion may play a role in some of the mild local effects that constitute the vast majority of clinical presentations after *B. irregularis* bites. The possible role of Type 1 hypersensitivity reactions in some patients bitten by *B. irregularis* and other colubroids is discussed in Section 4.6.

4.4.1.5   Conclusion and Assessment of B. irregularis

The profound ecological impact of *B. irregularis* has resulted in concurrent and significant medical repercussions in Western Pacific islands (especially Guam) invaded by this species. This snake exhibits remarkable durability as well as fecundity, and has presented a challenge to efforts focused on controlling its geographic expansion. It also displays disconcerting behavior suggestive of active predatory attempts on human infants. Only five documented cases of bites inflicted on infants have resulted in clinical features suggestive of systemic envenomation. The vast majority of bites have caused only mild local effects. The etiology of medically significant effects from these bites remains unclear. Although to date, the characterized postsynaptic neurotoxins in Duvernoy's secretion of *B. irregularis* are specific for avian and saurian prey, it is possible that other neurotoxins may contribute to the clinical syndrome in human infants. This possibility would be likely associated with protracted bites (allowing increased introduction of secretion) inflicted by smaller specimens on neonates or infants (due to low body weight, as well as vulnerability to bites and trauma to the airway via concomitant constriction). Smaller specimens would probably have a higher concentration of such neurotoxins in their secretion. On the other hand, an uncharacterized mammalian-specific neurotoxin could increase in concentration with size or age and thus play a role in the variable concomitant increase in murine toxicity with size or age. However, the ontogenetic/size-related variability in secretion components (especially detectable neurotoxicity) complicates analysis of the potential factors contributing to these cases. A possibly relevant consideration may be drawn from the highly specific neurotoxicity of distinctive neurotoxins from other ophidian species. For instance, the specificity and ontogenetic nature of the AchR-subunit composition at the murine motor end plate dictate the action of waglerin 1 from venom of the crotaline viperid, *Tropidolaemus wagleri* (Plate 4.87A and B; Aiken et al., 1992). Waglerin 1 specifically binds to the ε-subunit of the AChR. Therefore, it is active only in mature mice as neonate mice have AChR with γ-subunits that are later ontogenetically switched to ε with maturity. Thus, neonate mice are unaffected by waglerin 1 whereas the peptide is rapidly fatal to adult mice (i.p. LD50 of waglerin 1 [adult mice]=0.370 mg/kg). This peptide exhibits potent activity in the murine nerve-muscle assay. However, the venom has modal lethal potency in mice, and the purified peptide shows no AchRB activity when tested in assays using human or avian tissues (McArdle et al., 1999; Weinstein et al., 1991). Human envenomations by *T. wagleri* typically feature mild-to-moderate local edema and pain without manifestations of neurotoxicity (S.A Minton, personal verbal communication with SAW, March 1982). It is conceivable that *B. irregularis* may produce other neurotoxins yet to be identified that also exhibit target tissue ontogeny-dependent potency and specificity. Although irditoxin from *B. irregularis* Duvernoy's secretion is distinctive, it is highly specific for lizards and birds, and to date, there are no data to support the presence in this secretion of other neurotoxins that have significant toxicity for mammals.

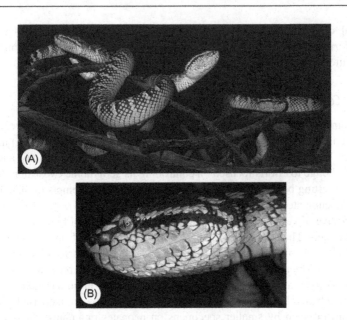

Plate 4.87 (A and B) Wagler's pit viper;Temple viper; ular kapak tokong; ular bakaw; djalimoo; others (*Tropidolaemus wagleri*), Penang Temple, Penang, Malaysia. The genus *Tropidolaemus* contains five species (*T. wagleri*, *T. huttoni*, *T. semiannulatus*, *T. laticinctus*, and *T. philippinensis*; Vogel et al., 2007) of distinctive arboreal crotaline viperids that are respectively found in Brunei, Indonesia, Malaysia, Philippines, Singapore, Thailand, and the Indian subcontinent. *Tropidolaemus wagleri* venom contains several unique, small peptide neurotoxins (e.g. the molecular mass of waglerin 1=2.5 kDa) that have ontogenetically determined murine AchR subunit specificity. Although two of these toxins have lethal potency for adult mice that approaches the toxicity of *Naja naja* crude venom, they are not active in neonate mice or humans. Bites by *T. wagleri* typically cause only mild-to-moderate local effects.
Photos copyright to David A. Warrell.

Therefore, in a medically relevant sense, it is premature and presumptive to consider this species "neurotoxic" without procurement of further clinical evidence.

Therefore, *B. irregularis* must be considered both an ecological threat and medically important species. This species produces the largest Duvernoy's secretion yield of any non-front-fanged colubroid studied to date. Large specimens should be approached with caution, and people living in areas affected by this invasive species should take careful precautions to protect infants, children, and domestic pets. Any infant or child bitten by a *B. irregularis* must be carefully monitored in a medical facility as systemic effects are possible and may occur as a result of the toxic effects from introduced Duvernoy's secretion, and/or the non-secretion-related effects of constriction-induced physical trauma.

Assessment of *B. irregularis* based on available evidence: Hazard Level 2/3 (see Table 4.3).

4.4.2 Malpolon monspessulanus

4.4.2.1 Background and Aberrant Features of Bites

The genus *Malpolon* (malpolon, hooded snakes) consists of two species, *M. monspessulanus* (Montpellier or yaleh snake; Plate 2.4D–F, p. 97) and *M. (Scutophis Padial, 2006) moilensis* (Moila's or hooded snake; Plate 4.33A and B). *Malpolon monspessulanus* (two subspecies, *M. m. monspessulanus* and *M. m. insignitus*; both are known as western Montpellier snakes) has purportedly been involved in >70 documented bites, the majority of which resulted in uncomplicated local wounds (puncture wounds/lacerations, mild edema, etc.; Plate 2.4G, p. 97; Table 4.1). Boulenger (1913) commented that *Malpolon* "poison" (secretion) had action "similar" to that of cobras. Three published cases have described systemic effects including ptosis and other cranial nerve palsies; peripheral neurotoxicity; and "drowsiness" (Table 4.1). It is important to emphasize that the identity of the snake responsible was unverified in many of the previous cases assigned to *M. monspessulanus*.

There is only one documented bite from the congener, *M. moilensis*, and that bite resulted in insignificant effects (Table 4.1).

4.4.2.2 Overview of the Duvernoy's Gland and Associated Dentition of M. monspessulanus

Boulenger (1913) reported that *M. (Coelopeltis) monspessulanus* have "maxillary teeth that are small and subequal, followed after a short interspace by one or two very large grooved fangs situated below the posterior border of the eye." Fry et al. (2008) noted that some of the posterior teeth of *M. monspessulanus* possessed a deep groove that ran most of their length. These authors also interpreted buccal mucosa associated with these teeth as a "fang sheath" (Fry et al., 2008). Examination of several living *M. monspessulanus* and osteological specimens show the notably enlarged, deeply grooved, recurved posterior maxillary teeth (Plate 2.4A–C, p. 13).

Taub (1967) described the Duvernoy's gland of *M. monspessulanus* as having a thick capsule and few thin trabeculae. The gland was composed of columnar cells, and about 10% of the tubular constituents had a lumen. The gland exhibited moderate vascularity and lacked mucous cells (Taub, 1967). However, Fry et al. (2008) reported that the *M. monspessulanus* "venom gland" (Duvernoy's gland) contained isolated mucoid cells or patches and a relatively large ovoid duct. They also described the presence of a "venom vestibule," defined as "a localized expansion of the venom duct," adjacent to the gland (Fry et al., 2008). The "venom duct" opened into both the oral cavity and the "fang sheath" (Fry et al., 2008).

4.4.2.3   Summary of the Properties and Toxinology of M. monspessulanus Duvernoy's Secretion

There are few data regarding yield of Duvernoy's secretion from *M. monspessulanus*, and no yield data for *M. moilensis*. Using fluothane for anesthesia and pilocarpine for parasympathomimetic stimulation of secretion, Rosenberg et al. (1985) reported a yield of 0.63 μL/g of snake body weight. Although solid yield was not reported, the liquid secretion contained 9.0 mg protein/mL. A later study compared extraction using fluothane with ketamine hydrochloride or fluothane alone (both methods included pilocarpine) and obtained contrasting volumes (Rosenberg et al., 1992). The former method yielded 0.44 μL/g snake body weight, while the latter obtained 5.2 μL/g snake body weight. Protein content was not reported (Rosenberg et al., 1992).

The two studies assaying enzymatic activities in secretion from *M. monspessulanus* described phosphodiesterase, alkaline phosphatase, acid phosphatase, caseinase, and/or PLA activities (Ovadia, 1984; Rosenberg et al., 1985).

There are also few data on lethal potency of Duvernoy's secretions from *M. monspessulanus*. Rosenberg et al. (1985) reported a murine i.v. LD_{50} of 6.5 mg/kg and noted that mice injected with lethal doses exhibited "paralysis."

Gel filtration chromatography of *M. monspessulanus* secretion yielded two lethal fractions (Rosenberg et al., 1985). One fraction ("IIIA") contained several components with molecular masses of 13 or 17 kDa. This fraction contained PLA_2 activity and had a murine i.v. LD_{50} of 2.75 mg/kg (Rosenberg et al., 1985). The other lethal fraction ("IV") lacked PLA_2 activity, contained components with molecular masses of approximately 13 kDa, and had a murine i.v. LD_{50} of 4.5 mg/kg (Rosenberg et al., 1985). An additional non-lethal fraction contained most of the phosphodiesterase activity detected in the secretion (Rosenberg et al., 1985). Further fractionation utilizing gel filtration and cation exchange procured a lethal hemorrhagic toxin ("fraction CM-6") with molecular mass of 24 kDa and a murine i.v. LD_{50} of 1.0 mg/kg. This toxin lacked proteolytic and procoagulant activities. Although negative in intradermal hemorrhagic assay, lethal and sublethal doses produced pulmonary hemorrhage in mice (Rosenberg et al., 1992).

4.4.2.4   Does M. monspessulanus *Produce Neurotoxic Envenoming?*

Among more than 70 medically documented bites thought to have been inflicted by this species, only three have reported neurotoxic effects (Table 4.1). A 36-year-old herpetologist was bitten by a large *M. monspessulanus* in southern France (Pommier and de Haro, 2007). Ninety minutes after the bite, his vision became blurred; some hours later, when he was admitted to the Poison Control Center in Marseille, there was bilateral ptosis, partial oculomotor paralysis, and loss of visual accommodation—all of which resolved over the next 6 days. This is convincing evidence of neurotoxic envenomation. Although there are a limited number of cases, it is likely several other people bitten by this species have developed similar features (Gonzáles, 1979, 1982).

Although the identification of the snake in the aforementioned case is not in question, consideration must be given to the lack of verified identity of the culprit snake in a large proportion of these cases. It must be pondered that in some cases the offending specimen was misidentified and actually was a viperid species. As an example, the aforementioned case featuring cranial nerve palsies occurred in southern France. However, in this case the victim reported having his finger deep inside the buccal cavity of the snake (formally identified as a *M. monspessulanus*) and thus received protracted contact with the posterior maxillary teeth (Pommier and de Haro, 2007). Neurotoxic populations of *Vipera aspis aspis* (asp viper) occur in southeastern France, and these snakes may produce the monomeric presynaptic neurotoxin, ammodytoxin B, and/or the heterodimeric postsynaptic neurotoxin, vaspin (Guillamen et al., 2003; Jan et al., 2002). Interestingly, neurological signs (mainly cranial nerve palsies) were reported after bites from *V. aspis* in three regions of France: Languedoc-Roussillon, Midi-Pyrénées, and Provence-Alpes-Côte d'Azur (Ferquel et al., 2007). However, *V. aspis*, including specimens from South France, have quite a different appearance than *M. monspessulanus* (see Plates 2.4D–F, p. 97 and 4.88A–D), and such misidentification is unlikely. On the other hand, a person unfamiliar with *M. monspessulanus* or *V. aspis* and experiencing anxiety after being bitten by a snake (see Section 4.5) could conceivably affirm an incorrect identity. Also, although the wounds produced by bites from these two species may appear different, the differences may not be distinctive. Occasionally, bites from species such as *H. nasicus* or *P. olfersii* (Table 4.1 and previous sections) produce local effects that resemble crotaline envenoming (see Plates 4.24D–J and 4.40A and B), while some bites from potently neurotoxic species, such as *Bungarus caeruleus* (Indian blue krait; Plate 4.64) or some specimens of *Crotalus scutulatus* [Mojave rattlesnake (Plate 4.89A and B); from those geographic populations that produce the PLA$_2$ subunit presynaptic neurotoxin, Mojave toxin, Type A populations; Glenn et al., 1983; Weinstein et al., 1985] may produce life-threatening envenoming without any significant local effects. Therefore, although there are data that support concerns regarding neurotoxicity in *M. monspessulanus*, lack of verified identity of the culprit snake in many cases ascribed to this species compels the need for caution when considering the potential risks from this taxa. As noted previously, when considering risk from possible neurotoxicity from *B. irregularis*, provision of an acetylcholinesterase inhibitor such as neostigmine after a bite from a verified *M. monspessulanus* could clarify the etiology of these reported effects.

4.4.2.5   Conclusion and Assessment of M. monspessulanus

The majority of reported bites from this species feature only mild local effects (many are medically insignificant). Although neurotoxic effects are questioned in two out of three cases because of uncertainty about the identity of the snake responsible, in one of these cases of neurotoxicity snake identification and clinical features of cranial nerve palsies were reliable. Therefore, large specimens of *M. monspessulanus* should be considered potentially dangerous, and any bites from this species should be reviewed promptly by a physician.

Assessment of *Malpolon monspessulanus* based on available evidence: Hazard Level 2/3 (see Table 4.3).

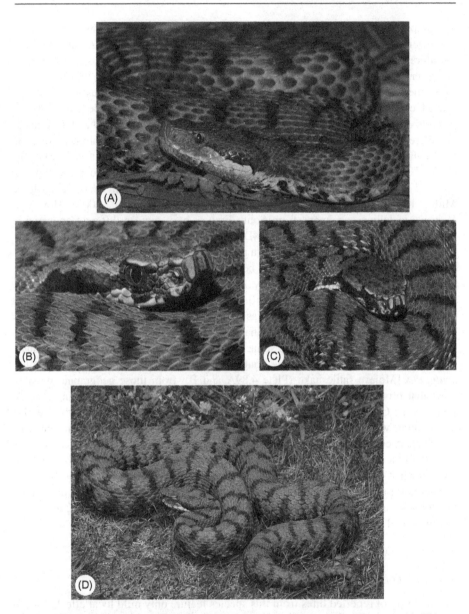

Plate 4.88 (A–D) European asp; juraviper, alpenviper, vipere aspic (*Vipera aspis*). This viperine viperid is found in France, Germany, Switzerland, Italy, Spain, and Slovenia. There are approximately five subspecies, and average adults may reach about 0.8 m in total body length. Although primarily nocturnal, it is diurnal in cooler months, and often found in open rocky hillsides, but also occurs in moist mountainous biotopes. Envenomations from this species may include mild-to-moderate local effects such as edema, ecchymoses, and pain (may be severe), and life-threatening systemic effects such as hypotension, respiratory distress, and cranial nerve palsies. Some populations found in southeastern France secrete

◄ **Plate 4.88** *(Continued)* venoms that contain the monomeric presynaptic neurotoxin, ammodytoxin B, and/or the heterodimeric postsynaptic neurotoxin, vaspin. Deaths have occurred, but are rare. Although it is reasonable to consider the possibility that some of the few medically significant bites by Montpellier snakes (*Malpolon monspessulanus*) that included cranial nerve palsies were cases of misidentified *V. aspis*, this is unlikely as these snakes differ markedly in appearance.
(A–C) *Vipera aspis*, **South France.** (Plate 4.88A, male; B, female).
(D) *Vipera aspis*, **Tuscany.** Plate 4.88A–C, photos copyright to Dave Nixon; Plate 4.88D, photo copyright to Wolfgang Wüster.

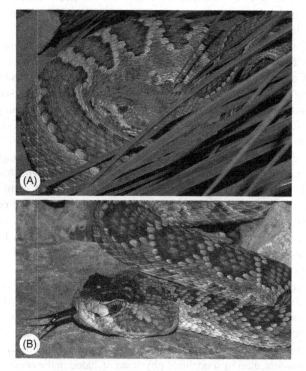

Plate 4.89 (A and B) Mojave rattlesnake (*Crotalus scutulatus*). Probably the most dangerous venomous snake of North America, *C. scutulatus* has highly variable venom that may contain the potent presynaptic dimeric neurotoxin, Mojave toxin. This crotaline species ranges from the southwestern USA through Mexico. The populations that produce venom containing Mojave toxin have been termed "Type A," while those without this toxin have been called "Type B." There are populations that appear to be intergrades of Types A and B. *Crotalus scutulatus* envenomations may present as those "typical" of most *Crotalus* spp. (moderate-to-severe local effects, coagulopathy, hypotension, myolysis, etc.), and/or with severe paralytic features. Tragically, the well-known American physician-herpetologist, Frederick Shannon (1921–1965), was fatally envenomated while working with a wild *C. scutulatus*.
Photos copyright to David A. Warrell.

4.4.3   Hydrodynastes gigas

4.4.3.1   Background of an Aberrant Case

Of the three species of *Hydrodynastes*[14] (false-water cobras, *H. gigas*; Plate 4.26A and B), *H. bicinctus* (Hermann's water snake, or double-banded false-water cobra; two subspecies, *H. b. bicinctus* and *H. b. schultzi*), and the recently described *H. melanogigas* (Franco et al., 2007), only *H. gigas* has figured in any documented cases of bites (Table 4.1). Three of the four reported cases featured only puncture wounds/lacerations, pain, edema, mild bleeding, and other minor local manifestations (Table 4.1; Plate 4.26E). One aberrant case, published as a brief abstract, describes mild local effects (minor swelling) that occurred shortly after the victim (an 18-year-old male pet shop worker who was maintaining the snake) received a protracted bite (≥ 1.5 min) on the left wrist. Due to the mild local edema, the victim ingested two diphenhydramine tablets. He had received several previous bites (presumably from this same species, or specimen) without any notable effect. The insignificant effects from this protracted bite were followed approximately 9 h later by expanding edema and reportedly serious systemic effects [dysarthria, "muscle paralysis," and "unsteady gait" ("causing him to fall ..."); Manning et al., 1999; Table 4.1]. He presented at an emergency room; noted were ECG changes consisting of premature atrial complexes (PACs) and a mild tachycardia of 105 bpm. The tachycardia resolved in 2 h, and all laboratory testing (including coagulation panels) remained unremarkable. The patient was observed overnight with his arm elevated/immobilized, and he was treated with ceftriaxone. The local symptoms persisted overnight, and the patient was discharged with a prescription for cephalexin. The patient later reported that the edema subsided after 5 days, but the "muscle pain and weakness" lasted for 2 months. The authors of this brief report concluded that "This is the first case reported of *H. gigas* envenomation causing significant local swelling, pain, muscle paralysis, and arrhythmias" (Manning et al., 1999).

Although not reviewed here, an anecdotal case published in an obscure amateur journal asserted that a *H. gigas* bite resulted in a "permanently disfigured arm" (Stevens, 2000). The multiple problems with these anecdotal reports are delineated in Section 4.5. As an example, many claims in such reports cannot be considered as evidence of sequelae assigned to the bite of any species, as there is no formal medical evaluation of the victim communicated by a qualified physician included in the account.

4.4.3.2   Overview of the Duvernoy's Gland and Associated Dentition of H. gigas

Specimens of *H. gigas* exhibit several enlarged deeply grooved posterior maxillary teeth with a broad depression spanning most of the width of the teeth at the edge of the buccal mucosum (Plate 4.26C and D). In contrast, Fry et al. (2008) described the posterior

---

[14] The taxonomy of *Hydrodynastes* is argumentatively unsettled as some authors assign the genus to the family Dipsadidae, subfamily Xenodontinae, while others consider this premature.

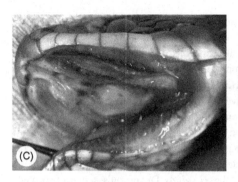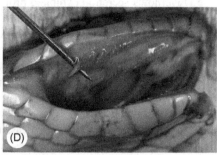

Plate 4.26 (C and D) False-water cobra (*Hydrodynastes gigas*). Shows the groove traversing almost the entire length of the enlarged posterior maxillary tooth.
Plate 4.26C and D, Brazilian specimens, photos copyright to David A. Warrell.

maxillary teeth of *H. gigas* as having a smooth surface. There are few additional data regarding the specific characteristics of the maxillary dentition of the genus.

The Duvernoy's gland of *H. bicincta* (Taub, 1967)[15] had a moderately thick capsule, many moderately thick trabeculae, and was composed of columnar cells (Taub, 1967). The glands were highly vascular and lumens were present in about 90% of gland tubules. There were no mucous cells in the gland, but there was an associated mucous supralabial gland (Taub, 1967). Fry et al. (2008) reported that the "venom gland" (Duvernoy's gland) of *H. gigas* contained isolated mucous cells or patches and exhibited a relatively large ovate duct. They also described a "venom vestibule" and "venom duct" that opened to both the oral cavity and "fang sheath" (Fry et al., 2008).

4.4.3.3 Summary of the Properties and Toxinology of H. gigas Duvernoy's Secretion

Glenn et al. (1992) reported a liquid yield ranging from 0 to 50 μL with a solid yield of 1.3 mg, reportedly from a single gland. Although protein content was not reported, these investigators noted that Duvernoy's gland of this species contained carbohydrate–protein complexes (Glenn et al., 1992).

Comparison of murine LD_{50} and proteolytic activities of buccal salivary secretions and Duvernoy's secretion highlighted the differences between these substances. The i.p. LD_{50} of *H. gigas* Duvernoy's secretion was 2.0 mg/kg, while the mixed buccal secretions s.c. LD_{50} was 11.5 mg/kg, respectively (Glenn et al., 1992).

---

[15] This is an ambiguous synonym for *H. bicinctus*, and has been used by several investigators in reference to thus labeled, catalogued American Museum of Natural History specimens (e.g. #88401 and #60822). Historically, major formal taxonomic descriptions beginning with Hermann (1804) have not included "*bicincta*" as a recognized species designation for *H. bicinctus*. Due to the fluid taxonomy of non-front-fanged colubroids, nomenclature can be complex and confusing. This again emphasizes the need for the physician to comprehend or investigate if necessary, the biological history of any colubroid species deemed responsible for a given snakebite presentation.

The Duvernoy's secretion exhibited proteolytic activity, while this was absent in the mixed buccal salivary secretions (Glenn et al., 1992).

In another comparison of *H. gigas* buccal secretions and Duvernoy's secretion, Hill and Mackessy (2000) used pilocarpine (see previous sections for details) in order to boost secretion yields. These investigators reported mean Duvernoy's secretion liquid and solid yields of 423 μL and 7.31 mg, respectively. Duvernoy's secretion contained a mean 67.1% protein, and the buccal secretions contained 30.9% protein (Hill and Mackessy, 2000). The total carbohydrate concentration of the Duvernoy's secretion ranged from 0.1% to 4.7%, and azocaseinase and caseinase, also present in the mixed buccal secretions, were the only enzymatic activities detected (Hill and Mackessy, 2000). Of the 12 non-front-fanged colubroid species studied, the *H. gigas* Duvernoy's secretion proteolytic activity was one of the two highest detected (Hill and Mackessy, 2000).

4.4.3.4 Analysis and Conclusions

Hydrodynastes gigas is a large, heavy-bodied, xenodontine colubroid popular in private collections. Although many are maintained in captivity, only four well-documented bites have been reported. Of these, only the single case described previously (Manning et al., 1999) featured symptoms suggestive of systemic effects such as PACs, "muscle paralysis," dysarthria, and "muscle weakness." The incident resulted in an extended convalescence, and "muscle weakness" that purportedly lasted almost 2 months (Manning et al., 1999). The major clinical features (particularly immobility, perceived muscular weakness, tachycardia, etc.) of this case, previously reviewed (Warrell, 2004), are most parsimoniously attributed to somatosensory amplification due to anxiety (see Section 4.5). As the snake reportedly inflicted a protracted bite, the mild-to-moderate edema may be due to the effects of a larger volume of Duvernoy's secretion introduced into the wound and/or hypersensitivity to the secretion, as well as other oral gland products (see Section 4.6). The patient indicated that he had received several insignificant bites previously, and these may have sensitized him. Thus, the protracted bite conceivably stimulated a notable anaphylactic response that resulted from acquired hypersensitivity.

Although the medical history of the patient is not available, there is no mention of any preexisting comorbidities or other factors predisposing to some of the reported effects (e.g., alcohol, prescription medications). However, a detailed analysis of this case may illustrate how consideration of alternative (and more likely) causes may clarify the origin of the observed effects. Therefore, the reported PACs are worthy of further consideration, as this was an objective finding. PACs are caused by generation of a premature impulse by the sinoatrial node (SA node). This impulse is conducted normally and results in a contraction; it is often asymptomatic, or experienced by the patient as a palpitation/"skipped beat." These arrhythmias are common and are most often benign in those without underlying cardiac disease. However, under pathological circumstances, some PACs may initiate atrial fibrillation (Narayan et al., 2008; Sra et al., 2001). Similarly, palpitations may also be caused by premature ventricular contractions (PVCs) that are caused by an ectopic cardiac pacemaker located in the ventricle, below the SA node. There are many causes of PACs and PVCs, including anxiety, numerous medications (pseudoephedrine, digoxin, etc.), alcohol, numerous street drugs (especially cocaine and amphetamines), and caffeine (excessive coffee intake is a common cause, and "energy drinks" also contain large amounts of caffeine as well as other stimulants such as guarana extract), hypoxia, electrolyte disturbances (e.g., hypokalemia), and other underlying asymptomatic and symptomatic arrhythmias, as well as myocardial infarction, myocarditis, cardiomyopathy, and others. In comparison to PACs, there are a few more data regarding the epidemiology of PVCs among certain populations. Available evidence indicates no increased mortality among patients with normal cardiac evaluation who report palpitations that are related to PVCs (Abbott, 2005; Kennedy et al., 1985). A large, multiple-community-based, cross-sectional analysis of 15,792 individuals (aged 45–65 years) suggested that PVCs were present in >6% of middle-aged American adults (Simpson et al., 2002). Increasing age, the presence of heart disease, faster sinus rates, African American ethnicity, male sex, lower educational attainment, and lower serum levels of some electrolytes (magnesium or potassium) were directly associated with PVC prevalence. Hypertension was independently associated with a 23% increase in the prevalence of PVCs (Simpson et al., 2002). This emphasizes the essential need for carefully collected and documented medical history, prescription medication regimens (and adherence or lack thereof to prescribed dosing frequency), and basic psychosocial background (especially alcohol and street drug use) of any patient presenting with a reportedly medically significant snakebite. These factors may play an integral part in the presentation, and thus related symptoms/signs may be independent of the circumstances. However, three cases of *Naja* spp. envenomings that included dysrhythmias have been reported. These occurred in India and Malaysia and included either ST segment depression with inverted T waves or atrioventricular juctional escape rhythm with left bundle branch block (Pahlajani et al., 1987; Reid, 1964). *Naja* spp. likely responsible for these envenoming (e.g., *N. kaouthia, N. naja*) secrete venoms that contain cardiotoxins and often produce serious or life-threatening envenoming. Therefore, some envenomings by highly venomous species may occasionally include dysrhythmias. Conversely, the clinician must remain cognizant of the possibility of exacerbation of comorbid illness (e.g., ischemic cardiac disease, generalized anxiety disorder, etc; see Sections 4.5 and 4.6) in the event of clinically significant effects from a bite inflicted by any colubroid species of unknown medical importance.

It must also be observed that although the patient in this aberrant case reported "paralysis" hours after sustaining the bite, and "muscle weakness" lasting for 2 months, there was no documented evidence of neuropathy, neurotoxicity, or myopathy. Regardless, due to the reported symptoms/signs, documentation of electromyographic testing, autoimmune serology, follow-up neurological examination, and imaging (if indicated) are all desirable (see the aberrant alleged *P. najadum* case; Sections 4.4 and 4.6).

Caution is advised when handling these snakes due to their large size, and their capacity for producing relatively substantial volumes of proteolytic secretion. Special precautions should be taken when feeding captive specimens or when performing captive maintenance after handling potential food items. Larger specimens are capable of inflicting a painful local wound. Currently, there are no data that provide acceptable evidence of systemic envenoming by this species.

Assessment of *H. gigas* **based on available evidence: Hazard Level 3/4** [Most bites feature uncomplicated local effects (typically, mild bleeding, limited edema, pain, etc.)]. Larger specimens may produce more extensive local effects, including ecchymoses and greater edema. Acquired hypersensitivity to Duvernoy's secretions [e.g., in those with a history of repetitive exposure to snakes (wild and/or captive), snake venoms/products, shed skins, etc.] may contribute to the clinical manifestations that occasionally are caused by bites from these snakes (see Section 4.6).

4.4.4 Philodryas olfersii latirostris

4.4.4.1 Background and Consideration of an Aberrant Case

The most commonly reported features of *P. olfersii* bites and the toxinology of members of this genus were described in Section 4.2 and Table 4.1. Of the three subspecies of *P. olfersii* (*P. o. olfersii*, *P. o. hebeus*, and *P. o. latirostris*), only *P. o. latirostris* figures in a documented report suggesting systemic effects (Peichoto et al., 2007a; Table 4.1). This case described the uncomplicated and medically insignificant bite of *P. o. latirostris* inflicted on a reportedly healthy 29-year-old herpetologist. Although the victim had been bitten by an indeterminate number of "colubrids" prior to this incident, no history of serious effects was reported. Also, the victim had no history of venomous snakebites and had never been given antivenom. The minor local effects of this bite quickly subsided, and the victim was asymptomatic for approximately 2 days following this incident, at which time he experienced a brief (an estimated 5 min) episode of dizziness. Four days later (6 days after the bite), the victim noted persistent dizziness, and presented at an emergency room with "severe rotatory dizziness," nausea, and vomiting (Peichoto et al., 2007a). The patient required assisted ambulation as he was reportedly "unsteady" on his feet. A CT scan of the head was unremarkable and otological and neurological examinations were within normal limits. There was no observed spontaneous or gaze-evoked nystagmus. The patient was treated with antihistamines and glucocorticoids. The nausea and vomiting subsided within 24 hours with a sustained vertigo for several days thereafter. Full resolution occurred within 2 weeks (Peichoto et al., 2007a). The authors remarked, "Although it is difficult to prove that the presentation of labyrinthine syndrome and the snakebite are actually associated, this case would have to be taken into account to alert professionals of the health care area about the necessity of attending carefully accidents involving colubrid snakes …" (Peichoto et al., 2007a). Thus, these workers "assumed" the vertigo and related symptoms were an "effect of ophitoxemia" (Peichoto et al., 2007a).

4.4.4.2 Commentary and Critique

This case offers another opportunity for detailed analyses that can highlight and emphasize the need for carefully prioritized, logical differential diagnoses when considering snakebite presentations that differ from the vast majority of formally documented cases. The assignment of this case to an "effect of ophitoxemia" is unsupported by available data and is unlikely, considering the 48-h delay after the bite to a transient episodic vertigo, followed thereafter in approximately 4 more days by vertigo and other related vestibular symptoms. The symptoms resulted in an emergency-room review. These symptoms constitute some of the most common presenting complaints in general medicine. A well-grounded interpretation of this case requires a carefully and accurately considered differential diagnosis. The duration of discrete vertiginous events comprises the foundation for a likely diagnosis.

Vertiginous symptoms and signs are categorized as peripheral or central. These have been reviewed in detail elsewhere (Fauci et al., 2007), but an important distinguishing feature is the paroxysmal onset of vertigo of peripheral etiologies [vestibular neuronitis, benign paroxysmal positional vertigo (BPPV), cervical vertigo, Ménière's syndrome, etc.] versus the gradual onset of vertigo from central causes (vertebrobasilar insufficiency, cerebellar, pons or medullary lesions, multiple sclerosis, migraines, etc.; Chan, 2009; Karatas, 2008; McPhee and Papadakis, 2009). Peripheral vertigo often includes horizontal nystagmus and may also feature tinnitus and/or some abnormal auditory testing. Central vertigo usually does not cause abnormal auditory testing. Recommended investigations include MRI of the brain with gadolinium, electronystagmography, and videonystagmography.

The authors reported a negative CT of the head (MRI was unavailable in their facility), an absence of nystagmus, and unremarkable neurological exam, as well as auditory testing (Peichoto et al., 2007a). Although, as the imaging study was not optimal, there is a chance of an undetected central lesion, the published medical history and symptoms/signs of the patient suggest that the described course is most likely related to a vestibular neuronitis. This form of labyrinthitis is often of unknown etiology and results from a disruption of afferent neuronal input from one of the two vestibular apparatuses. In some cases, a viral etiology has been demonstrated (unspecified enterovirus; Ergul et al., 2006), while in others it is strongly suspected (adenovirus; Zannolli et al., 2006). Reactivation of latent herpes simplex-1 in vestibular ganglia may account for some cases of this syndrome (Gacek, 2008). Paroxysmal vestibular neuronitis (PVN) frequently occurs over several days to a week or two with gradual clearing. In some patients, a brief prodrome occurs days or hours prior to sustained episodes (Lee et al., 2009). Nystagmus may be present (often it is not) and an absent response to caloric stimulation is noted. It is not clear if such testing was performed in this case, although many features of this syndrome are compatible with the history as reported.

Another differential that must be considered is BPPV, which may present similarly to PVN except that it tends to occur in cluster episodes lasting several minutes or longer, following specifically provoking head movements/position. The etiology probably is related either to canalithiasis or cupulolithiasis that results in abnormal stimulation of the crista ampullaris (for details of the proposed pathophysiological models; see Schuknecht, 1969 and Epley, 1992). Some surgical data lend support to the canalithiasis theory (Parnes and McClure, 1991). The presentation of BPPV may be variable and its onset described quite differently by various patients (SAW, personal observations). Diagnosis may be assisted by response to and/or reproduction of the transient vertigo by Hallpike, Epley, or Semont canalith repositioning maneuvers. The transient episode of vertigo experienced by the patient several days prior to the persistent vestibular symptoms could be related to an exacerbation from a provoking head movement.

Although toxic insult may produce such responses, these would most frequently be immediate or would occur shortly after exposure (e.g., tetrodotoxin ingestion, Ahasan et al., 2004; injection of castor bean extract (*Ricinus communis*), Coopman et al., 2009). Dizziness occasionally associated with bites inflicted by viperids and elapids occurs within minutes or hours after the envenoming and is probably due to hypovolemia, pain, and autonomic responses (Warrell, 2004; White and Dart, 2008; www.toxinology.com). Also, while several snake venom toxins have been characterized that produce vestibular disturbances in mice ("gyroxin" or "gyrotoxin"), to date all of these have been either identified in or isolated from crotaline viperid venoms [e.g., tiger rattlesnake, *Crotalus tigris* (Minton and Weinstein, 1984; Weinstein and Smith, 1990), tropical rattlesnake, *C. durissus terrificus* (Alexander et al., 1988), bushmaster, *Lachesis muta* (da Silva et al., 1989; Magalhaes et al., 1993), *B. asper* (terciopelo, barba amarilla, or cuatro narices; Perez et al., 2008), *B. jararacussu* (jararacuçu; Perez et al., 2007) and others; see Plates 2.2, 4.73, 4.74A and B, and 4.86]. Further, these toxins produce distinctive axial gyrations in mice injected with lethal doses of venom or isolated toxin. Interestingly, gyroxin from *C. d. terrificus* venom (and others) has been characterized as a thrombin-like enzyme with fibrinogenase and fibrinase activities (Maruñak et al., 2004). It may appear tempting to some to speculate that some of the fibrinogenases/proteases characterized from *P. olfersii* Duvernoy's secretion might be similar to gyroxins. However, there have been no reports of such signs in experimental animals injected with any *Philodryas* spp. Duvernoy's secretion, and there are no reports of thrombin-like activity in Duvernoy's secretion of any *Philodryas* spp. studied to date (see Section 4.2).

Management of either PVN or BPPV may include antihistamines, such as meclizine or promethazine, and glucocorticoids. Although considered controversial, glucocorticoids (e.g., 100 mg/day for 3 days followed by a 20 mg/day taper) have been reported to decrease the duration of the episodes associated with vestibular neuronitis and Ménière's syndrome (Cope and Bova, 2008; Fauci et al., 2009; McPhee and Papadakis, 2009). BBPPV often responds to Epley, Semont, or Brandt-Daroff maneuvers. Although evidence-based studies are limited, some data suggest that canalith repositioning maneuvers have greater therapeutic efficacy than medications (Clinch et al., 2010). Most presentations of either PVN or BPPV resolve in 1–3 weeks (Fauci et al., 2009; Kerber, 2009; Lee et al., 2009; McPhee and Papadakis, 2009). The response to some of these treatments, and the duration of signs/symptoms, is compatible with the outcome of the reported case.

The delay between the *P. o. latirostris* bite and the development of the presenting symptoms (about 6 days) strongly argues against any specific linkage of the bite and the episodic vertigo. The possibility of sequestered Duvernoy's secretion causing a delayed clinical effect may be contemplated. However, this is an extremely remote, unlikely possibility, as the vast majority of *P. olfersii* bites are medically insignificant, with some significant bites resulting in only mild-to-moderate local effects (Table 4.1; Section 4.2). Isolated reports of abnormal laboratory tests suggestive of systemic symptoms (i.e., coagulopathy; Orduna et al., 1994) require further documentation, as there is little current evidence of any substantial risk of such effects from bites from this species. In addition, an occasional report of nausea, dizziness, and/or vomiting associated with patients presenting with *Philodryas* sp. bites (e.g., in a 2-year-old patient bitten by *P. olfersii*, Ribeiro et al., 1999, and in 7 out of 297 patients bitten by *P. patagoniensis*, de Medeiros et al., 2010), cannot be accepted as sole evidence of systemic effects as snakebites of any kind are frequently accompanied by autonomic symptoms related to anxiety or somatosensory amplification (White and Dart, 2008; Section 4.5).

4.4.4.3   Conclusion and Assessment of P. o. latirostris

There are few cases of bites from *Philodryas* spp. that are assigned to subspecies. As was noted in considering the medical importance of the genus, *Philodryas* spp., medically significant bites from *P. olfersii* most frequently result in mild-to-moderate local effects. Most bites are likely medically insignificant, although uncommon cases of extensive ecchymoses have been documented (see Section 4.2). The reviewed case includes an unsupported presumptive connection between a medically insignificant bite from a specimen of *P. o. latirostris* and a vestibular syndrome most likely due to a vestibular neuronitis or BPPV. In fact, these appear unrelated and are probably coincidental. Therefore, the patient's presentation should not be assigned to what by all available information was an inconsequential bite. There are no current data supporting systemic effects from this subspecies. However, as stated previously, it is reasonable to carefully assess victims of *Philodryas* spp. bites due to the uncommon risk of systemic effects that to date have been limited to extensive ecchymoses, as well as the possible clinical role of fibrinogenolytic enzymes and myotoxins that have been isolated from Duvernoy's secretions of these snakes (Section 4.2).

Assessment of *P. o. latirostris* based on available evidence: Hazard Level 3 (see Table 4.3).

4.4.5   Platyceps (Coluber) najadum: A Fatal Case of Progressive Neuropathy from a Colubrid Bite?

4.4.5.1   Analysis and Critique of an Aberrant Report

The single clinically documented case of a purported *P. najadum* (family Colubridae, sub-family Colubrinae; Plate 4.13A–C) bite occurred in Greece and presents a concerning clinical history of segmental muscle spasms that progressed to flaccid quadriplegia and a fatal outcome in less than 6 months (Chroni et al., 2005; Table 4.1). The patient, a 67-year-old woman, reported receiving multiple bites on the lower extremities from an approximately 80 cm *P. najadum*. The authors did not indicate how the identification of the snake was established and/or if it was verified by a qualified individual. Therefore, this case must be considered one of presumed identity. The patient was initially treated with antibiotics and steroids, and provided with tetanus toxoid. It is noteworthy that the authors commented, "… antivenom therapy was not considered necessary …" (Chroni et al., 2005) as there is no reason to have any antivenom available for snakes of this genus (see Section 4.2; Table 4.1), and therefore there is no antivenom against any *Platyceps* spp. Also, from information in the presenting history, there is no basis to contemplate antivenom administration even if it was available.

Shortly after the aforementioned treatments were initiated, the patient developed generalized muscle aches and hyperpyrexia that were attributed to wound site infection. The patient improved, was discharged, then gradually exhibited body aches as well as severe stiffness of the back, upper arms, and neck. She was re-admitted 20 days after the initial episode and on admission persistent stiffness with muscle spasm and hyper-reflexia were noted (Chroni et al., 2005). Although laboratory tests were within normal limits, needle electromyography of affected muscles showed sustained motor unit activity with reduction induced by i.v. diazepam. The authors then treated the patient for suspected tetanus with antitetanus immunoglobulin, antibiotics, and diazepam (Chroni et al., 2005). Shortly thereafter (2 months after the initial admission), the patient developed flaccid paraparesis. A nerve conduction study indicated the presence of axonal motor neuropathy. A cerebral spinal fluid (CSF) analysis was acellular, but with markedly elevated protein (110mg/dL; Chroni et al., 2005). There was no evidence of neuromuscular junction failure, and a tentative diagnosis of Guillain–Barré syndrome (GBS) was considered. The patient was treated with i.v. administration of immunoglobulin, resulting in mild improvement. However, over the following month, the patient developed quadriplegia without cranial nerve involvement and with intact sensation. Magnetic resonance imaging, autoimmune screening, and comprehensive blood tests were all negative (Chroni et al., 2005).

The patient was given a course of 60mg of prednisone/day and was discharged tetraplegic. She was again re-admitted 1 month later and deteriorated during this admission. The patient expired 5.5 months after the alleged *P. najadum* bite; death was ascribed to massive mesenteric thrombosis (Chroni et al., 2005).

The authors stated that the case was inconsistent with tetanus (due to a lack of trismus and facial muscle involvement as well as the progressive autonomic dominant neuropathy) or GBS (due to the irreversible progression to quadriplegia and fatal outcome; Chroni et al., 2005). The results of numerous tests were not consistent with myasthenia, myasthenic syndrome, or polymyositis (Chroni et al., 2005). They also considered that administration of tetanus toxoid may have caused a polyradiculitis, although previously documented cases have usually involved multiple doses and this patient received only a single dose (Chroni et al., 2005; Reinstein et al., 1982). However, while considering the aforementioned likely etiologies, the authors suggested that this complex and unfortunate case might be due to "… an immune reaction against neural antigens generated by the snake toxins." This was hypothesized to have caused a widespread inflammatory disease in the nerve roots (Chroni et al., 2005).

These complex polyneuropathies often are a diagnostic and management challenge. Their features, natural history, diagnosis, and management are far too extensive to discuss here and have been thoroughly reviewed (Goetz, 2007; Longmore et al., 2001). Some of these neuropathies can be associated with comorbidities, but the authors asserted an unremarkable medical history of their patient (Chroni et al., 2005). The possibility of GBS can be briefly considered, as it is often associated with a recent history (usually within weeks) of infection [e.g., viral upper respiratory infection, atypical pneumonia (e.g., *Mycoplasma pneumoniae*), herpes zoster reactivation,

Epstein–Barr virus], recent surgery, and occasionally immunization (Keenlyside et al., 1980; Longmore et al., 2001; Sindern et al., 2001). Features supporting a diagnosis of GBS include (but are not limited to): progression up to about 4–5 weeks; closely symmetric signs/symptoms; mild sensory symptoms, if present at all; bilateral facial weakness; autonomic dysfunction, and early recovery at about 2 weeks at the completion of the progressive symptoms (Longmore et al., 2001). Although the patient did not exhibit facial weakness or apparent facial nerve involvement, many other features are consistent with GBS or a related, less-defined polyradiculitis. Even though recovery from these syndromes commonly occurs, fatalities certainly are well documented, and mortality from GBS has been estimated at approximately 10% (Longmore et al., 2001). Therefore, although the authors fairly rigidly define their analysis of the patient's etiology, the basic presentation and features, as well as the fatal outcome, can be compatible with GBS or a closely related polyneuropathy.

In this regard, it is also reasonable to briefly consider acute polyradiculitis, possibly related to the provision of tetanus toxoid. Acute polyradiculitis often initially presents as a paresthesia that begins from the lower extremities and develops into a symmetrically ascending myasthenia. The symptomatology is variable and may feature mild asthenia or complete tetraplegia, as was seen in the reviewed case (Chroni et al., 2005; Kärppä, 2009). These symptoms may be accompanied by autonomic dysfunction, cranial nerve palsies, or asphyxia (Kärppä, 2009). Areflexia, ataxia, and ophthalmoplegia can be noted in the rarer Miller Fisher syndrome (Longmore et al., 2001). Although there are no specific laboratory tests for acute polyradiculitis, a common finding is acellular CSF containing elevated protein (Kärppä, 2009). Prognosis is usually good, but up to 20% may have functional impairment and fatalities are well documented (Kärppä, 2009). Thus, in the reviewed case, the patient's course, test results, and outcome are consistent with GBS or another less-defined acute polyradiculitis.

Interestingly, there are a few documented cases of GBS or related polyneuropathy postenvenoming from elapids or crotaline viperids (Chuang et al., 1996; Ekenback et al., 1985). These are readily distinguishable from the case reported by Chroni et al. (2005), as they all involved serious envenoming. However, although these are likely related to the reported post-envenoming polyneuropathy, it still must be considered that even these cases may have alternative explanations (e.g., an unreported recent viral infection).

The patient in this case did not have a postmortem (Chroni et al., 2005). An autopsy might have facilitated an improved understanding of the neuropathy. Neuropathological investigation of a 36-year-old male who succumbed to an inflammatory polyradiculopathy (posthepatitis B vaccination) showed severe axonal loss with peripheral nerve demyelination and mononuclear cell infiltration in nerve roots and spinal ganglia (Sindern et al., 2001). Therefore, with the available information regarding this case, the authors' proposed linkage between the *P. najadum* bites and the fatal progressive neuropathy is far less likely than the probability of GBS or another related polyradiculopathy resulting from tetanus toxoid or a coincident unreported viral infection. Although there are no data regarding the properties of Duvernoy's secretions of *P. najadum*, to date, there is no evidence that bites by this species produce any significant medical effects in humans. The lack of verified identification of the culprit snake must be considered, but as the bites were insignificant, there is still no link that can be confidently established between the bites and the fatal progressive neuropathy.

4.4.5.2 Conclusion and Assessment of P. najadum

Chroni et al. (2005) documented an unfortunate case of fatal progressive neuropathy and proposed possible linkage with bites from a presumed *P. najadum* as the precipitating cause (i.e., immune response "against neural antigens generated by snake toxins"; Chroni et al., 2005). Although several rare instances of GBS have been documented postenvenoming from elapids or crotaline viperids, even these cases may have alternative etiologies and this case involved medically insignificant bites from a colubrid species that has no documented medical importance or known appreciable toxicity. Due to the fatal outcome and the apparent insignificance of the purported *P. najadum* bites delivered to the patient, there is no evidence sufficient to assign this fatal case to the bites from this colubrid. This case highlights the need for thorough documentation of these cases including verification of identity of the involved snake and scrutiny of any other factors (e.g., recent/concomitant immunizations, infections, family history) potentially contributing to the etiology of such progressive and life-threatening neuropathies.

Assessment of *P. najadum* based on available evidence: Hazard Level 3 (see Table 4.3).

4.4.6 Hierophis (Coluber) viridiflavus: A Case of Neurotoxic Colubrine Bite or a More Common Etiology?

4.4.6.1 Analysis and Critique

This single case of a purportedly medically significant bite from a *H. viridiflavus* (family Colubridae, subfamily Colubrinae; Plate 4.16A–D) occurred near Bordeaux, France. Published as an abstract, this brief report summarizes the events that ensued after the 20-year-old male victim was allegedly bitten by a 100-cm *H. viridiflavus* (Bedry et al., 1998; Table 4.1) after placing the wild-caught snake around his neck. It is important to note that the victim did not express awareness of being bitten. Rather, his companions informed him that he had received a bite from the snake. The patient had ingested "a few pints" of an alcoholic beverage (presumably beer) prior to this incident. Approximately 30 min later, the victim reported dizziness and was "affected by a major muscular weakness" (Bedry et al., 1998). After 3 h, the victim, anxious and drowsy, was admitted to the ICU. Shortly thereafter, he experienced vertigo and vomiting. Neurological examination revealed "an inability to open his eyes and lifting his head off the bed" (Bedry et al., 1998). Laboratory results were unremarkable (although specific details of the tests included were not mentioned) aside from a blood alcohol level of 2.1 g/L (Bedry et al., 1998). The reported neurological signs "declined" within 90 min and the vomiting ceased within 24 h. The authors considered two possible causes for the observed syndrome: ethanol intoxication or an "envenomation with an incomplete curare-like syndrome (ptosis, muscle weakness of the head)" (Bedry et al., 1998). These investigators added that two necessary conditions would be needed for this snake's bite to be responsible for the observed effects: "a venomous saliva" and "a minimal time of contact between it and the wound" (Bedry et al., 1998). They concluded that the "... exceptional circumstances of this accident explain a poisoning by *Coluber viridiflavus* ... raises the question of a real toxicity of snakes described as nonvenomous as they are fangless" (Bedry et al., 1998).

Assessment of this case is hindered by the brevity of the report and its limited detailed information. However, the available data raise significant questions regarding the possible assignment of envenomation as the cause of the reported syndrome. First, although the authors inferred that a sustained bite would be necessary in order to account for medically significant effects, available information suggests "minimal contact" between the victim and the snake. This argues against a protracted bite that would raise the likelihood of a secretion volume sufficient to cause the serious effects as reported. This is particularly noteworthy as it is likely that, similar to members of the genus *Coluber*, these snakes do not possess any dentition clearly adapted for grasping prey or possibly allowing increased entry of associated secretions into inflicted wounds (see Section 4.1). Such brief contact could be sufficient to cause a medically significant bite if this species had a highly toxic secretion (i.e., see *R. tigrinus* and *R. subminiatus*; Section 4.3). However, there are no available data indicating that this species produces such a toxic secretion. Although there are no specific data regarding the presence of any Duvernoy's glands in this species, similar colubrine taxa such as *Coluber constrictor* (Plate 4.80A and B) have been reported to contain a "venom gland" associated "venom duct" (Fry et al., 2008). As noted in Section 4.1, there are no well-documented cases of medically significant bites from any *Coluber* spp. and numerous bites witnessed or experienced personally by several of us were insignificant.

It is important to recognize that Bedry et al. (1998) assumed in their report that the bite did in fact occur. As this critical assumption is based on the comments of the victim's companions, all who may have been ingesting significant amounts of alcohol, the specific basis for this case must be considered tentative at best. Unfortunately, the case report lacks any information regarding examination of the purported bite site. The most likely cause of the reported presentation is a result of alcohol intoxication, possibly with somatosensory amplification (Section 4.5.2). The victim's reported blood level (2.1 g/L or 210 mg/dL) is well over the level predictive of gross intoxication (120–160 mg/dL; Trevor et al., 2008). This level is notable because behavioral, cognitive, and psychomotor changes can occur at blood alcohol levels as low as 20–30 mg/dL, a level achieved after ingestion of just one or two standard drinks (Fauci et al., 2009). The level is also over four times the legal blood alcohol limit in France [0.05% (50 mg/dL) for drivers of a noncommercial vehicle (http://www2.securiteroutiere.gouv.fr/ressources/conseils/l-alcool-au-volant.html)]. Review of these basic calculations suggest that the victim ingested a large volume of alcohol and the detected blood alcohol level was metabolically decreased from the time of the incident, as these levels decrease by approximately 0.01%/40 min (www.cdc.gov). Therefore, at the time of the reported bite, it is likely that the victim had even higher blood alcohol level. The body weight and habitus of the victim (these details were not included in the case report) would also be important factors influencing the degree of intoxication per the ingested volume.

The pharmacology of ethanol is complex and only partially characterized. It is known to act as an agonist of Type A γ-aminobutyric acid ($GABA_A$) receptors and inhibits glutaminergic activation of N-methyl-D-aspartate (NMDA) receptors as well as modifies functions of adenyl cyclase, phospholipase C, and some types of ion channels (Trevor et al., 2008). This complex pharmacology can be expressed in the multiple organ involvement typically observed with significant intake of ethanol. Thus, almost all of the reported clinical course could be ascribed to acute ethanol intoxication that may include signs/symptoms such as nausea, vomiting, and neurosensory effects including blurred vision, headache, stupor, confusion, slurred speech, and fine motor tremors. Nystagmus associated with cranial nerve palsies may also occur (American Psychiatric Association, 2000). The "major muscle weakness" may have been due to somatosensory amplification (e.g., compare with the *H. gigas* case reported by Manning et al., 1999; Table 4.1 and Section 4.3.3) and/or intoxication-induced immobility.

4.4.6.2 Conclusion and Assessment of H. viridiflavus

As noted in a significant number of these cases, this report describes a concerning clinical course that was hypothetically considered a result of a bite from a non-front-fanged colubroid species without any documented medical risk. In evaluating the limited evidence provided in the report, it must be noted that the reviewer cannot have confidence that any bite did in fact occur, and the victim had a very substantial blood alcohol level that was in excess of four times the legal driving limit in France. Therefore, the likelihood of acute alcohol intoxication ± somatosensory amplification provides a far more probable explanation for the reported signs/symptoms than a medically significant bite from *H. viridiflavus*. The nature of the oral glands and properties of any associated oral secretions of *H. viridiflavus* require study and characterization. As discussed earlier, the use of the term "venom gland" and "venom ducts" for oral structures of allied taxa such as *C. constrictor* is premature and misleading.

A presentation reported in a little-known journal featured ophthalmoplegia, facial nerve (cranial nerve [CN] VII) palsy and right-sided hemiparesis was described as possible sequelae of a snakebite from an unidentified species locally named, "kyzl ilan" (Aleksankin, 1968). The aforementioned clinical course reportedly developed in the previously healthy patient approximately 4 years after the bite. Some have speculated that the snake responsible was a *Dolichophis*[16] (*Hierophis* Nagy et al., 2004a) *schmidti* (Nagy et al., 2004b). As discussed in Section 4.5, the lack of any substantial information regarding the snake allegedly involved in such an atypical case as well as the obscurity of the report compels rejection of any linkage of the described clinical presentation with a non-front-fanged colubroid bite. Although it is unlikely that the patient's reported palsies were due to the alleged snakebite (that has no verifiable description or documentation), the remote possibility of GBS following a serious envenoming from a front-fanged species (e.g., the lebetine or blunt-nosed

---

[16]Another genus split from the previous inaccurate grouping of several colubrine taxa within the genus, *Coluber, Dolicophis* contains four species. Two of these, *D. jugularis* and *D. caspius*, are respectively illustrated in Plates 4.70A and B and 4.91.

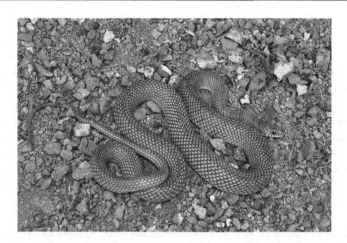

Plate 4.90 European or Caspian whip snake (*Dolicophis caspius*). Like other colubrine taxa (e.g., *Hierophis*, *Platyceps*, *Hemmorhois*) previously included in the genus *Coluber*, this fast-moving species of the genus *Dolicophis* has a generalized diet including lizards, small mammals, nestling birds, etc. It is found in Eastern Europe and Russia. There are no known medically significant bites by this species.
Photo copyright to Daniel Jablonski.

viper, *Macrovipera lebetina*, Plate 4.72) could be contemplated with the acquisition of further detail/evidence (see Section 4.4.5).

As in any case of a bite inflicted by an ophidian species of unknown importance, a proviso must be raised regarding the possibility of undocumented clinically significant toxic potential. However, based on available data, this case cannot be utilized as evidence of any medical risk from *H. viridiflavus*.

Assessment of *H. viridiflavus* based on available evidence: Insufficient to assign a specific ranking; likely Hazard Level 3/4 [Most bites feature uncomplicated local effects (typically, mild bleeding, limited edema, pain, etc.). Larger specimens may produce more extensive local effects].

4.4.7 "Venomous" Bites by Nonvenomous Lizards?

Although two species of venomous lizards (Family, Helodermatidae), the Gila monster (*Heloderma suspectum*) and beaded lizard (*Heloderma horridum*),[17] have caused life-threatening envenomations, recent reports have described toxins and/or toxin transcripts in oral secretions of some lizards of several families including Iguanidae (iguanas and their allies), Agamidae (chisel-toothed lizards), and Varanidae (monitors and goannas; Fry et al., 2006, 2009b). One of these, the Komodo monitor or dragon (*Varanus komodoensis*), the largest extant lizard species [reaching

---

[17] For reviews and discussion of the biology of *Heloderma*, their venoms, and the rare envenomations by these inoffensive lizards, see Bogert and Del Campo (1956), Mebs (2002), Campbell and Lamar (2004), and Beck (2005).

documented lengths up to (and possibly exceeding) 3.4 m],[18] has caused human fatalities.[19] As a result of the discovery of toxins in the oral secretions of these lizards, they have been prematurely labeled "venomous." This information has been sensationalized and accepted by the press (and some of the established scientific community) without further verification. Consideration must be given to the current consensus definition of venom (see p. 32), and the need for evidence supporting the use of venom in the subjugation/capture of prey and/or as an antipredator strategy. Although there are toxins of several classes common to venomous snakes present in the oral secretions of these lizards, there is no evidence verifying the use of these in prey capture. Their function may be a result of "preadaptation" (also referred to as "exaptation"; Gould and Vrba, 1982), an evolutionary phenomenon that assigns previous characters of ancestors in one biological role being co-opted to new biological roles in later descendants (Gould, 2002). Toxins that occur in oral secretions, when biochemically documented in colubroid snakes and basal squamates, do not automatically qualify the reptile as venomous. Instead, these toxins may play different biological roles in basal groups, later to be co-opted into a new role in the true venom system of derived snakes (Weinstein et al., 2010). Therefore, these genes and their products (in these cases, toxins) are "exapted" (adapted at a later date) from earlier phylogenetic roles into new derived roles (Arthur, 2002). The only way to confirm a toxin's biological role in basal squamates is by experimental confirmation and/or extensive, well-documented field observations.

There is also no evidence of medical significance of these saurian secretions. While it is agreed that the oft proposed and popular theory of *V. komodoensis* prey capture via sepsis[20] is most likely incorrect, to date the few well-documented cases of bites inflicted on human victims by this endangered species have only included infection, physical trauma, and blood loss. In the most recent documented attack (the first fatality documented in approximately 33 years), an 8-year-old boy was tragically killed after being bitten on the "waist," and "tossed viciously from side-to-side," he "died from massive bleeding half an hour later" (*The Guardian*, Monday, June 4, 2007). Auffenberg (1981) reported two uncomplicated aseptic bites inflicted by 1.0–1.2 m specimens. Interestingly, a recent consideration of the potential role of oral bacterial flora of *V. komodoensis* contemplated a new model ("lizard–lizard epidemic"), partly based on field observations, in which bacteria spread epidemically among lizards via oral

---

[18] According to the US National Zoological Park, Smithsonian Institution (http://nationalzoo.si.edu), the largest verified specimen reached a length of 3.13 m and weighed 166 kg (this may have included the weight of a recent undigested meal). More typical weights for the largest wild dragons are about 70 kg. A recent study found average snout–vent lengths (SVL) ranged between 74.7 and 92.1 cm and mass between 7.9–23.5 kg among a significant sampling of specimens from four islands in the Komodo National Park. Maximal *V. komodoensis* SVL and mass were strongly correlated with prey density [specifically, Timor deer (*Cervus timorensis*)] on a given island (Jessop et al., 2006).

[19] See Auffenberg (1981) for a detailed, fascinating discussion of the biology and predatory behavior of *V. komodoensis* and historical examples of fatal attacks by this imposing species of giant lizard.

[20] Multiple taxa of pathogenic bacteria have been identified and cultured from the oropharynx of *V. komodoensis*. These included several taxa of *Streptococcus*, *Staphylococcus*, *Pasteurella multocida*, and a number of other organisms. The colonizing flora between captive and wild lizards was notably different, with wild specimens containing a preponderance of potential pathogens (see Montgomery et al., 2002).

exposure from prey that escape an initial attack. Escaping prey infected with organisms from the attacking lizards thereby serve as vectors and spread the infection among the lizards' oropharynx, possibly through communal feeding (Bull et al., 2010). As noted by Bull et al. (2010), there is a paucity of knowledge about the natural history of these lizards and their oral flora. Therefore, the functional role(s), if any, of oral bacteria, as well as proposed toxin-induced shock and/or coagulopathy in bitten prey (Fry et al., 2009b), requires confirmatory biomedical evidence in addition to careful field observations of predatory behavior, and the subsequent effects on prey such as buffalo, deer, pigs, and the like.

There are two reports of "toxic" bites from one species of varanid lizard, the desert monitor, *V. griseus* (Ballard and Antonio, 2001; Sopiev et al., 1987). These reports described "toxic effects" such as dysphagia, dyspnea, chest discomfort, and other signs/symptoms (Ballard and Antonio, 2001). However, these and similar cases require careful evidence-based and physician-based evaluation (Weinstein et al., 2010). Bites from large lizards may cause painful, freely bleeding wounds due to physical trauma from the powerful jaws, and this certainly can induce anxiety with additional somatic manifestations (see Section 4.5). Varanid, agamid, and iguanid lizards are very common in private collections, and bites from some of these are reasonably common. However, there are no well-documented reports from medical facilities recording the clinical evolution of such "toxic effects." Instead, medically verified clinical sequelae of varanid and iguanid bites feature mechanical trauma (severity may be related to the involved anatomical region) and infectious complications (Weinstein et al., 2010). Presentations may include severe lacerations, extensive soft tissue injury/cellulitis, and type I hypersensitivity (Bibbs et al., 2001; Hsieh and Babel, 1999; Kelsey et al., 1997; Levine et al., 2003; Merin and Bush, 2000). Increased relative bite performance is selectively favored in lizards and is associated with increasing cranial size as well as ontogenetically related growth of jaw adductor muscles (Herrel and O'Reilly, 2006). Therefore, larger specimens inflict correspondingly more serious wounds. This is consistent with the greater than 12 cases of bites inflicted by large varanids (Nile monitor, *V. niloticus*, Bengal monitor, *V. bengalensis*, water or Salvator monitor, *V. salvator*, and lace monitor, *V. varius*) that were personally experienced, medically managed, or observed firsthand by one of the authors (SAW). These cases presented as purely local wounds of varying severity with reactive erythema and mild edema. Increased size of the varanid responsible for the bite was associated with increased severity of the resulting injury. Broad-spectrum antibiotic coverage (amoxicillin/clavulanate, 875/125 mg, twice per day) was prescribed in one of three cases managed by SAW. None of these three cases had any clinically significant sequelae (Weinstein et al., 2010).

Some investigators have noted the regional beliefs that have anecdotally assigned toxicity to several taxa of lizards including varanids (Smith, 1935); geckos (leopard gecko, *Eublepharis macularis*; Minton, 1964), and agamids (Ruppell's agama, *Agama ruppelli orientalis*; MacCabe, 2009). The fearsome and factually unsupported reputation of some of these may rival that of well-known medically important venomous snakes. The innocuous gekkonid, *Eublepharis macularis*, is one of the most popular pet lizards in Europe, the USA, Canada, and parts of Asia. However, it is dreaded among the Sindhis of West Pakistan, referred to as "khan" or "hun khun," and is believed to cause instant death (Minton, 1964). Its body fluids are equally feared as being lethal on contact (Minton, 1964). Fear of geckos is reasonably common among some indigenous people in Africa and Asia (Schmidt and Inger, 1966; Frembgen, 1996). In the Turkana region of northern Kenya, bites by Ruppell's agama lizard (*Agama ruppelli orientalis*) are feared even more than bites by *Echis pyramidum* (Geoffroy's carpet viper, Kenyan carpet or saw-scaled viper; MacCabe, 2009; see pg. 198).

As noted elsewhere in this book, unless the defining interpretation of the term "venom" is modified by consensus, a rigorous body of evidence should be expected prior to referring to any squamate oral secretion as venom. Agamids and iguanids do not have any obvious need for the use of toxins in subjugation of their prey, and many iguanids as well as some agamids are omnivorous with strong preferences for vegetarian diet. It is interesting that aside from local perceptions in West Papua about the hazards of blue-tongued skinks (*Tiliqua gigas*; see pg. 198) there are no similar reports of such toxins or concerns about scincid lizards. The possibility of prey-specific, digestive and/or other functions of toxins present in the oral secretions of these species requires firm biomedical confirmation and ethological support (e.g., observations of active use in prey capture and/or digestion). The proposed/implied clinical importance of these secretions is not established or medically documented. Only in the event of well-documented and clinically verified cases of recognizable envenomation by any of these lizards (e.g., varanids, agamids) can the medical risks of these species receive any due consideration.

4.5   Pitfalls Noted in Documented Cases: Differentiating Perceived Versus Evidence-Based Risk

"... וּמִתּוֹךְ זֶה, אַתָּה מְצַיֵּיר אֶת הַמַּסְקָנָה?" ... and from this, you are drawing a conclusion?

Mishnah

Get your facts first, and then you can distort 'em as much as you please.

Mark Twain

4.5.1   Examples of Pitfalls Noted in Documented Cases

4.5.1.1   Lack of Verified Identity of Snakes Responsible for Reported Bites

Because of the uncertain medical importance of the majority of these diverse colubroids, identification of snakes involved in documented bites is an essential cornerstone of risk assessment. Accounts of bites by numerous non-front-fanged colubroid species have been negatively impacted by a lack of verified identification of the snakes involved. Notably, the series of >70 bites attributed to *M. monspessulanus* includes probably >60 cases in which the snake was not satisfactorily identified (Table 4.1; Section 4.4.2). As the victims in two of these cases had paralytic features, accurate identification is essential and requires appropriate confirmation. Assigning the risk of neurotoxic envenoming to a given species may equate a bite to serious envenomation or may even permanently label the species responsible as presenting a life-threatening hazard. Although there is only a single well-documented neurotoxic envenomation by *M. monspessulanus*, it does provide evidence of the neurotoxic effects that may result from a bite from this species. However, the presumed neurotoxicity ascribed to bites by *B. irregularis* does not have such unambiguous supporting evidence. Therefore, although it may be prudent on occasion to "err on the side of caution," risk assignment must be founded on sound, verifiable evidence.

Similarly, incorrect identification may result in assignment of medical importance to the wrong species. In a case documenting the mild local effects that resulted from a bite inflicted by *Stenorrhina freminvillei*, the author published a photo of the snake involved (Cook, 1984). Several years later, Johnson (1988) published a commentary on the case correcting the identification to *Conophis lineatus* (Table 4.1).

Incorrect identification carries the potential for other serious consequences. Nonvenomous species or those of unknown medical importance may be mistaken for venomous species. This can lead to inappropriate provision of antivenom, thereby subjecting the patient to unnecessary and even life-threatening adverse effects (Ariaratnam et al., 2009; Viravan et al., 1992). For example, in their review of 91 cases of nonvenomous snakebite that were recorded in a teaching hospital in Brazil, Silveira and Nishioka (1992) reported several cases of provision of antivenom for nonvenomous bites. In one example, these authors documented life-threatening anaphylaxis in a patient given anti-*Bothrops* spp. antivenom after being bitten by a nonvenomous colubrine, *Drymarchon corais* ssp. (cribo; subspecies was not indicated). A bite from a *Sibynomorphus mikanii* (South American slug-eating snake or Mikan's tree snake) that reportedly caused a prolonged clotting time was treated with anti-*Bothrops* spp. antivenom (Silveira and Nishioka, 1992; Table 4.1). Similarly, a child bitten by a *Boiruna maculata* (mussurana; culebra de sangra; others; the name "mussurana" is also commonly used for *Clelia* spp.; see Table 4.1) presented with mild-to-moderate local effects and "discrete cyanosis" was also treated with anti-*Bothrops* spp. antivenom (Santos-Costa et al., 2000; Table 4.1). As this child also had a tourniquet applied to the affected limb, the described "cyanosis" may be a result of inappropriate and incorrectly applied first aid. It is noteworthy that of 43 patients reviewed in a Brazilian retrospective study of *P. olfersii* bites (see Section 4.1), six (14%) presented with a tourniquet that had been previously applied proximal to the bite (Ribeiro et al., 1999). Similarly, approximately 29 of 297 patients bitten by *P. patagoniensis* in São Paulo, Brazil, had received a tourniquet prior to presentation at the hospital, and this was significantly associated with the presence of local edema (de Medeiros et al., 2010). Misidentification of a *Chrysopelea pelias* (twin-barred tree or flying snake) for a *Bungarus* spp. (krait) resulted in unnecessary administration of antivenom. In addition, the antivenom did not even have efficacy for any of the medically important species of the region (Malaysia; Ismail et al., 2010; Table 4.1). Similarly, a herpetologist with mild local effects from a bite by a *Pliocercus elapoides* (false-coral snake) was treated with polyvalent antivenom incorrectly and uselessly administered intramuscularly in aliquots (Seib, 1980; Table 4.1). There are several reports of patients with mild-to-moderate local effects after receiving bites from *Philodryas* spp. that were treated with anti-*Bothrops* spp. antivenom (Table 4.1).

It is also conceivable that a venomous species might be misidentified as a nonvenomous colubroid with the result that appropriate antivenom treatment would be withheld. However, this very concerning consideration has not been well-documented and is less likely than the opposite, thoroughly documented scenario.

Although almost wholly relevant to only bites by captive specimens in private collections, an additional consideration is the recognition of genetic variants or different color phases of some colubroid species. There is a wide array of genetically selected variants ("sunset," albino, leucistic, melanistic, etc.) of selected snakes including elapid species (e.g., monocellate, or monocled cobra, *Naja kaouthia*), crotaline viperids (e.g., western diamondback rattlesnake, *Crotalus atrox*; eastern diamondback rattlesnake, *C. adamanteus*; Plate 4.91A), and non-front-fanged colubroids such as the western hognose snake (*H. nasicus*; Plate 4.91B–F). Therefore, victims of bites from venomous or nonvenomous snakes may present with a snake specimen that is not readily recognizable to those unfamiliar with genetic variants. The treating clinician must remain aware of this possibility and, if unfamiliar with these variants, seek well-informed consultation for accurate identification of the specimen.

Conclusions and Recommendations

When determining the medical importance of little-known ophidian species, documented and verified identification is an essential and fundamental necessity. Using stringent safety precautions, and whenever possible, any specimen involved in a bite should be procured and brought to a recognized institution for confirmation of identity. This could allow precise documentation of the specimen, confirming attribution of the case and aiding future study. If the specimen is not captured or sacrificed, photographs (even cell phone photos) can sometimes establish the identification.

With the exception of a handful of toxinologists and specifically trained medical professionals, most clinicians should not attempt to identify specimens brought by patients. This may include phase/pattern variants of common species that are selectively bred for the commercial trade. Unfortunately, such identifications by medical staff are frequently incorrect for snakes (Ariaratnam et al., 2009; Viravan et al., 1992), and for spiders assumed to be responsible for skin lesions incorrectly identified as necrotic araenism (Vetter, 2009). In a study examining the ability of a cross-section of Australians to identify venomous and nonvenomous snakes, only approximately 25% of medical students and physicians in the study could accurately identify a given ophidian species (Morrison et al., 1983). Identification must be verified by a herpetologist or appropriately trained toxinologist.

4.5.1.2   Lack of Qualified Medical Assessment/Review

One of the most common flaws in reports of purportedly significant medically significant non-front-fanged colubroid bites is lack of formal medical review. Any case of snakebite with medical effects that are perceived as significant requires evaluation by a medically qualified professional. This is important for the patient's care based on a carefully collected and analyzed history. This includes verification of identity of the snake (see previous section); consideration of sympatric alternative species potentially responsible for the bite if identity cannot be established; review of the medical history, allergies, and any medications that might influence or account for the presentation; and, if

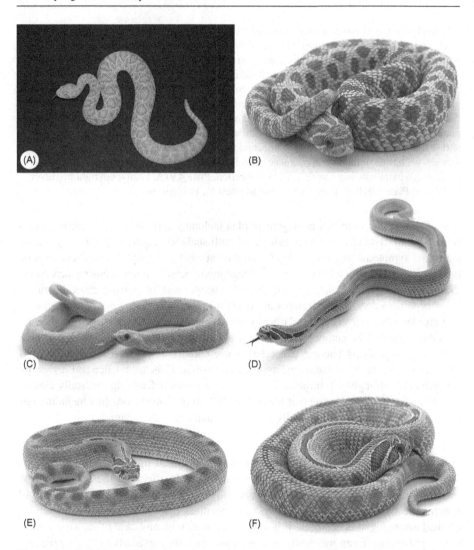

Plate 4.91 (A–F) Pattern/phase variants of representative ophidian species popular in private collections.
(A) Eastern diamondback rattlesnake (*Crotalus adamanteus*), albino phase. Clinicians treating patients presenting with snakebites must remain aware of the increasing availability (in Europe, the USA, and parts of Asia) of captive bred genetic variants of common venomous species. Victims may present with snakes that appear markedly different from the normal phase of a given species such as the albino *C. adamanteus* pictured here. Albinos, leucistics, melanistics, or other genetically selected phases such as "sunset" can be unfamiliar and confusing to the treating clinician. It is important to verify the identity of any snake involved in a presenting snakebite, as this guides critical management decisions that frequently will directly impact the outcome.
(B and C) Western hognose snake (*H. nasicus*), albino phase variants. Western hognose snakes are very popular in private collections, and a variety of phase/pattern variants are

(*Continued*)

◄ selectively bred by commercial breeders and "herpetoculturists." *Heterodon nasicus* have rarely caused medically significant bites (see Plate 4.24D–J) and are phlegmatic captives. Almost all of the seven documented cases occurred when offering a captive specimen food, or shortly after contacting food items before handling the snake (see text and Table 4.1). **(D–F) Western hognose snake (*H. nasicus*), breeder-selected pattern variants.** These phases are variously called "anaconda" (in reference to the numerous spots reminiscent of the green anaconda, *Eunectes murinus*, a boiid member of the Henophidia), striped, reduced pattern, hypomelanistic, etc. The physician must remain aware of such variants if presented with a snake deemed responsible for a bite, and the specimen is identified as a familiar species, yet has an unfamiliar appearance. This is particularly relevant in the case of a presenting victim who has a private snake collection. Plate 4.91A, photo copyright to Trevor D. Keyler; Plate 4.91B–F, photos copyright to Brent W. Bumgardner.

indicated, establishment of a management plan including appropriate tests and investigations. The understandable anxiety associated with snakebite regularly creates a group of signs and symptoms that can mislead both patients and their physicians. These include tachycardia, palpitations, sweating, overbreathing/hyperventilation (causing acroparesthesia, tetany, lightheadedness, faintness, and syncope) and, in extreme cases, histrionic conversion disorders. These features are often misinterpreted as signs of envenomation and are described naïvely and uncritically in accounts of snakebites written by the victims themselves or by authors without medical training. Autonomic responses to even a medically insignificant bite can exacerbate some comorbidities, such as ischemic heart disease (angina) or generalized anxiety disorder (panic). Thus, attendance and review by a physician is strongly recommended in any case reportedly featuring medically significant effects. It is disconcerting that fewer than 35% of published cases (not including retrospective reviews) feature medically qualified evaluation of the victim.

Conclusions and Recommendations

Anyone bitten by a snake of known or unknown medical importance that develops signs/symptoms and/or is concerned regarding possible effects of the bite should be promptly reviewed by a medical professional. As many non-front-fanged colubroid species are likely to be unfamiliar to most medical personnel, consultation with a clinical toxinologist is desirable if not mandatory, as with any case of unusual intoxication/poisoning. Even medically insignificant bites may exacerbate some preexisting comorbidities, and patients so affected should be managed appropriately.

4.5.1.3   Frequent Authorship ("Auto-Reporting") of Snakebite Cases by Victims

Another profoundly serious flaw in many of these reports is authorship by the victims themselves. Not only is this unacceptably subjective, but it reinforces the grave drawback posed by a lack of clinical acumen/training of these authors. Even a clinically trained victim/author should not function as the senior contributor to their own snakebite case report.

Lack of medically qualified review often amplifies clinically insignificant signs/ symptoms that are uncritically reported (see Table 4.1 and Section 4.5.1.4 for representative examples). Thus, unqualified commentary may subjectively sensationalize the mild, local effects of the bite (see Sections 4.5.1.4, 4.5.1.5, and 4.5.2). This is not surprising when the victim gives a report describing their pain, edema, and other sensations experienced after the bite, as the description will more likely be colored by effects felt rather than observed. These deficiencies can also result in unrecognized subtle, yet significant, alternative explanations for the observed symptoms and signs. Lack of analysis by an experienced clinician may result in failure to recognize medically important signs/effects or misinterpretation of the results of investigations. The importance of this flaw should not be underestimated. For example, as described previously, bites by *B. irregularis* have, based on inadequate observations, been thought to occasionally cause neurotoxicity, including cranial nerve palsies (see Sections 4.4.1 and 4.4.2). Similarly, the neurotoxicity of *M. monspessulanus* had little documented support until the recent strong case reported by Pommier and de Haro (2007; see Section 4.4.2). However, even though cranial nerve testing is robust, traditional, and well-established, under some circumstances even experienced clinicians can have difficulties with objective assessment of some cranial nerve functions. Modification of several scales designed for assessment of cranial nerve VII (facial nerve) has been proposed in order to aid objective examination of CN VII function and decrease subjective interpretation (Kang et al., 2002). Thus, as experienced physicians may have difficulty interpreting some clinical signs, it is clear that such signs would be subject to probable misinterpretation by a casual observer.

Adding to this serious issue of excessively subjective and often medically unqualified authorship is the common tendency to publish these reports in nonmedical journals, thus escaping review by medically qualified referees. Many reports have been published in herpetological or natural history journals, and these are often obscure periodicals. Obviously, without appropriate and qualified review, errors such as those outlined above are published and perpetuated. Therefore, incorrect interpretation of signs and symptoms may be introduced into the literature and gain provisional validity. This may propagate incorrect assignment of risk, and obfuscate evidence-based assessment of the medical importance of a given colubroid species. Unfortunately, cases of snakebite are often rejected by mainstream medical journals because this subject is considered to be esoteric, only peripherally important, or irrelevant. Therefore, although this limitation does not obviate the need for mandatory standards imposed on these published cases as they would be for any clinical report, it is necessary to recognize this unfortunately narrowed access to appropriate outlets for these reports.

Conclusions and Recommendations

It has been long recognized that the art of medicine injects subjectivity into the interpretation of the results of physical examination (Clarke and Fries, 1992; Joshua et al., 2005; Leder, 1990). It is essential that the attending physician maintains as much objectivity as possible in reporting a patient's presenting signs/symptoms. In the event of a lack of appropriate clinical training, as well as authorship of one's own case report, this inherent subjectivity is exaggerated by lack of medical acumen. This can result in misrepresentation of the objective effects of a bite. Even trained clinicians may excessively personalize their own symptoms and signs. Cases should be prepared by trained medical professionals (even if properly trained, the senior author should not be the victim/patient), and reviewed by appropriately medically qualified referees.

Due to space constraints and an unfortunate lack of interest, most medical journals do not accept these case reports. Since many of these reports describe clinically insignificant bites, this is to some extent understandable. Journals must devote most of their content to cases of greater interest, excitement, and general importance. However, a body of reports for a given species, even if indicating only minimal or minor effects of negligible medical significance, are very valuable in establishing the correct risk profile for that species. This will direct appropriate management of future cases and can be just as worthy of publication as cases showing severe envenoming. Regrettably, editors of medical journals may not fully comprehend this. Regardless of this prejudice, case reports should be submitted to clinical toxicology/toxinology journals, as these periodicals will provide review by qualified medical professionals familiar with envenomation.

4.5.1.4   Lack of Established Linkage Between Reported Serious Symptoms and the Snakebite

Any snakebite case study that describes serious or life-threatening signs/symptoms should provide data/clinically confirmed observations that support a causal relationship between the bite and the reported effects. In the vast majority of published reports describing serious envenoming inflicted by viperids, elapids, and atractaspidids such linkage is well established based on the temporal relationship between the bite and ensuing evolution of clinical features of envenomation. Envenomation from these snakes produces unmistakably serious effects such as coagulopathy, paresis, myotoxicity, vasculotoxicity, and many others (Minton, 1974; Russell, 1980; Warrell, 1995a, 1995b, 2004; White and Dart, 2008). Envenoming from Burmese (Myanmarese) populations of Russell's viper (*Daboia russelii*) can produce specifically distinctive pathology, such as pituitary infarct resulting in panhypopituitarism (Sheehan's syndrome; Warrell, 1995a).

In contrast, very few colubroids of the former colubrid assemblage have an established linkage between reported serious signs/symptoms and their bites. The local effects that usually occur after bites by most non-front-fanged colubroids are medically insignificant. Some species may rarely inflict bites causing moderate local effects that can resemble mild-to-moderate crotaline envenomation (Plates 4.24D–J and 4.40A and B). However, these effects are not clinically comparable to the severity of moderate-to-severe crotaline envenomation (Plate 4.92A–F). Only cases involving several members of the tribe, Dispholidini, and family, Natricidae, exhibit a clearly established linkage between reported life-threatening effects and their bites (see Section 4.3; Tables 4.1 and 4.3). Other species are associated through multiple reports with serious signs/symptoms, but without clear causal relationship established between the bite and reported effects (e.g., *B. irregularis*; see Section 4.4.1 and Table 4.1). Furthermore, the literature contains occasional reports of bites with serious effects inflicted by species of unknown medical importance (Table 4.1; Section 4.4). Several examples summarized below highlight significant flaws in these reports.

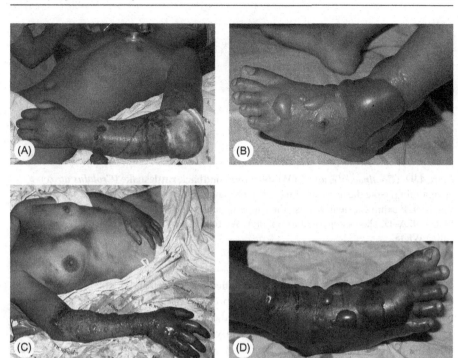

Plate 4.92 (A–F) Examples of local effects of crotaline viperid envenomations. Moderate-to-severe envenomation by most crotaline viperids produces local effects that are readily distinguishable from the comparatively milder local effects of some non-front-fanged colubroids. Aside from all hazard level 1 and two species of hazard level 2 (*P. olfersii* and *Malpolon monspessulanus*) "colubrids," there are no documented systemic effects associated with bites by the vast majority of non-front-fanged colubroids.
(A) Common lancehead (*Bothrops atrox*) envenoming, Pulcalpa, Peru. Note the marked edema, bleeding, ecchymoses, seepage of serosanguinous fluid, and evidence of extensive inflammation.
(B) Jararaca (*Bothrops jararaca*) envenoming, São Paulo, Brazil. The patient has large bullae, cellulitic changes, and edema.
(C) Malayan pit viper (*Calloselasma rhodostoma*) envenoming, Chantaburi, Thailand. The patient has severe blistering, edema, and early necrotic changes.
(D) Malayan pit viper (*Calloselasma rhodostoma*) envenoming, Trang, Thailand. Note the severe blistering, edema, and early necrotic changes.

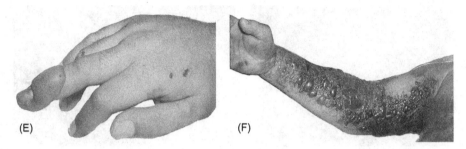

Plate 4.92 (*Continued*)(**E and F**) **Western diamondback rattlesnake (*Crotalus atrox*)** **envenoming.** Note the necrosis of the distal phalangeal skin in Plate 4.92E. The patient in Plate 4.92F exhibits extensive blistering, superficial necrosis, edema, and lymphadenopathy. Plate 4.92A–D, photos copyright to David A. Warrell; Plate 4.92E and F, photos copyright to Julian White.

Philodryas olfersii latirostris—As detailed in Section 4.4.4, this case described a vertiginous syndrome that developed 4–6 days after a bite from this species that caused no signs of envenomation. Due to the natural history of common causes of vertigo, this case report cannot be confidently linked to a medically insignificant bite after the aforementioned timeline (see Section 4.4.4). Evidence-based clinical analysis is essential when considering a case involving a species of unknown medical importance. As discussed in Section 4.4.4, common causes of vertigo are far more likely etiologies than the delayed effects of an otherwise inconsequential snakebite. These should be given first consideration and emphasized unless clear evidence for alternative causes is procured.

Hydrodynastes gigas—Initially minor local effects of a bite from a captive specimen were reportedly followed 9 h later by a series of concerning symptoms and signs, including an alleged movement disorder/transient paresis (Table 4.1; Section 4.4.3). This case contains features strongly suggesting somatosensory amplification precipitated by stress/anxiety (see Section 4.5.2). Aside from the local edema and pain, there are no data or information in the report that links the reported symptoms/signs (particularly the much delayed "paralysis," dysarthria, etc.) causally to any specific effects of the bite. One must distinguish between association, which may be coincidental or circumstantial, and causation. The brief tachycardia and premature atrial complexes spontaneously resolved and the local edema was said to have lasted about 5 days, although the patient reported (via telephone follow-up only) that the "muscle pain and weakness" persisted for almost 2 months. Since there was no further formal follow-up/medical review including physical examination, and investigations (see Section 4.4.3), these symptoms cannot be properly evaluated. Therefore, this unusual case does not provide sufficient evidence to support systemic effects of a bite inflicted by this species. In the few other documented cases, only mild-to-moderate local effects resulted from bites by this species (Table 4.1).

Macropisthodon rhodomelas (**blue-necked keel-back**)—The single report of a bite from this species was authored by a zoologist bitten by a specimen approximately

35 cm in total length collected on a nature reserve in Singapore (Subaraj, 2008; Table 4.1). The bite was protracted with penetration by a single enlarged maxillary tooth. He reported immediate local effects (paresthesia, mild bleeding, and pain) as well as concerning systemic symptoms including giddiness, "massive headache," "collapse," tachycardia, diaphoresis, dyspnea, and chest pain (Subaraj, 2008; Table 4.1). Speech difficulties and mild cognitive dysfunction persisted for almost 24 h. Although the author was attended by paramedics called by his companions, he refused transport to hospital or formal medical review (Subaraj, 2008).

This report is suggestive of an autonomic (anxiety-driven) response to this incident (see Section 4.5.2). The author indicated that *M. rhodomelas* was "not known to be venomous" and allowed the snake to maintain a grasp during the bite until it became increasingly painful. All of the symptoms/signs suggesting systemic effects spontaneously resolved in less than 24 h. This case lacks any objective assessment apart from a borderline tachycardia (pulse 100/min) measured by an ambulance paramedic. Therefore, it cannot be accepted as any evidence of medical risk from this species. As the data are insufficient to provide a thorough risk assessment of *M. rhodomelas*, careful handling of these snakes is advisable until further documentation is available.

Conclusions and Recommendations

Case reports describing bites from colubroids of unknown medical importance may include descriptions of serious symptoms/signs that lack a causative linkage with the bite, or with envenomation. It is imperative that these cases be analyzed using an evidence-based approach. Common, alternative etiologies should be carefully considered. Case reports are frequently excessively subjective and carry, or imply, unsupported speculative conclusions. A carefully formulated and clinically astute differential diagnosis is more likely to clarify the natural history and true etiology of the illness, as opposed to anxiety-driven responses to a bite that may well be medically insignificant.

4.5.1.5 Insufficient or Irrelevant Documentation of History and Clinical Features/Analysis

Many reports contain incomplete or irrelevant details with a concomitant lack of critical, clinically knowledgeable analysis. Consideration of a representative case featuring multiple flaws illustrates the difficulty in assessing the risk assigned to a given species.

Phalotris trilineatus (Argentine black-headed snake; Plate 4.37A–C) has been considered as a species of possible medical importance based on anecdotal evidence. Several reports have suggested significant medical effects resulting from bites by this species, but they have appeared in limited-circulation or institution-based, obscure periodicals (Table 4.1). In one of only two documented cases, the herpetologist victim/author was presented with a juvenile specimen of this species after having "a lot of barbecue and beer at lunch" (de Lema, 2007). The author was bitten while he identified the specimen. He reported that his curiosity led him to allow a protracted bite until a "strong growing burning sensation ... became unbearable," at which time the snake was removed (de Lema, 2007). The author eventually drove himself to the hospital, took an unknown dose of aspirin, and reported having fairly constant gingival bleeding. He described a serious clinical course that spanned 5 days. Within 67 h postbite, he reported experiencing headache, "strong maxillary hemorrhage," "right radial arm bone pain," and drowsiness (de Lema, 2007). Over the next few days he reported fatigue, "strong gingivorrhage," hematuria, bone pain in upper and lower limbs, "anuria," and "left kidney failure" (de Lema, 2007). He precisely detailed his diet and stool character. It is noteworthy that during a period of presumed AKI that would have been expected to be associated with uremia, he reported that his appetite remained unabated and commented on his enjoyment of his meals.

The author indicated that a "well-known toxicologist" was consulted and recommended left nephrectomy with "graft of an artificial kidney" (de Lema, 2007). However, shortly thereafter, the author added that tests indicated normal kidney function and that "surgery was not necessary ... but it was missing a stimulant factor of the kidneys because they were almost inert ... it was not noticed jaundice nor anemia ..." (de Lema, 2007). Earlier in the account, without including specific laboratory values, the author reported coagulopathy and anemia. Treatment reportedly consisted of multiple blood transfusions, vitamin K, and five ampoules of "global anti-ophidic serum" (de Lema, 2007). The author also took large quantities of a homeopathic botanical mixture containing three plant species. The reported symptoms/signs fully resolved approximately 7–10 days following the incident (de Lema, 2007).

Conclusions and Recommendations

This case account, based on the author/victim's case notes, contains a mixture of conflicting terminology, misinformation (e.g., "graft of an artificial kidney"), incorrect interpretations, speculation, and inappropriate personal details. As the author is a well-regarded herpetologist, the identification of the snake was probably accurate. Also, although the author's genuine desire to precisely describe his experience is unquestioned, there is no clear linkage between the described clinical course and the bite. Included also are incorrect diagnoses, management that is unsupported by information regarding the disease described in the report, and use of nonallopathic therapeutics of unproven efficacy.

Basic requirements of any clinical case report include clarity, accuracy, inclusion of information directly relevant to the case, well-reasoned consideration of a differential diagnosis, and practical clinical acumen. While it is recognized that English was not the author's first language, and that this and/or poor translation may have contributed to a lack of clarity, this report exhibits multiple flaws. Informed analysis of any snakebite case study must be followed by equally measured and accurate written communication of relevant, important features of the case. As the case reported by de Lema (2007) lacks these essential components, this report cannot be used to assess the medical importance of *P. trilineatus*.

4.5.2   Perceived Versus Evidence-Based Risk: Human Response to Trauma and Somatosensory Amplification

Human response to any medical effect from *any* bite inflicted by a snake may lead to disproportionate concerns. In this, the individual physiological response to minor

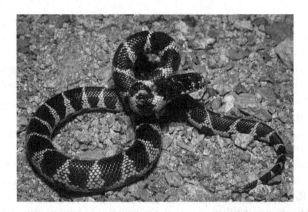

Plate 4.93 Desert kingsnake (*Lampropeltis getula splendida*). The colubrine genus *Lampropeltis* contains approximately nine species (with >40 subspecies). Many of these are attractively patterned and are popular in private collections. Some of these snakes have plasma α_1-albumins that probably antagonize the vascular endothelial receptor for crotaline venom proteolytic hemorrhagins, and thereby provide resistance against some crotaline venoms (Weinstein et al., 1992). This allows some species of *Lampropeltis* to opportunistically prey on sympatric crotaline snakes. These snakes lack Duvernoy's glands as well as any specialized dentition, and bites are medically insignificant.
Photo copyright to Julian White.

trauma (e.g., penetration of a steel nail in a digit, or mild blunt impact) may produce variable erythema, reactive edema, and ecchymoses. Therefore, even minor trauma without any toxic insult may be interpreted subjectively when such trauma is inflicted by a snakebite. For example, de Haro and Pommier (2003) reported a case of *Lampropeltis* spp. (king or milk snake species, e.g., Plate 4.93) bite that featured pain, edema, and lymphangitis. In contrast, Weed (1993) reported a *Lampropeltis* spp. bite without any significant effects. Several of us have personally experienced and observed numerous bites from various *Lampropeltis* spp. without any significant effects. Members of the tribe Lampropeltini either lack Duvernoy's glands or exhibit structures interpreted by some investigators as "atrophied" Duvernoy's ("venom") glands (Fry et al., 2008), and any effect from their bites can be ascribed to minor physical trauma and/or individual atopic tendencies towards ophidian saliva. It is noteworthy that in the cases cited above, the individuals bitten by *Lampropeltis* spp. were concerned enough by the experience to present at a local emergency room. Thus, a significant anxiety-driven somatosensory amplification component is probably present in a number of these cases (e.g., *H. gigas*, Manning et al., 1999; *M. rhodomelas*, Subaraj, 2008; Table 4.1). Some authors have opined that a bite from any ophidian species can frighten the victim so profoundly that a bitten patient may appear "half-dead with fear" (Saha and Hati, 1998). Although this may seem extreme, a substantial number of people in Western and Third World cultures are deeply influenced by snakes, and the prospect of snakebite is perceived as tantamount to a death sentence.[21] This can present

---

[21] As noted previously (see section 4.4.7), even innocuous lizards such as the leopard gecko (*Eublepharis macularis*) may be viewed as causing "instant death" on contact.

tangible risk as some studies enrolling patients with baseline generalized anxiety disorder (GAD) found a highly significant independent association of GAD with markedly increased (74%) cardiovascular event rate (Martens et al., 2010). Therefore, such fear of snakebite can conceivably precipitate a serious cardiovascular consequence in those with GAD. Additionally, some may suffer localized trauma from unobserved bites or stings from other nonophidian sources, and attribute the symptoms to a bite from a snake because they are known to inhabit the geographic region.

Somatosensory amplification and symptom attribution influencing clinical presentation are common phenomena and can be culturally influenced (Duddu et al., 2006; Kirmayer et al., 1994). Symptom attribution style and concomitant cultural mores may contribute to the interpretation of a given somatic complaint (Kirmayer et al., 1995; Robbins and Kirmayer, 1991). Some evidence suggests that somatosensory amplification is neither sensitive nor specific to somatizing states, and other factors—such as anxiety and/or additional circumstantial factors such as depression—may have influence (Duddu et al., 2006).

Brief consideration of some representative case scenarios may help illustrate the potential role of anxiety in somatosensory amplification. Among a series of patients with minor injuries on the arms or shoulder sustained from grazing bullet wounds or superficial knife lacerations, several complained of a broad spectrum of symptoms, including low back pain, chest pain, palpitations, "severe" headache, abdominal pain/nausea, and lower-limb "numbness"/paresthesia (SAW, personal observations). Clearly, assessment of these patients should not lead to the inclusion of these symptoms as likely direct consequence of either a grazing bullet wound or minor laceration from a knife. Rather, these are individual autonomic, anxiety-driven responses (some with somatosensory amplification) to traumatic events that had a marked psychological effect on the patient (i.e., being shot or attacked by a knife-wielding assailant in a street altercation). It is noteworthy that in several of these cases, the patients had previously experienced similar wounds. This did not alter their acute psychological response. Although the physical pathology was clinically mild, and the patient's psychological response was partly anxiety driven, the need for clinical management of the primary presenting complaint remains. Similarly, in the case of an apparently medically insignificant snakebite inflicted by a species of unknown medical importance, the physician must evaluate the symptoms with careful systems-based physical examination and supporting investigations as indicated. The majority of the cases reviewed here (Table 4.1) suggest a significant degree of subjective interpretation by nonmedically qualified authors, and an absence of appropriate formal clinical review (Table 4.1; see Section 4.5.1). Therefore, it is likely that some of these cases carry marked subjective bias toward symptoms interpreted (or misinterpreted) by the victims themselves and, in some cases, with an anxiety and/or somatosensory amplification contribution to the presentation. Although this may simply be reported as "severe" local effects, occasionally serious disproportionate symptoms/signs without clear linkage to the inflicted bite are reported (e.g., see Sections 4.4 and 4.5.1; Table 4.1). Even experienced field herpetologists may exhibit anxiety after sustaining a bite from an ophidian species of unknown medical importance. Possibly, having knowledge of the enlarged dentition and presence of Duvernoy's glands in a given taxa may provide fuel for concerns regarding unknown clinical potential. Also, the majority of these bites occur during intentional contact with the snake. Therefore, the inherent curiosity of many professional biologists and interested amateurs occasionally results in a protracted bite due to interest in "what might happen" (e.g., see Sections 4.5.1, 4.5.1.4, and 4.5.1.5 and Appendix A). This subjective experiment projects uncertainty regarding possible effects and thus can generate anxiety regarding an unforeseen response perceived as clinically significant.

4.6 Recommendations for Management of Medically Significant "Colubrid" Bites

4.6.1 General

Most victims bitten by non-front-fanged colubroid snakes report mild, usually medically insignificant effects (Table 4.1; previous sections). However, as detailed in Sections 4.3 and 4.4, bites by some taxa prove serious and occasionally cause fatal envenomation. Therefore, as the majority of these diverse colubroids are of unknown medical importance, specific management guidelines cannot be provided for most species. Table 4.3 assesses the medical risk of species for which sufficient information is available to evaluate their potential hazard index. Table 4.3 also summarizes recommendations for management of medically significant bites inflicted by these species. Significant envenomation from taxa assigned with a level 1 hazard index require admission, extended observation, investigations/serial monitoring focused on hemostatic and renal functions, supportive measures as indicated (see later), and specific antivenom as available (Table 4.3; Section 4.3). Although comprehensive coagulation panels can help further characterize the nature of the hemorrhagic diathesis, evidence suggests that a combination of the PT and aPTT is a sufficient and cost-effective endpoint for treating venom-induced consumptive coagulopathy (Isbister et al., 2006). Some patients bitten by hazard level 1 colubrids may exhibit gingival bleeding as is observed in envenomings by front-fanged colubroids such as the Malayan pit viper (*Calloselasma rhodostoma*; see Plate 4.94). As noted previously, observations made during management of some life-threatening *R. tigrinus* envenomations have suggested that simple urine dipsticks may detect proteinuria and/or hemoglobinuria, thereby providing an early indicator of systemic envenomation (see later). In rural medical facilities without access to any instrumented testing, the bedside 20-min whole blood clotting test provides a reasonably reliable guide to the presence of coagulopathy (Warrell, 1995a, 1995b). Early discharge of these patients is strongly discouraged.

Those with level 2 or 2/3 hazard indices often only require local wound care, but occasional bites may produce systemic effects of unclear etiology, especially in pediatric and, possibly, geriatric patients (see Sections 4.4.1 and 4.4.2 and Tables 4.1 and 4.3). Species with a level 3 hazard ranking commonly produce minor local effects, but may produce moderate local effects (Table 4.3). Some may have the potential for

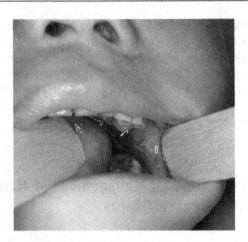

Plate 4.94 Bleeding gingival mucosa after envenoming by the Malayan pit viper
(*Calloselasma rhodostoma*), **Chantaburi, Thailand.** As is observed in victims envenomated by
some venomous species such as the crotaline viperid, *C. rhodostoma*, and the viperine viperid,
Echis spp., patients with serious envenomation by hazard level 1 colubrids may present with (or
later develop) bleeding from numerous anatomical sites including the gingival sulcus.
Photo copyright to David A. Warrell.

mild systemic effects, but to date there are insufficient data to establish this risk (see
Table 4.1 and Sections 4.4 and 4.5). The majority of bites from these species require
only wound care and simple supportive measures as indicated (i.e., tetanus prophylaxis; Table 4.3). An overview of evidence-supported symptoms and signs reported
in documented bites of non-front-fanged colubroids is provided in Table 4.4. As indicated above, most commonly only mild local effects are reported, but moderate local
edema, ecchymoses, and occasionally lymphadenopathy may occur after bites from a
handful of species (Tables 4.1 and 4.4).

4.6.2 Specific

4.6.2.1   First Aid

There is no recommended *specific* first aid other than the globally applicable WHO
recommended use of immobilization of the bitten limb and patient as universally
safe first aid for all snakebites. There is no direct evidence to support the use or
benefit of pressure-immobilization (PI)[22] or pressure pad for acute management of
hazard 1 colubrid bites. However, as many of these bites are not generally associated with significant local tissue injury, there is no clear contraindication for use of
PI either. Also, since limited Australian experience may indicate a possible benefit
for PI in delaying onset of envenoming, it is reasonable to consider PI for hazard
level 1 colubrid bites, with the understanding that this is unproven first aid in this
setting. Although rapid onset of non-front-fanged colubroid (principally, hazard level

[22] The use and correct application of PI is detailed at www.toxinology.com

1 colubrid) envenomation has not been described, this consideration may assume greater weight when the bite occurs in a remote location and/or there is anticipation of an extensive delay for transport to a medical facility. Further cases of neurotoxic envenomation from species such as *M. monspessulanus* would be required in order to support the use of PI in bites from these species. As in any snakebite, harmful and/or useless practices must be avoided [e.g., tourniquets, cut/suction, venom extractors, electric current, ligature/cryotherapy, application of permanganate or other oxidizing agents or proteases (e.g., meat tenderizers such as papain), etc.], and the patient should be counseled, with efforts to keep the patient as calm and still as possible. The patient should avoid any unnecessary movements and be carried on a litter if possible (transport by ambulance is obviously strongly recommended). Expeditious transport to a Level 1 (if possible) trauma facility is mandatory. Although many hazard level 1 colubrid bites are serious, most cases may produce significant bleeding and complications but are not fatal.

4.6.2.2 Evaluation of the Patient

Patient assessment should follow standard protocol as in any presentation with careful attention to medication regimens [especially NSAIDS, warfarin, some antidepressants (particularly mixed reuptake inhibitors such as venlafaxine that predispose to ecchymoses), platelet inhibitors, etc.]; medical history [e.g., comorbidities such as diabetes may predispose to more serious local wounds and delayed healing with increased risk of infection; psychiatric illnesses may increase anxiety and somatosensory amplification as well as potential exacerbation of cardiovascular comorbidities (see previous section), neurological history (i.e., seizures), etc.]; drug and alcohol use and previous history of snakebites (including nonvenomous); maintenance/husbandry of captive reptiles and exposure to lyophilized venoms (potential risk for sensitization/anaphylaxis; see later). Also, recent surgical wounds, dental work, tattoos or piercings, and even trauma-induced bruises should be carefully examined, as in some cases these may be subject to persistent bleeding (especially after envenoming from hazard level 1 species; Table 4.2). Patients presenting after being bitten by hazard level 1 colubrids must be observed and monitored for as long as necessary in order to rule out coagulopathy, that may have a delayed onset (e.g., several days).

4.6.2.3 Confirmation of Snake Identification

The identity of the snake must be verified and taxonomically documented. If the snake is a captive specimen, its identity will often be known to the victim. However, this requires evaluation on a case-by-case basis. For instance, consider issues regarding confusion between potentially life-threatening species and those without medical importance (e.g., *Amphiesma stolata* and *R. tigrinus*; see Section 4.3 and Plates 4.45A and B, 4.46A and B, and 4.84A–E), as well as specimens incorrectly identified by vendors or incorrect information obtained via the Internet. Identification often requires professional verification (see Section 4.5.1.1).

Although exotic snakebite victims/owners usually know the identity of the snake responsible for biting them, they may use misleading common names for it. For example, the "Western hog-nosed viper" is strictly a Central American pit viper (*Porthidium ophryomegas*), but this name has been used mistakenly for a North American non-front-fanged colubroid, the Western hog-nosed snake (*Heterodon nasicus*). A "South American Parrot snake" could be a pit viper *Bothrops* (*Bothriopsis*) *bilineata*, but this name is usually applied to the non-front-fanged colubroid, *Leptophis ahaetulla*. "Mangrove snake" could mean a South Eastern Asian pit viper (*Cryptelytrops/Trimeresurus purpureomaculatus*), but usually refers to non-front-fanged colubroids, either the South Asian *Boiga dendrophila* or the North American natricid from Florida, *Nerodia clarkii compressicauda* (Minton, 1996; Warrell, 2009).

4.6.2.4 Toxinologist Consultation

In cases that involve significant local effects, consultation with a clinical toxinologist is at the discretion of the attending physician. In cases with expanding local effects or systemic effects, consultation is strongly recommended. However, determining expertise in clinical toxinology is currently problematic, as there is no registered medical college/board specifically standardizing qualification in clinical toxinology, a subspecialty of medical toxicology. As a bare minimum, anyone claiming to be a clinical toxinologist should: (a) have an appropriate medical qualification, and preferably a postgraduate medical qualification as well, relevant to toxinology; (b) have undertaken at least some recognized and tested training in clinical toxinology (currently there is only one such international-level training course available), or has direct mentored training with a recognized authority in the field; and, ideally, (c) have clear peer acceptance of expertise (this might be through a body of published work, or through accreditation with a poisons information center or clinical toxicology center).

4.6.2.5 Wound Care

Any significant wound and related local effects require meticulous decontamination, irrigation, and careful observation. Aspiration of blisters is typically unnecessary, as these very rarely yield any significant cultures. Although sometimes difficult to distinguish from local effects of envenomation, whenever possible antibiotics should only be used with evident signs of infection such as spreading erythema, presence of purulent discharge, and pyrexia (see Section 4.6.2.15). Concerns regarding potential wound contamination (e.g., by saprophytic or marine organisms) may justify prompt initiation of an appropriate antibiotic regimen. If antibiotics are deemed necessary, broad-spectrum coverage can be accomplished with amoxicillin/clavulanate. Doxycycline or clindamycin may be used in penicillin-allergic patients (Weinstein and Keyler, 2009), and other combinations have been recommended (see later). Patients with comorbidities such as diabetes mellitus require particularly close scrutiny of significant wounds sustained from any snakebite.

4.6.2.6 Basic Supportive Measures

Any patient reportedly bitten by a colubroid snake presenting with clinically significant symptoms should be provided with basic supportive measures. These are outlined in

Table 4.3 and include i.v. access and fluid resuscitation as needed, wound evaluation, and management as noted previously, and attention to case-specific requirements (e.g., nasal cannula and oxygen). Need for insertion of central lines and/or repeated venipuncture must be cautiously considered in any case suggestive of possible coagulopathy due to the risk of uncontrollable bleeding (see Tables 4.1 and 4.3 and Section 4.3). Arterial puncture and/or lines are contraindicated.

Patients with comorbidities such as ischemic heart disease may require admission to a cardiac telemetry unit, as the anxiety/elevated catecholamine stimulation may exacerbate cardiac symptoms (e.g., angina, dyspnea). Similarly, patients with psychiatric disorders (particularly generalized anxiety disorder or psychotic illnesses) may require reinforced reassurance and mild sedation. Supportive management is determined on a case-by-case basis due to individual levels of anxiety, the nature of the bite and its effects, and the extent of comorbid pathology.

4.6.2.7 Antivenom

The only antivenoms available for non-front-fanged colubroid snakes are prepared against two hazard level 1 species (*D. typus* and *R. tigrinus*; Table 4.3). As noted, there are no commercial antivenoms against any species of *Thelotornis*, and antivenom against *D. typus* venom does not cross-react with or paraspecifically neutralize *Thelotornis* venoms (Atkinson et al., 1980; Du Toit, 1980; Visser and Chapman, 1978).

Antivenom Against *D. typus*

Effective antivenom against *D. typus* was first documented by Grasset and Shaafsma (1940). These investigators also reported lack of efficacy of South African Institute for Medical Research (SAIMR; now, South African Vaccine Producers, SAVP) polyvalent antivenom for *D. typus* envenoming (Grasset and Shaafsma, 1940). Anti-*D. typus* antivenom has been used in a significant number of serious envenoming cases, and it clearly reverses the life-threatening coagulopathy that characterizes the venom disease from this species (Table 4.1). For example, Lakier and Fritz (1969) administered four ampoules of anti-*D. typus* antivenom to a patient with life-threatening coagulopathy. The antivenom effectively reversed the patient's consumptive coagulopathy and DIC. It is important to note that this patient still received dialysis due to probable microangiopathic hemolytic anemia (MAHA) with concomitant AKI due to hemoglobinuric nephropathy (Lakier and Fritz, 1969). A thromboelastographic analysis indicated reversal of an evolving consumptive coagulopathy following administration of two ampoules of *D. typus* antivenom in a 10-year-old patient envenomed by a *D. typus* (Aitchison, 1990). A similarly rapid reversal was noted in a delayed presentation after a life-threatening *D. typus* envenoming. The patient presented 60 h after a bite from a snake tentatively identified as either a "birdsnake or a boomslang" (Du Toit, 1980). It is noteworthy that the patient, a native "snake charmer," incorrectly identified the snake as a green mamba (Eastern green mamba, *Dendroaspis angusticeps*; although these snakes look significantly different, a casual or excited observer could mistake their identities; see Plate 4.95A and B, and compare with Plate 4.20A–C). The patient was semicomatose on arrival and exhibited marked anemia and consumptive coagulopathy (Du Toit, 1980). Two vials of anti-*D. typus*

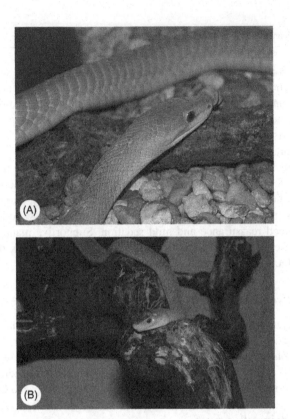

Plate 4.95 (A and B) Eastern green or common mamba; Groen Mamba, Ilumangiu
(*Dendroaspis angusticeps*). The African genus *Dendroaspis* contains four species of fast-moving, distinctive elapids. *Dendroaspis angusticeps* is medically important throughout its range (mid-East Africa-eastern South Africa), but is a shy and retiring species that attains an average adult length of approximately 1.80 m. However, its bite can be fatal; numerous life-threatening and fatal cases have been well documented. Its venom (i.p. murine LD_{50} ranges between 0.25 and 0.70 mg/kg) has been thoroughly studied, and several three-finger-fold postsynaptic muscarinic neurotoxins/α_2-adrenocepter antagonists, natriuretic peptides as well as novel potassium ion channel/mixed agonist/antagonizing toxins (dendrotoxins that sequentially suppress, then enhance acetylcholine release, thereby excessively facilitating and ultimately "exhausting" synaptic transmission resulting in paralysis), acetylcholinesterase inhibitors (fasciculins), and other components have been characterized. These toxins are useful biomedical tools and may hold some potential as therapeutics. Although these snakes have a distinct appearance, a casual observer may mistake (especially from a distance) for *D. angusticeps* other similarly colored ophidian species such as the green or "jungle phase" hazard level 1 colubrid, *D. typus* (compare Plate 4.95B with Plate 4.20A–D), or one of the medically unimportant arboreal colubrines, such as the African green, bush, forest, wood, or tree snakes, *Philothamnus* spp. (approximately 18 species). It is worth noting that one of the other members of the genus *Dendroaspis*, the black mamba (*D. polylepis*), has been subjected to much misinformed sensationalism. Although the body color of this snake is variable, it typically is gray, and the common name is derived from the dark color of the buccal mucosa. It is a large species (occasionally exceeding 3.5 m) with highly toxic venom (equal to the common Asian cobra, *Naja naja*; the i.p. murine LD_{50} averaging 0.30 mg/kg) can be aggressive if molested; fatal bites are well documented. The venom apparatus of these snakes is representative of the "proteroglyphous" condition with fixed, erected, canaliculated fangs.
Photos copyright to Julian White.

antivenom were provided 86h postenvenoming. Reversal was dramatic and immediate. The patient showed almost full clinical recovery 30h after antivenom administration (Du Toit, 1980; see also sections 4.1.1.6 and 4.13).

As demonstrated by these representative cases, although additional therapies directed at correction of anemia and afibrinogenemia have been used (see later and Table 4.1), antivenom is the only evidence-based effective treatment for life-threatening *D. typus* envenoming. Clearly, delayed presentation (even up to approximately 5 days postenvenoming) is not a contraindication to administering this antivenom, if available, provided that there is persisting evidence of systemic envenomation (WHO AFRO, 2010). Availability is a significant issue, but delay to provision of antivenom should not influence any effort to procure at least two ampoules for use in serious cases. Table 4.3 outlines a recommended approach to administering antivenom for treatment of *D. typus* envenoming.

Reactions to SAVP (SAIMR) Anti-*D. typus* Antivenom

Authors of several case studies of *D. typus* envenoming treated with monospecific antivenom have raised concerns regarding reportedly frequent hypersensitivity reactions, including anaphylaxis associated with this antivenom (Du Toit, 1980). A limited retrospective review reported that treatment for anaphylaxis was required in three out of five patients who received anti-*D. typus* antivenom (Du Toit, 1980). However, like all antivenoms, SAVP equine $F(ab')_2$ monospecific boomslang antivenom has occasionally caused early anaphylactic reactions, but the danger of these reactions must not be exaggerated. Although they may, on rare occasions, be life threatening, there have been very few reported deaths and even the most severe reactions are eminently controllable by the early use of i.m. epinephrine. The terminology and perceived mechanism of early antivenom reactions have been plagued by confusing and incorrect terminology, made worse by a consensus review of definitions of allergic phenomena (Johansson et al., 2004). The use of terms, such as "allergic," "sensitization," or "hypersensitization," implying that early anaphylactic reactions to antivenoms were the result of prior sensitization to animal serum proteins ignored abundant published evidence of lack of specific IgE as a basis for these reactions. According to the classic Gell and Coombs (1963) classification, Type I immediate hypersensitivity reactions are IgE-mediated. However, skin tests, the most sensitive means of detecting specific IgE hypersensitization, are negative in the vast majority of patients who suffer early antivenom reactions (Cupo et al., 1991; Malasit et al., 1986), hence the futility of skin (or conjunctival) testing with antivenom before therapeutic use as these tests have no predictive value. Early antivenom reactions usually consist of pruritus and/or urticaria, but in about 10% of cases more severe features of anaphylaxis develop. They were formerly designated "anaphylactoid" reactions to distinguish them from cross-linked IgE-mediated anaphylaxis, but nomenclatural revisions now include them in the term "anaphylactic reactions" (Johansson et al., 2004). Reactions to any particular antivenom are dose dependent (Reid, 1980) in a positively monotonic fashion, like reactions to macromolecules and *N*-acetylcysteine that occur in patients not previously exposed and lacking detectable specific IgE. Comparison of the low reactogenicity of single vial treatment with antivenom that is sufficient for most cases of envenoming by scorpions, spiders, and European *Vipera*, with the high reactogenicity of the larger doses of antivenom required to treat some snakebites (Cardoso et al., 1993) further illustrates this important point (Chippaux and Boyer, 2010). The mechanism of the vast majority of antivenom reactions has nothing to do with acquired hypersensitivity or IgE, but to complement activation by aggregates of IgG or its fragments, or to osmotic effects of the large intravenously administered bolus of antiserum protein. In a prospective review of 147 patients who presented with snakebites in a rural South African hospital, 13 out of 17 treated with SAVP/SAIMR polyvalent antivenom developed early, potentially severe anaphylactic reactions (including urticaria, bronchospasm, angioedema, and hypotension; Moran et al., 1998).

Current evidence contraindicates pretreatment with epinephrine, antihistamines, or glucocorticoids (Table 4.3; Weinstein et al., 2009). However, a recent low-power study compared the incidence of early reactions in envenomed patients given pretreatment with i.v. hydrocortisone and diphenhydramine and in whom diluted antivenom was infused over 1 h, to historical controls prior to slow infusion of equine-derived antivenom with those who had no premedication and in whom undiluted antivenom was given via i.v. push injection over about 10 min (Caron et al., 2009). This investigation suggested that premedication combined with slow administration of diluted antivenom might reduce the frequency and severity of antivenom-related reactions. In reviewing the literature, the authors found no convincing evidence that corticosteroid, histamine (H-1) blockers, or epinephrine, used singly or in combination, significantly decreased the incidence of antivenom reactions (Caron et al., 2009). Another study reported that discretionary use of premedication did not reduce the frequency of reactions (Isbister et al., 2009). Therefore, until further study clarifies this issue, antivenom is best administered with slow i.v. infusion following a standard dilution (see Table 4.3). In the event of a reaction (urticaria, wheeze/rhonchi, angioedema, laryngospasm, hypotension, GI symptoms, etc.), the infusion should be discontinued and the patient should immediately be given i.m. epinephrine urgently, followed by an i.v. antihistamine H-1 blocker such as chlorpheniramine, and i.v. hydrocortisone. Patients with severe bronchoconstriction/spasm should be given nebulized salbutamol (or another β_2-agonist) for rhonchus/wheeze. When the reaction has subsided, the antivenom infusion can be resumed at a slower rate in order to complete the full dose, but with continued close vigilance for any signs of further reaction. The risk of early anaphylactic reactions is one reason why use of antivenom by nonmedically qualified persons outside of a medical facility is discouraged. It emphasizes the need to provide antivenom in a hospital setting (e.g., Level I–II trauma facility) that is fully equipped to manage a patient with life-threatening anaphylaxis.

A Further Comment on Thelotornis Envenoming and the Lack of Commercial Antivenom

As there is no anti-*Thelotornis* antivenom commercially available, it is fortunate that envenoming from *Thelotornis* spp. is so rare. In any case of serious *Thelotornis* envenoming, consultation with an experienced clinical toxinologist via a poison control center is mandatory. Treatment must therefore focus on managing hemostatic deficiencies resulting from the consumptive coagulopathy and hemorrhagic diathesis. Although rapidly falling hemoglobin must be addressed, it is crucial to remain cognizant of possible hemoglobinuric nephropathy and resulting ARF that may be poorly responsive to diuretics or dialysis (Table 4.1; Mebs et al., 1978). Therefore, hematocrit should be maintained with concomitant serial evaluation of renal function (i.e., infuse PRBCs sufficient to sustain low normal hemoglobin in the setting of an evolving nephropathy). Thrombocytopenia can be addressed with platelet transfusion. There are no data regarding treatment of *Thelotornis* or any other consumptive coagulopathic envenoming with medications used for endotoxin-related DIC such as the recombinant antithrombotic, α-drotrecogin. Similarly, use of FFP/cryoprecipitate is controversial and of unproven efficacy, but could be considered in life-threatening cases (see later). Heparin and fibrinolytics can cause further uncontrolled bleeding and are absolutely contraindicated, although some data suggest possible efficacy (see later).

Antivenom Against *R. tigrinus*

This antivenom first became available in 1986 and was raised in both rabbits and goats (Kawamura et al., 1986). The rabbit- and goat-derived antivenoms (The Japan Snake Institute, Japan) were tested in small groups of mice and reportedly neutralized 60 µg [24 murine minimal lethal doses (MLD)] and 200 µg (80 MLD) of *R. tigrinus* venom, respectively (Kawamura et al., 1988). Shortly after production and initial animal testing, the rabbit-derived antivenom was used to successfully treat a serious case of *R. tigrinus* envenoming with DIC (Wakamatsu et al., 1986). There was dramatic reversal of a consumptive coagulopathy similar to the previously discussed cases of *D. typus* envenoming treated with anti-*D. typus* antivenom (see previous section and Table 4.1). Another similarity with management of *D. typus* envenoming is the efficacy of anti-*R. tigrinus* antivenom used in treatment of envenoming with delayed presentation. The patient in the case noted earlier presented some 50 h after the bite and was effectively treated with antivenom (Wakamatsu et al., 1986).

Similar efficacy was reported with anti-*R. tigrinus* antivenom used in two cases documented by Kikuchi et al. (1987). In one of these cases, a pediatric patient was treated almost 48 h after a bite from a presumed *R. tigrinus*. The patient presented with consumptive coagulopathy, hematuria, and hemorrhagic diathesis (Kikuchi et al., 1987). The coagulopathy was reversed within approximately 12 h after infusion of one ampoule of antivenom (Kikuchi et al., 1987). Assessment of several cases of *R. tigrinus* envenoming suggested that there was notable variability in time between the bite and development of systemic clinical effects (4–30 h; Kikuchi et al., 1987; Ogawa and Sawai, 1986; Wakamatsu et al., 1986). Kikuchi et al. (1987) observed that microhematuria, detected 1 h after the bite in one case, might be an early sign of developing systemic hemorrhagic diathesis. Thus, careful clinical evaluation of patients bitten by *R. tigrinus* may facilitate early recognition of an evolving systemic envenomation and thereby expedite procurement and administration of antivenom.

Another pediatric case featured consumptive coagulopathy and hemorrhagic diathesis (Akimoto et al., 1991). The patient was treated 21.5 h postenvenoming with one ampoule of caprine-derived anti-*R. tigrinus* antivenom. Within 5 h, the coagulopathy and hemorrhage had been controlled, and the patient showed rapid clinical improvement (Akimoto et al., 1991).

Both rabbit- and goat-derived antivenoms were clinically effective, and none of the patients developed antivenom reactions. Available data suggest that one ampoule of either goat- or rabbit-derived antivenom should be sufficient to treat most serious envenomations by R. tigrinus. In the setting of a life-threatening envenomation from this species, procurement of two ampoules is recommended. However, this antivenom is in short supply and difficult to obtain.

Treatment of R. subminiatus Envenoming

Although there is no commercial antivenom against R. subminiatus venom, Kawamura et al. (1988) reported that 0.1 mL of anti-R. tigrinus rabbit-derived antivenom neutralized 46. 2 μg (10.8 MLD) of R. subminiatus venom. This suggests that anti-R. tigrinus antivenom can provide paraspecific protection against R. subminiatus envenomation.

To date, no documented case of R. subminiatus envenomation has been managed with R. tigrinus antivenom. Some cases have resolved without any specific treatment (Hoffmann et al., 1992), while others have been managed with supportive measures consisting of infusions of fibrinogen, low-dose heparin (this is strongly discouraged; see later) and exchange blood transfusion (Zotz et al., 1991) or comprehensive replacement therapy (i.e., repeated infusions of packed red blood cells (PRBCs), fresh frozen plasma (FFP)/cryoprecipitate, fibrinogen ± platelets; Cable et al., 1984; Mather et al., 1978). In a recent case of R. subminiatus envenoming in the Netherlands, the patient's severe bleeding diathesis had resolved spontaneously by the time R. tigrinus antivenom had arrived from the Japan Snake Institute (DAW, personal communication). Another recent case of a European victim bitten in Thailand while handling a wild-caught R. subminiatus was managed without antivenom (DAW, personal communication).

In the case reported by Zotz et al. (1991), repeated exchange blood transfusion, fibrinogen, and low-dose heparin resulted in intermittent cessation of bleeding. The bleeding recurred between treatments, and the course of this hemorrhagic diathesis continued for about 10 days. Hemostatic parameters remained abnormal for over 1 month (Zotz et al., 1991). With replacement therapy, a patient envenomed by a R. subminiatus had undetectable fibrinogen for 1 week after the bite (Cable et al., 1984). The patient's bleeding ceased, but similar to that reported by Zotz et al. (1991) did not have normal hemostatic parameters for 2 weeks after discharge (Cable et al., 1984).

Serious cases of R. subminiatus envenomation should be treated in the same way as recommended for R. tigrinus. As noted when considering R. tigrinus envenomation, procurement of antivenom is the primary issue complicating optimal management of envenomation by these snakes.

Polyvalent Antivenoms Should Not Be Used for Treating Colubrid Bites

A substantial number of colubrid bites from species of unknown medical importance have been inappropriately treated with polyvalent antivenoms (Table 4.1; Section 4.5.1.1). This has been most commonly documented in bites from South American species, particularly Philodryas spp. (Table 4.1; Sections 4.1.1 and 4.5.1.1), and South Asian species (Ariaratnam et al., 2009; Viravan et al., 1992).

Aside from possible efficacy of *R. tigrinus* antivenom for envenomation by the congener, *R. subminiatus*, no data currently available support provision of any non-specific antivenom for any non-front-fanged colubroid bite. As detailed in the previous sections, the only antivenoms available against any of these snakes are prepared against two hazard level 1 species (*D. typus* and *R. tigrinus*; Table 4.3). There is no clinical evidence of paraspecific protection afforded by any polyvalent or nonspecific monovalent antivenom against the effects of any non-front-fanged colubroid species. Further, as summarized in Table 4.1 and in Section 4.1, the vast majority of bites from many of these species feature only mild local effects. In addition, even medically significant bites from species that occasionally produce moderate local effects (e.g., *Philodryas* spp., *H. nasicus*; Table 4.1 and Section 4.1), would not merit the risks of antivenom therapy if specific antivenoms were available. As described in Section 4.5.1.1, inappropriate provision of antivenom for insignificant, nonvenomous snakebites have sometimes produced life-threatening anaphylaxis.

It is also important that medical personnel (particularly in regions where such bites more frequently occur) should realize that no specific antivenoms are available, and that non-front-fanged colubroid bites rarely if ever justify the risk of this treatment. For example, in the case of a *Boiruna maculata* bite in Brazil, the pediatric patient was given polyvalent anti-*Bothrops* spp. antivenom although the snake had been positively identified (Santos-Costa et al., 2000; Table 4.1 and Section 4.5.1.1). Similarly, a 17-year-old male bitten by a *P. patagoniensis* presented with moderate edema, erythema, and mild ecchymoses of the right hand was given eight ampoules of anti-*Bothrops* spp. polyvalent antivenom (Correia et al., 2010). This unfortunate patient then suffered a moderately severe antivenom reaction due to an unnecessary and useless treatment for this bite.

Polyvalent antivenoms are often used to treat serious envenomation inflicted by a "presumed" species of unidentified elapid or viperid. In many cases, as long as the likely species responsible is covered by the antivenom and/or established paraspecific protection has been determined and is inclusive of the suspected species, this would be a reasonable approach barring a firm identity of the snake. The main concerns regarding this approach are whether the antivenom contains a significant neutralizing titer of antibody against medically important toxins present in the venom of the envenomating species and the likely larger volume required for effective treatment (greater risk of antivenom reactions, etc.). However, treatment of a presumed hazard level 1 colubrid species such as *D. typus* must be based on a careful history, clinical assessment, and investigations, as effective treatment is founded on monospecific anti-*D. typus* antivenom therapy. In one case of presumed *D. typus* envenomation, provision of SAIMR polyvalent antivenom was predictably ineffective (Bajaj et al., 1980), as it was when also used to treat *T. capensis* envenomation (Beiran and Currie, 1967).

A few investigators have described *in vitro* antigenic cross-reactivity between various non-front-fanged colubroid Duvernoy's secretions and commercial antivenoms against viperid and elapid venoms (Boquet and Saint Girons, 1972; Minton and Weinstein, 1987; Weinstein and Smith, 1993). However, it was uncertain whether these immunological cross-reactions had any clinically protective value and therefore were of any medical importance. Assakura et al. (1992) reported that hemorrhagic activity of Duvernoy's gland secretion from *P. olfersii* was neutralized by commercial horse antivenoms against *Bothrops* spp., as well as by rabbit antisera specific for hemorrhagic factors isolated from several *Bothrops* venoms. Notably, no immunoprecipitation was detected, and this suggested that there were few shared epitopes with *P. olfersii* hemorrhagin. In addition, Kamiguti et al. (2000) described a 65-kDa protein from *D. typus* venom that cross-reacted with polyclonal antibody raised against a class P-III snake venom metalloprotease with hemorrhagic activity from *B. jararaca* venom.

Despite these reports describing antigenic cross-reactivity and limited *in vitro* neutralization of hemorrhagins, there is no current clinical basis for treating any non-front-fanged colubroid bite with polyvalent antivenoms.

4.6.2.8 Replacement Therapy

Blood Transfusions and PRBCs

As described in detail in Section 4.3, DIC and hemorrhagic diathesis are characteristic of the clinical effects that occur after hazard level 1 colubrid envenomation. Prior to the development of antivenom against *D. typus* and *R. tigrinus*, the primary treatment for envenomation by these species was replacement therapy. This strategy has continued for those species for which there is no antivenom. Due to the lack of commercial antivenom, treatment of *Thelotornis* spp. envenoming is managed with replacement therapy only, while *R. subminiatus* envenoming has to date been managed with replacement therapy because antivenom was not available. Anti-*Rhabdophis tigrinus* antivenom now affords a potentially effective cornerstone of treatment for *R. subminiatus* envenoming.

There is an inherent dilemma in managing consumptive coagulopathic envenomation with factor replacement in the absence of antivenom. Some of the venom toxins that cause coagulation factor consumption, particularly the direct or indirect consumption of fibrinogen, may have an extended half life. Therefore, as long as these toxins remain in the circulation, infusion of blood products (including FFP, cryoprecipitate, and whole blood) that contain toxin-targeted clotting factors provides more substrate for the toxins, producing ever higher levels of degradation products and the risk of fibrin clot deposition in the microvasculature. Fibrin degradation products are generally cleared by the kidneys, so that increasing the load may theoretically further imperil the increasingly stressed kidneys (see later for a proposed outlined model of venom coagulopathy-induced renal pathophysiology). Treatment with clotting factors might therefore increase the severity of the pathophysiology of coagulopathic envenomation. On the other hand, failure to restore minimal levels of clotting factors increases the risk of severe or fatal hemorrhage. Similarly, if there is persisting hemolysis, infusing further RBC (either as whole blood or PRBCs) will potentially add more substrate for the pathologic process, leading to an increasing load of hemoglobin and other products of hemolysis that may damage the kidneys. Yet failure to replace critically depleted RBC carries a clear and lethal risk.[23] The

---

[23] Rapidly developing anemia may cause hypoxia, and in those with preexisting comorbidities (e.g., ischemic heart disease, congestive heart failure) this can result in life-threatening decompensation.

decision to give replacement therapy is therefore a balancing act between competing adverse outcomes. There is no clear formula to maintain the patient (or the physician) safely on the highwire.

Replacement therapy has often included repeated blood transfusions or infusions of PRBCs (Blaylock, 1960; Kono and Sawai, 1975; Nakayama et al., 1973; Table 4.1). Repeated transfusions are frequently necessary in these cases due to the marked anemia that develops in most patients envenomed by these species because of massive and continuing intravascular hemolysis (Section 4.3; Table 4.1). Some of these cases report provision of large volumes of PRBCs or blood. For example, Mather et al. (1978) transfused 10 units each of whole blood, platelets, FFP, and 4.2 g of fibrinogen for a patient envenomed by a *R. subminiatus*. In another case of *R. subminiatus* envenoming, Cable et al. (1984) gave 11 units of PRBCs, 12 units of FFP, and 3 units of plasma. These authors discontinued attempts to replenish clotting factors, but continued PRBCs infusions in order to maintain a normal hematocrit (Cable et al., 1984). In a serious case of *T. capensis* envenoming, Beiran and Currie (1967) provided 6 units of whole blood with a positive outcome. Similarly, Du Toit (1980) gave 5 units of fresh blood and 3 units of FFP in a life-threatening case of *D. typus* envenomation. Clearly, transfusion should be dictated by clinical need, bearing in mind the increasing recognition of the potential danger of all blood products.[24] Patients with significant anemia must be given blood and/or PRBCs sufficient to maintain an acceptable hematocrit. The physician must remain aware of the risk of venom-induced intravascular hemolysis and related hemoglobinuric nephropathy. Therefore, hematocrit should be maintained just below or at the low normal range unless a patient's individual comorbidities dictate otherwise.

FFP and Cryoprecipitate

As described previously, FFP and/or cryoprecipitate are commonly given in the management of envenomation by hazard level 1 species (Tables 4.1 and 4.3). The primary basis for infusion of plasma or plasma products is the restoration of clotting factors. A secondary benefit is increasing circulating volume. Treatment of coagulopathic envenoming with replacement therapy comprised of FFP, cryoprecipitate, and/or specific clotting factors has remained controversial since the late 1980s (Burgess and Dart, 1991; White, 2005). One limited low-powered study reported no evidence of efficacy of FFP in treatment of *Pseudonaja affinis* (dugite) coagulopathic envenomation in the canine model (Jelinek et al., 2005). Consumptive coagulopathy induced by white-lipped pit viper, *Cryptelytrops* (*Trimeresurus*) *albolabris* envenomation was refractory to FFP therapy (Yang et al., 2007). However, Isbister et al. (2009) reported that early (within 4 h postenvenomation) administration of FFP may shorten the time to recovery from Australian elapid snakebite-induced coagulopathy,

---

[24] Any patient receiving blood products must be counseled, and consented, about the aforementioned risks as well as the risk of exposure to blood-borne pathogens (HIV, hepatitis B and C, etc.), leukocyte "ghost"(disrupted leukocyte membranes)-induced febrile episodes, and Type IV hypersensitivity reactions. Although the risks of blood-borne pathogens have been substantially lowered in most "First World" countries, it remains a serious concern in countries with limited facilities for plasma screening.

provided that antivenom had been administered. Further confirmation of these findings is essential.

Therefore, the role of FFP and cryoprecipitate in the treatment of coagulopathic envenoming remains unclear. Although current data suggest similar mechanisms of coagulopathy induced by elapid, viperid, and hazard level 1 colubrid snakes, there is insufficient evidence regarding the utility and safety of FFP/cryoprecipitate therapy in serious coagulopathic envenomations. Thus, caution should be exercised as prodigious volumes of plasma products may comprise replacement therapy in these cases. For example, during an admission for severe *R. subminiatus* venom-induced consumptive coagulopathy/DIC, a patient was given 2 units of PRBCs, 59 units of FFP, and 76 bags of cryoprecipitate (Seow et al., 2000).

In sepsis-related DIC (see Appendix C), replacement therapy is rarely helpful and seems likely to aggravate microvascular thrombosis (Marino, 2009). The primary goal of management is to treat the specific cause of the DIC. This is crucial as advanced cases of DIC may exhibit a mortality rate exceeding 80% (DeLoughery, 2005; Marino, 2009). It is important to note that some investigators are questioning whether snake venom-induced coagulopathic effects and DIC are truly comparable. Isbister (2010) has suggested that as the coagulopathy overlaps with thrombotic microangiopathy, the combined effects are mistakenly interpreted as DIC. Although this definition remains to be fully settled, optimal management for envenomation-related DIC as currently defined is provision of specific antivenom if available. In cases of severe bleeding, replacement treatments may have a role at the discretion of the attending physician as determined by individual patient characteristics and the clinical course of the venom disease. The role of FFP/cryoprecipitate in less severe cases requires further study in order to evaluate its effectiveness as well as potential risks (e.g., perpetuation of microthrombi formation) associated with this therapy.

Platelets

Thrombocytopenia is a common feature of coagulopathic envenomation (Warrell, 2004; White, 2005; White and Dart, 2008) including from hazard level 1 colubrids (Table 4.1). In a review of several *D. typus* envenomations, Du Toit (1980) remarked that although thrombocytopenia was not ubiquitous in these cases, it could be severe. Four vials of anti-*D. typus* antivenom did not have any effect on the development of venom-induced thrombocytopenia in a patient with consumptive coagulopathy from a *D. typus* envenomation. It took 1 week for platelet counts to be restored from 10,000/cu. mm to 300,000/cu. mm (Lakier et al., 1969). Atkinson et al. (1980) reported that platelet levels returned to "near-normal values" over a 7-day period following a *T. capensis* envenoming in a pediatric patient treated with only limited replacement therapy. In a case of *T. c. oatesii* envenoming, thrombocytopenia developed over 4–5 days followed by a gradual rise in platelets from 6 days postenvenoming (Muguti and Dube, 1998). The patient was treated with PRBCs, platelets, vitamin K, and hydrocortisone (Muguti and Dube, 1998).

It is possible that hazard level 1 colubrid envenomations may cause MAHA (see pg. 243). This may contribute to the profound and prolonged thrombocytopenia as well as the anemia that occurs in some envenomations by these species. The deposition of fibrin on activated vascular epithelium (possibly damaged by proteolytic rhexic hemorrhagins and other venom components) can alter erythrocyte morphology (e.g., schistocytes or helmet cells) and produce MAHA. This complication of venom-induced DIC has been reported after envenomations by western brown snakes (*Pseudonaja nuchalis*), the desert horned viper (*Cerastes cerastes*), the African lowland or swamp viper (*Proatheris superciliaris*), and others (Keyler, 2008; Schneemann et al., 2004; Warrell, 2005; White, 2005).

Similar to the case of *D. typus* envenoming reported by Lakier et al. (1969), the following case of *R. tigrinus* envenoming suggests that antivenom therapy may not influence venom-induced thrombocytopenia. Akimoto et al. (1991) reported a gradual rise in platelets over a 9-day period following a serious *R. tigrinus* envenoming treated with anti-*R. tigrinus* antivenom. The rate of recovery of normal platelet levels reported by those authors is similar to that of a 20-day history reported for a patient also envenomated by a *R. tigrinus* and treated with exchange blood transfusion and plasmapheresis (Mori et al., 1983). However, a patient with hemorrhagic diathesis following a *R. subminiatus* envenoming maintained a normal platelet level throughout the course of the venom disease (Hoffmann et al., 1992).

Available data indicate that although common, thrombocytopenia is not inevitable in envenomation from hazard level 1 colubrids. Therefore, there is no universal recommendation for platelet replacement in serious envenomation by *D. typus*, *Thelotornis* spp., *R. tigrinus*, and *R. subminiatus*. Severe thrombocytopenia should be corrected by platelet infusions as clinically indicated. When available, specific antivenom is the most effective therapy for reversing the coagulopathy, although doubts have been expressed regarding efficacy of antivenom in some coagulopathic envenomings (specifically, envenoming by Australian elapid snakes with types C and D prothrombin-activators[25]; Isbister et al., 2009). Also, as noted above, thrombocytopenia can persist in some coagulopathic envenomings (i.e., from some crotaline viperids) regardless of provision of antivenom with platelet infusions (Odeleye et al., 2004).

Analogous to some of the reported cases of envenomation by *Thelotornis* spp. (Table 4.1 and previous sections), Mebs et al. (1998) reported that platelet therapy with fibrinogen infusions appeared to stabilize a patient within 2 days postenvenomation by *Atheris squamiger* (African green bush viper), a species for which no specific antivenom is available. A patient with coagulopathic envenoming from another species for which there is no antivenom, *Proatheris superciliaris*, developed thrombocytopenia and was successfully managed with platelet infusions, FFP, and hemodialysis (Valenta et al., 2008). It must be noted that these cases may suggest also that although seriously envenomated, these patients might not have received a potentially fatal dose of venom.

---

[25] Group C (e.g., pseutarin, from Eastern brownsnake, *P. textilis* venom) and D prothrombin activators (e.g., notecarin and trocarin, from venoms of the common tiger snake, *Notechis scutatus* and the roughscaled snake, *Tropidechis carinatus*, respectively) are structural and functional homologues of factor Xa and the prothrombinase complex, respectively (see Joseph et al., 2002 and Rao et al., 2003).

Therefore, with or without antivenom therapy, provision of platelets is at the discretion of the physician and the need for platelet therapy should be determined by close serial monitoring of platelet counts and other hemostatic variables (see Table 4.3) balanced with the clinical status of the patient (especially evidence of active spontaneous systemic bleeding and consumptive coagulopathy, etc.).

4.6.2.9 Heparin, Antifibrinolytics, Vitamin K, and Adrenocorticotrophic Hormone

Attempts to inhibit the envenomation-induced DIC from hazard level 1 species have included administration of heparin, antifibrinolytics (specifically, ϵ-aminocaproic acid or transexamic acid), or adrenocorticotrophic hormone (ACTH; Table 4.1).

Heparin

The strategy of heparinization has been advanced as a means to prevent perpetuation of the consumptive coagulopathy in a patient treated with replacement therapy (provision of fibrinogen through FFP, whole blood or isolated fibrinogen, etc.; see section 4.2.6.8). Hoffmann et al. (1992) suggested that thrombin inhibition with heparin or hirudin would probably provide the most "logical" means of treating *R. subminiatus* envenoming. Their view was couched in their proposed coagulopathic mechanism of *R. subminiatus* venom toxins. This mechanism consisted of potent prothrombin activation along with concomitant activation of protein C and, possibly, factor X (Hoffmann et al., 1992). These authors did not weigh the risks/benefits of heparinization versus the possibility of cross-neutralization of *R. subminiatus* venom by anti-*R. tigrinus* antivenom, and effectiveness of heparin assumes that (1) venom-induced thrombin is susceptible to heparin, and (2) there is adequate circulating antithrombin III to complex with heparin.

Heparin has been included in the treatment strategy of several documented cases of hazard level 1 colubrid envenomations (Table 4.1). For example, in discussing two published cases of *D. typus* envenomation, Du Toit (1980) observed that heparin apparently afforded little clinical benefit, while antivenom administration produced rapid improvement. Similarly, the course of coagulopathy appeared unaffected by low-dose heparin given to a patient with severe hemorrhagic diathesis from a *R. subminiatus* envenoming (Zotz et al., 1991).

Several clinical trials have assessed heparin therapy for treatment of coagulopathic envenomation (primarily from viperid envenomation; Myint-Lwin et al., 1989; Paul et al., 2007; Warrell et al., 1976b). Most of these studies have not demonstrated any efficacy of heparin, and some have revealed the dangers of this treatment (Schneemann et al., 2004). However, in a small study of patients envenomed by *Echis carinatus* (Indian saw-scaled viper), Paul et al. (2007) reported that bleeding and hypotension were reduced in patients receiving low molecular weight heparin (LMWH). AKI was observed more commonly in the test subjects than in the controls, and mortality was less in the test group. However, none of the differences were found to be statistically significant, and these investigators called for a larger trial in order to confirm their results (Paul et al., 2007). The authors opined that the potential efficacy of LMWH in comparison to unfractionated heparin (UFH) was due to their differing activities as "LMWH exerts its anticoagulant effect by inactivating factor Xa, while UFH has effect on factors IIa, Ixa, xIa, XIIa, and XIIIa" (Paul et al., 2007). These authors also stated that unlike UFH, LMWH has "no effect on platelets," and that due to these differences in action, speculated that there is "less chance of severe bleeding when LMWH is used" (Paul et al., 2007).

A common property of many venoms that contain prothrombin-activators or thrombin-like enzymes is the venom-induced generation of thrombin that is uninhibited or only partially inhibited by antithrombin III or antithrombin–heparin complex (Marsh and Williams, 2005; Salazar et al., 2008; Schneemann et al., 2004). Zotz et al. (1991) reported that an extract from Duvernoy's glands of *R. subminiatus* contained a powerful prothrombin-activator that generated thrombin with antithrombin III and antithrombin–heparin complex resistant properties. Therefore, although a lack of antithrombin III consumption has been noted in *R. subminiatus* envenoming (Zotz et al., 1991), UFH would not likely achieve any therapeutic advantage in these cases. Similarly, although LMWH exhibits an approximately 4:1 action in relation to binding to Factor X:thrombin, respectively, it would probably still be ineffective in envenomings from hazard level 1 colubrids that possess similar venom properties.

The main risk of heparin, even in low doses, is its exacerbation of bleeding. For this reason its use for ancillary treatment of a number of diseases, such as severe falciparum malaria and dengue hemorrhagic syndrome, has been abandoned. An additional consideration is the risk of heparin-induced thrombocytopenia (HIT). Heparin can bind to platelet factor IV and this may induce an antibody response against those platelets. This can result in aggregation and subsequent clearance of large numbers of platelets resulting in thrombocytopenia (Napolitano et al., 2006). The antiplatelet IgG populations are usually transient, and last for approximately 3 months (Ahmed et al., 2007). Although HIT is significantly less frequent with LMWH therapy compared to UFH therapy, it still may occur and is a risk (Jang and Hursting, 2005; Shuster et al., 2003). Therefore, the assertion of Paul et al. (2007) regarding the lack of effect of LMWH on platelets is inaccurate. The risk of HIT must be considered an additional concern due to the possibility of HIT compounding the venom-induced thrombocytopenia associated with some hazard level 1 colubrid envenomings. The paradoxically increased prothrombotic tendency in some patients when treated with heparin for several days may comprise additional risk (Warkentin, 1999).

The preponderance of current evidence suggests that heparin probably increases the risk of hemorrhage in patients afflicted with viperid venom-induced coagulopathy, and its use is therefore contraindicated in these cases (Mahasandana et al., 1980; Schneemann et al., 2004). Also, UFH and, to a lesser extent, LMWH, carry significant risk in a number of clinical presentations and have uncertain benefit in the management of coagulopathic envenoming. Therefore, current evidence indicates that the risks of heparin therapy outweigh any marginal benefit demonstrated to date. Thus, heparin therapy cannot be endorsed for use in hazard level 1 colubrid envenomation and is positively contraindicated.

Antifibrinolytics, Vitamin K, and ACTH

Antifibrinolytic therapy, often combined with vitamin K, was used in several cases of presumed or verified *R. tigrinus* envenomation (Mandell et al., 1980; Mittleman and Goris, 1974). Mandell et al. (1980) reported clinical improvement in observed clotting after i.v. administration of aminocaproic acid and hydrocortisone to a pediatric patient envenomed by a presumed *R. tigrinus*. Earlier treatment with vitamin K was ineffective. Similarly, in one case retrospectively summarized by Mittleman and Goris (1974), a patient was given i.v. vitamin K_1, ε-aminocaproic acid, and hydrocortisone. This treatment reportedly resulted in stable clot formation. Continued infusion of ε-aminocaproic acid for an additional 8 h was said to cause further improvement in clot formation and cessation of superficial bleeding (Mittleman and Goris, 1974). A patient with consumptive coagulopathy/DIC and renal failure following *R. tigrinus* envenoming exhibited no clinical benefit from i.v. administration of transexamic acid (Mittleman and Goris, 1978).

Provision of i.v. vitamin K for *R. subminiatus* venom-induced hemorrhagic diathesis did not produce any clinical benefit (Cable et al., 1984). Administration of i.v. ACTH to a patient with *R. tigrinus* venom-induced consumptive coagulopathy/DIC was ineffective, while blood transfusion reportedly corrected aberrant coagulation (Mittleman and Goris, 1974).

The lysine analogs, transexamic acid and aminocaproic acid, prevent fibrinolysis by inhibiting plasminogen and the binding of plasmin to fibrin (Slaughter and Greenberg, 1997). Although these have variable utility in controlling perioperative bleeding and menorrhagia (Schouten et al., 2009; Wellington and Wagstaff, 2003), their use in management of envenomation is limited to a few isolated cases without formal clinical evaluation or testing. Therefore, these are contraindicated.

Vitamin K_1 (phytonadione) is used in the prevention and treatment of hypoprothrombinemia caused by vitamin K deficiency, oral anticoagulants, or other factors which impair the absorption or synthesis of vitamin K. Phytonadione is also used in the prevention and treatment of hemorrhagic disease of newborns. Its mechanism of action remains unclear, but it is necessary for hepatic synthesis of factor II (prothrombin), factor VII (proconvertin), factor IX (thromboplastin), and factor X (prothrombinase). Aside from a limited retrospective review of seven cases (Dabo et al., 2002), the use of vitamin K in management of envenoming is without any formal testing or evaluation. It has no proven benefit and may carry risk, and is therefore contraindicated. Similarly, the previously documented use of ACTH or hydrocortisone has no apparent clinical strategic benefit and is also contraindicated.

4.6.2.10   Prothrombin and Direct Thrombin Inhibitors

There are no data regarding the use of prothrombin inhibitors such as α-drotrecogin, direct thrombin inhibitors (DTI; e.g., argatroban, bivalirudin, and hirudin), or Factor Xa inhibitor (fondaparinux) in hemorrhagic–coagulopathic envenoming. Some data obtained from studies of antithrombotic therapy during percutaneous cardiac intervention (cardiac catheterization) suggest that the DTI, bivalirudin, may offer reduced bleeding risk in comparison with some other assessed antithrombotics (Bonaca et al., 2009).

However, the risk/benefit profile for use of these agents in coagulopathic envenoming is unestablished. Therefore, no evidence-based assessment of these possible therapies for use in hazard level 1 colubrid envenoming is currently feasible.

4.6.2.11   Plasmapheresis/Exchange Transfusion

Exchange transfusion or plasmapheresis was used to treat several cases of severe envenoming by *R. tigrinus* (Table 4.1). Mori et al. (1983) reported recovery of "hemostatic function" after exchange transfusion of a pediatric patient with *R. tigrinus* venom-induced consumptive coagulopathy/DIC. The authors indicated that the procedure was used due to lack of antivenom availability. Despite this treatment, the patient had chronic renal failure for several months (Mori et al., 1983). Another case of severe *R. tigrinus* envenoming was treated with exchange transfusion due to unavailability of antivenom (Ogawa and Sawai, 1986). The comatose patient reportedly exhibited improved coagulation parameters, but the procedure did not alter the fatal outcome (Ogawa and Sawai, 1986).

Envenomation by *D. typus*, *R. tigrinus*, or *R. subminiatus* should be treated with antivenom, as noted above. Consumptive coagulopathy from envenomation by species without available antivenom (e.g., *Thelotornis* sp.) should be treated with supportive measures such as conservative replacement therapy as clinically indicated. There is no clear clinical benefit from exchange transfusion/plasmapheresis in these cases. This has been similarly noted in management of some consumptive coagulopathic envenomations from Australian elapids (e.g., *Pseudonaja* spp.; Isbister et al., 2007).

4.6.2.12   Diuretics and Dialysis: The Causes and Management of Acute Kidney Injury (AKI) after Bites of Hazard Level 1 Colubrid Species

Venom-induced consumptive coagulopathy/DIC often cause acute and chronic (and, occasionally, acute on chronic) renal failure and thus are frequent sequelae after envenomation by hazard level 1 colubrid snakes (Table 4.1; Section 4.3). The AKI observed in these cases is primarily due to prerenal effects of hypovolemia and shock (hypotension) as well as intrarenal effects (tubulointerstitial disease) due to hemoglobinuric nephropathy/acute tubular necrosis (Table 4.1; Section 4.3 and later). Direct toxin-induced nephropathy is a possible additional etiology. Figure 4.4 illustrates some of the causes of AKI caused by hazard level 1 colubrid envenomations.

Some cases of hazard level 1 colubrid envenomation feature AKI that is poorly responsive or nonresponsive to diuretics and dialysis (Table 4.1; Section 4.3). In the case reported by Lakier et al. (1969), a patient with *D. typus* venom-induced consumptive coagulopathy/DIC developed renal failure 4–5 days postenvenoming. Hemodialysis was performed four times over a 2-week period (Lakier et al., 1969). This patient exhibited the triad characteristic of hemolytic–uremic syndrome (HUS): ARF, thrombocytopenia, and hemolytic anemia with altered erythrocyte morphology (schistocytes) (Date et al., 1986). However, as noted in Section 4.3, encompassing these effects under the specific term, HUS, may be misleading. Renal

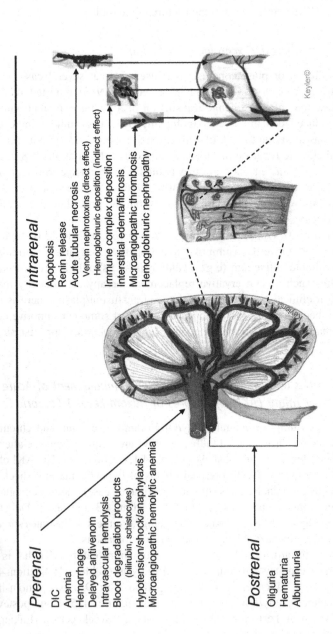

Renal complications and colubroid envenomations
Associated with Hazard Index I Species
(*Dispholidus typus, Thelotornis capensis, T. kirtlandii, Rhabdophis tigrinus, R. subminiatus*)
Venom/Toxin-induced effects

Prerenal

DIC
Anemia
Hemorrhage
Delayed antivenom
Intravascular hemolysis
Blood degradation products
(bilirubin, schistocytes)
Hypotension/shock/anaphylaxis
Microangiopathic hemolytic anemia

Intrarenal

Apoptosis
Renin release
Acute tubular necrosis
Venom nephrotoxins (direct effect)
Hemoglobinuric deposition (indirect effect)
Immune complex deposition
Interstitial edema/fibrosis
Microangiopathic thrombosis
Hemoglobinuric nephropathy

Postrenal

Oliguria
Hematuria
Albuminuria

Keyler©

Figure 4.4 Renal complications and non-front-fanged colubroid envenomations. Envenomation from bites by several non-front-fanged colubroid species may cause acute kidney injury (AKI). Venom- or venom toxin-induced effects may impact physiological systems (blood and vascular) causing prerenal insults that lead to AKI, while other venom components may have direct effects (intrarenal) on specific kidney structures (renal cells, glomerulus, tubules). Venom-induced prerenal and intrarenal toxicity will result in reduced or abolished glomerular filtration, and thus decrease diuresis (postrenal effect). This will produce renal insufficiency that may progress to renal failure and uremia. Some victims with hazard level 1 colubrid envenomation-associated AKI respond poorly to dialysis. *D. typus*, photo copyright to Julian White; renal figure copyright to Daniel E. Keyler.

biopsy revealed hemoglobinuric nephropathy, tubular necrosis, and marked interstitial edema. The patient's complicated course required extended inpatient management; he was discharged 48 days after admission. Notably, this patient also had a markedly elevated bilirubin (with a high ratio of unconjugated bilirubin) during the course of the venom disease. Although likely due to intravascular hemolysis related to the venom-induced erythrocyte membrane fragility, the authors considered fibrin thrombi and/or direct hepatotoxicity as additional factors contributing to the hyperbilirubinemia (Lakier et al., 1969).

In a fatal case of *T. kirtlandii* envenoming, daily hemodialysis had an insignificant effect on the clinical course (Mebs et al., 1978). Similarly, *R. tigrinus* envenoming can feature ARF and anuria that are unresponsive to dialysis (Mittleman and Goris, 1978). A patient with *R. tigrinus* venom-induced consumptive coagulopathy/DIC developed anuria and also showed evidence of digital ischemia 48 h postenvenoming (Nakayama et al., 1973, reported by Mittleman and Goris, 1978). The patient remained in renal failure and required almost daily dialysis. Ten days after admission, left renal biopsy revealed "chestnut-sized" lumps, a softened cortex, and subcapsular "bloody swellings" (Mittleman and Goris, 1978). Extensive, severe hemorrhage and necrosis were noted in the glomeruli and tubules. Biopsy of the right kidney performed 1 month after admission showed "almost complete destruction" of the majority of glomeruli, hyalinization of remaining glomeruli, and extensive interstitial fibrosis (Mittleman and Goris, 1978). In their translation of this case, Mittleman and Goris (1978) interpreted the impression of Nakayama et al. (1973) that the patient had "no possibility" of regaining normal function of the left kidney, while the right kidney showed evidence of some cortical tubular regeneration. At 62 days postenvenoming, the patient's urinary output increased to 100–200 mL/day and dialysis was performed twice weekly. Unfortunately, the patient expired shortly thereafter following two episodes of acute pulmonary edema. Autopsy findings included renal atrophy (Mittleman and Goris, 1978).

These representative cases of AKI following life-threatening or fatal envenomation by some hazard level 1 colubrids are very similar to those seen in coagulopathic viperid or elapid envenoming. For example, Thein-Than et al. (1991) reported renal effects in 15 out of 24 patients envenomed by *D. siamensis* (Eastern Russell's viper) in Burma (Myanmar). Ten of these patients exhibited mild renal dysfunction, while five developed ARF. It is noteworthy that patients with ARF were oliguric on admission, developed ARF despite treatment with appropriate antivenom, and showed a positive clinical response to peritoneal dialysis (Thien-Than et al., 1991). These authors identified albuminuria as a possible early marker of evolving venom-induced nephropathy (Thien-Than et al., 1991). This is similar to the observation of Kikuchi et al. (1987) regarding microhematuria as a potential early marker of systemic envenoming by *R. tigrinus*. Therefore, after envenoming from some hazard level 1 colubrid species, even a urine dipstick assay may facilitate early recognition of systemic involvement with possible impending renal dysfunction.

Markers of renal function [e.g., blood urea nitrogen (BUN) and/or creatinine] have been used to assess the risk of complications after coagulopathic envenomation. In a retrospective study of 68 cases of *Echis coloratus* (Middle Eastern saw-scaled viper or Burton's carpet viper) envenoming in Israel, Porath et al. (1992) evaluated symptoms/signs as predictors of bleeding and azotemia. These investigators reported that clinical complications were unlikely in patients with hemoglobin ≥ 13 g/dL; platelet count $\geq 100,000/mm^3$; blood urea ≤ 7 mmol/L; and an absence of proteinuria or bleeding (Porath et al., 1992). Importantly, these authors found that treatment on admission with monovalent antivenom was associated with a shorter duration of hemostatic dysfunction, while provision of FFP did not appear effective in preventing complications (Porath et al., 1992).

In a prospective survey of 100 patients envenomed by *Crotalus durissus* (tropical rattlesnake) in Brazil, other biochemical disturbances were identified as precursors of AKI (Pinho et al., 2005). These authors reported that among the 29 patients in their series who developed AKI, 24% required dialysis, and 10% died. The patients with AKI had smaller body area in comparison to envenomated patients without AKI; lower urinary output on admission; a marked CK increase; and had received antivenom later than other patients and/or received a lower dose (Pinho et al., 2005). Patient age <12 years, provision of antivenom >2 h postadmission, and a CK >2000 U/L were all identified as independent risk factors for AKI. Diuresis ≥ 90 mL/h was deemed a protective factor (Pinho et al., 2005).

Coagulopathic envenoming from some elapids also present with a similar set of concerns. For instance, among 32 cases of *Pseudonaja* spp. (Australian brown snakes) envenoming with severe consumptive coagulopathy enrolled in the Australian snakebite project, four had thrombotic microangiopathy (Isbister et al., 2007). These patients exhibited thrombocytopenia that was most severe 3 days postenvenoming and required 1 week to normalize. All showed erythrocyte fragmentation, and most developed AKI that persisted for 2–8 weeks and required dialysis (Isbister et al., 2007). These authors included two additional cases of *Pseudonaja* spp. envenoming that had features shared with those in their enrolled series. Importantly, although all six patients received antivenom, provision of antivenom was delayed in comparison to other *Pseudonaja* spp. envenoming cases studied. Four patients were treated with plasmapheresis that did not appear to provide any significant clinical benefit (Isbister et al., 2007).

These brief representative cases involving viperids and elapids suggest venom-induced renal sequelae similar to that from some hazard level 1 colubrids. In all of these cases, thrombocytopenia, anemia, probable intravascular hemolysis, altered erythrocyte morphology, possibly, microangiopathic thrombosis, and delayed or absent antivenom provision all are associated with serious renal dysfunction. Although some authors report improvement in a sampling of patients treated with dialysis or plasmapheresis (Mori et al., 1983; Pinho et al., 2005), many patients with consumptive coagulopathy/DIC from envenomation by colubroids with venoms that contain prothrombin-activating or thrombin-like enzymes do not respond to these measures and often have extended periods of renal dysfunction (see previous sections and Table 4.1). This can have long-term implications for envenomed patients. Several studies have demonstrated a significant association between AKI and long-term morbidity and mortality (Bihorac et al., 2010; Coca et al., 2009). An additional retrospective matched cohort study concluded that acute renal injury requiring dialysis was significantly associated with increased risk of end-stage renal disease, but unrelated to all-cause mortality (Wald et al., 2009). Therefore, although long-term mortality risk associated with AKI is arguably controversial, it is probable that risk of end-stage renal disease is greater in those who have had a renal insult requiring dialysis. This must be considered in the long-term prognosis of patients who have experienced ARF requiring dialysis from coagulopathic envenoming, including those from hazard level 1 colubrids.

Experimental pathophysiological study of venom-induced AKI has provided some correlation between renal pathology in the rat model and clinical manifestations in envenomed humans. Glomerular, tubular, interstitial, and vascular lesions have been described. Experimentally, some venoms (e.g., from viperids) cause mesangiolysis, and this may be a significant factor in the pathogenesis of some venom-induced glomerular disease (George et al., 1987). Burdmann et al. (1993) studied ARF induced in rats by i.v. injection of *B. jararaca* (jararaca) venom. Noted were acutely decreased glomerular filtration rate, diuresis and renal plasma flow; intravascular hemolysis; and hypofibrinogenemia. Histopathology revealed massive fibrin deposition in glomerular capillaries, proximal and distal tubular necrosis, and tubular deposition of erythrocyte casts (Burdmann et al., 1993). The authors emphasized ischemia due to glomerular coagulation and intravascular hemolysis as the most important factors influencing renal damage. Direct venom nephrotoxicity could not be excluded, as has been noted by other authors who have reported that some venom-induced renal lesions appear to reflect a direct action of venom toxins on kidney parenchyma (George et al., 1987; Burdmann et al., 1993). These findings resemble those determined from renal biopsy performed in patients with AKI caused by severe envenoming from *D. typus* or *R. tigrinus* (Lakier et al., 1969; Mittleman and Goris, 1978; Nakayama et al., 1973).

Generally, available data suggest the following basic mechanisms of consumptive coagulopathic envenoming-induced AKI: generation of microthrombi, development of hypofibrinogenemia, anemia (probably mainly due to hemolysis and splenic clearance of schistocytes, etc.), and intravascular hemolysis. Some of these processes cause a rapid deposition of hemoglobin and erythrocyte casts in the renal tubules and result in acute tubular necrosis. Simultaneously, microthrombi accumulate in glomeruli, and probably in the afferent and efferent vasculature. Additionally, it is likely that the decreasing erythrocyte population causes increased stimulation of the peritubular and/or tubular capillary endothelial cells to produce erythropoietin in order to replenish the sudden drop in erythrocytes and restore the concomitantly decreased transport of oxygen. The oxygen deficiency could also stimulate the rate of adenosine formation, thereby lowering the rate of glomerular filtration by constriction of afferent arterioles, particularly in superficial nephrons, thus lowering the salt load and renal transport workload (Vallon and Osswald, 2009). Likewise, in response to hemorrhage and concomitant hypotensive effects, renin secretion from the juxtaglomerular cells (as well as other recruited renal cells in the circumstance of a growing threat to homeostasis) will predictably increase. These simultaneous processes will likely exert greater metabolic stress on renal function within a developing ischemic state. It is possible that this may stimulate acute tubular apoptosis as opposed to strictly defined acute tubular necrosis, as has been suggested for mechanisms contributing to Gram-negative, sepsis-induced renal failure (Wan et al., 2003). Therefore, dynamic and progressive combinations of prerenal and intrarenal pathophysiological processes comprise the renal effects observed in these envenomations (Figure 4.4). Although the AKI and chronic renal dysfunction may be largely due to these proposed mechanisms, there is a strong possibility of a direct nephrotoxin in some of these venoms as have been detected in venoms of other colubroids. For example, direct nephrotoxicity of *D. russelii* venom has been demonstrated in the perfused rat kidney (Ratcliffe et al., 1989). A basic 7.2-kDa nephrotoxin has been isolated from *D. r. russelii* venom (Mandel and Bhattachuryya, 2007). The authors suggested that this toxin ("RVV-7") was renally concentrated and its accumulation resulted in necrotic destruction of the tubular epithelium (Mandel and Bhattachuryya, 2007). A recent review suggested that renal cell-adhesion molecules (cadherins, catenins, etc.) may be important early targets for nephrotoxic venom components (Prozialeck and Edwards, 2007).

AKI from venom-induced consumptive coagulopathy/DIC should be managed initially by the early administration of specific antivenom if available, and careful fluid resuscitation (with adjustment for any individual comorbidities, e.g., congestive heart failure). Some medications used for renal protection under certain circumstances (e.g., during provision of contrast media) such as *N*-acetylcysteine may be considered on a case-by-case basis. However, the putative protective effects of medications such as *N*-acetylcysteine are unclear and unproven when used in the setting of AKI caused by different ischemia-related etiologies (e.g., elective aortic aneurysm repair; Macedo et al., 2006). There are no trialed, tested, or well-documented data regarding the use of *n*-acetylcysteine or other renally protective medications in management of coagulopathic envenoming. The use of angiotensin-converting enzyme inhibitors (ACEI) in these cases is worthy of study, although ACEI can precipitate AKI in some patients, and there is a report suggesting ACEI exacerbation of venom-induced hypotension (Svensson et al., 1993). Emerging data also suggest a potential protective role in LPS-induced AKI of protein C due to its modulatory effects on renal inflammation. This includes downregulation of renal inducible nitric oxide synthase and reduction of the mRNA expression involving the renin–angiotensin system, renal ACE-1 as well as angiotensin II (Gupta et al., 2007). The possible therapeutic application of activated protein C in coagulopathic envenoming such as those from hazard level 1 colubrids may be worthy of careful investigation.

Additional management should follow standard protocol and include careful placement of a Foley catheter in order to closely monitor diuresis (being mindful of concomitant coagulopathy-related risks in such a procedure); serial assessment of electrolytes and treatment of hyperkalemia as indicated; judicious use of loop diuretics along with careful hydration (choice of i.v. fluid is at the discretion of the attending physician); provision of oral and i.v. amino acids and oral fluids (volume of urinary output + 500 mL/day); and increased carbohydrate intake in order to minimize catabolism. Nephrology consultation is strongly recommended. Dialysis should be performed as necessary, although, as noted, response is often suboptimal in serious cases. Some studies have suggested that hemodialysis has a more favorable outcome in venom-induced AKI than peritoneal dialysis (Wiwanitkit, 2005), although the choice of the method used may be governed by availability. Patients should be counseled regarding the potential for loss of function despite correct therapy, as well as the possibility of extended need for dialysis and/or additional supportive measures.

4.6.2.13   Imaging Studies

There are no general indications for imaging of patients with medically significant colubroid envenoming. However, some patients envenomated by hazard level 1 colubrids may require imaging, as brain hemorrhage has been reported in several cases [e.g., from *R. tigrinus* and *T. kirtlandii* envenomations; Ogawa and Sawai, 1986 (see Plate 4.46D), and Mebs et al., 1978, respectively; see Table 4.1 and Section 4.3]. Therefore, CT (computerized axial tomography) of the head without contrast should be performed on patients that exhibit consumptive coagulopathy with altered sensorium ± other neurological signs or at the discretion of the attending physician. There are no data supporting the need for other imaging aside from the assessment of secondary effects from exacerbations of preexisting comorbidities or specific complications (e.g., chest films for suspected pulmonary edema or congestive heart failure, venous and/or arterial Doppler ultrasound imaging of an bitten extremity with history of vascular insufficiency).

4.6.2.14   Additional Investigations

Other investigations that may be considered could include fecal occult blood (guaiac) serial assays; 24-h creatinine; renal sonogram; continuous cardiac monitoring/echocardiogram (as indicated); and esophageal gastroduodenoscopy (in the setting of posttreatment unexplained bleeding). However, any invasive investigation, including those listed above, should be carefully considered from a risk–benefit perspective, if there is active coagulopathy still present.

4.6.2.15   Microbiology of the Ophidian Oropharynx and the Use of Antibiotics for Medically Significant Colubrid Bites

Overview of Microbial Flora

The buccal cavity of snakes contains a wide array of microorganisms, some of recognized medical importance (Goldstein et al., 1979, 1981; Lam et al., 2010; Parrish et al., 1956; Theakston et al., 1990; Williams et al., 1954). Clinically important species of crotaline viperids and elapids studied to date harbor numerous strains (in some cases >400) of up to 72 bacterial taxa (including Gram-negative, Gram-positive, facultative and anaerobic flora; Lam et al., 2010; Shek et al., 2009; Theakston et al., 1990). Some bacterial species present in the ophidian oropharynx (e.g., *Stenotrophomonas maltophilia*) are also relevant to the veterinary care of captive snakes, as well as human medicine (e.g., *Aeromonas hydrophila*; Angel et al., 2002; Hejnar et al., 2007; Jacobson, 2007).

The oropharynx of non-front-fanged colubroid snakes contains a similarly broad variety of bacterial species. A study of 50 specimens of four *Thamnophis* spp. [*T. s. sirtalis*, *T. couchi* (Western aquatic, or Sierra garter snake), *T. radix*, and *T. sauritus*] found 126 strains of aerobic and facultative bacteria. The potential pathogens included *Pseudomonas aeruginosa*, *Klebsiella oxytoca*, *Arizona hinshawii*, *Acinetobacter calcoaceticus* (var. *anitratus*), and *Shigella* spp. (Goldstein et al., 1981). A similar spectrum of bacterial species have been cultured from the oropharynx, venom glands, and venom of several species of crotaline viperids and captive

Australian elapids (Goldstein et al., 1979; Parrish et al., 1956; Williams et al., 1954). In a study of 100 taxa of venomous and nonvenomous snakes, 406 strains of 72 bacterial species were cultured (Lam et al., 2010). The Chinese cobra, *N. atra*, harbored the greatest number of microbial species.

Does *Clostridium tetani* Occur in the Ophidian Oropharynx?

Some authors assert no evidence of *C. tetani* in the ophidian oropharynx (Daley and Alexander, 2010), while others state that it does occur and tetanus prophylaxis (in Western countries tetanus toxoid booster and wound care) should always be provided to victims of snakebites (Akubue, 1997; Omogbai et al., 2002). The perceived absence of *C. tetani* is also asserted in a pharmaceutical company information insert that was supplied with anti-Eastern coral snake (*Micrurus fulvius*) antivenom[26] (Wyeth Inc., Philadelphia, PA, USA). However, several cases of tetanus after serious envenomation by *N. nigricollis* (black-necked spitting cobra), *Echis ocellatus* (West African saw-scaled or carpet viper), and *Cryptelytrops* (*Trimeresurus*) *albolabris* have been reported (Habib, 2003; Suankratay et al., 2002). Fatal cases of tetanus have been reported after Malayan pit viper (*Calloselasma rhodostoma*) envenomings (Reid et al., 1963; Tantanun, 1957), and Parrish (1957) reported a case complicating a water moccasin (or cottonmouth, *Agkistrodon piscivorus*) envenomation. Although 10 taxa of *Clostridium* spp. were isolated from the oropharynx of *T. albolabris*, *C. tetani* was not found (Suankratay et al., 2002). It can be observed that microbial surveys of the ophidian oropharynx are far from complete, and detection as well as culture of anaerobic organisms can be difficult. Another consideration is the microbiological shifts/population changes in the colonizing bacterial flora (Blaylock, 2001). Snakebite-related tetanus may also be a result of wound contamination, or inoculation with organisms derived from prey that has transiently colonized the snake's dentition. Rare cases of tetanus complicating snakebites might have been due to the relatively infrequent presence of *C. tetani* in the ophidian oropharynx, but whatever the source of the pathogen, deep and necrotic snakebite wounds are an ideal medium for this and other anaerobic organisms. Thus, potential exposure to tetanus toxin[27] justifies provision of tetanus toxoid in cases of medically significant snakebite. This includes bites inflicted by colubroids that produce significant local effects. In Third World communities or in the event of other circumstances in which previous immunization may be lacking, treatment, whenever possible, should include administration of tetanus γ-globulin (250–500 U, i.m., in the opposite extremity in which toxoid is administered, or 3,000–10,000 U if clinical tetanus is suspected).

---

[26] Aside from archived ampoules, this antivenom is no longer available, and a new anti-*Micrurus* antivenom (Coralmyn®) is under review for possible use in treatment of *Micrurus* envenoming in the USA.

[27] Tetanus results from the action of tetanus toxin, a 150-kDa heterodimeric metalloprotease that hydrolyzes some of the major proteins that regulate exocytosis of neurotransmitters from inhibitory interneurons of the central nervous system. The toxin causes tonic skeletal muscle spasms followed by contractions. The initial muscle stiffness often involves the jaw ("lockjaw") and/or neck, followed by generalized contractures that may result in respiratory paralysis and death.

Antibiotics Should Not Be Used Prophylactically for Nonnecrotic Snakebites

Several observational studies/reviews have reported a low incidence of wound infection after most snakebites (e.g., several *Crotalus* spp. and others; Clark et al., 1993; LoVecchio et al., 2002; White and Dart, 2008). In a prospective controlled trial with 114 patients, there were no statistically significant differences in outcome in terms of the number of abscesses that occurred between antibiotic-treated and untreated patients. On the basis of these results, the authors declined recommending routine use of prophylactic antibiotics for prevention of infectious complications of crotaline envenomation (Kerrigan et al., 1997). Similarly, a retrospective review of snakebites (number unclear) that presented during 2003–2008 to the Jawaharlal Institute of Postgraduate Medical Education and Research Hospital in Pondicherry, India, identified 43 cases that included infections. The snakes involved were not specifically identified, but the bacteria isolated included *Staphylococcus aureus, Enterococcus faecalis, Streptococcus* spp., *Escherichia coli, Klebsiella pneumonia, Pseudomonas aeruginosa*, and others (Garg et al., 2009). The authors indicated that broad-spectrum antibiotics should be used only in the event of clinical evidence of infection after snakebites (Garg et al., 2009).

The only double-blinded randomized study addressing this question enrolled 251 patients with proven envenoming by *Bothrops* spp. that were admitted to two hospitals in Brazil between 1990 and 1996 (Jorge et al., 2004). The potential role of prophylactic antibiotics in preventing local infections or abscesses among these patients was studied by providing chloramphenicol to 122 patients ("group 1"), while 129 were given placebo ("group 2"). There were no significant differences in the occurrence of abscesses (six patients in each group, or a combined incidence of 4.8%) or necrosis (seven in group 1, and five in group 2, or a combined incidence of 4.8%). It was concluded that the use of orally administered chloramphenicol for victims of *Bothrops* envenomation with signs of local envenoming on admission was not effective for the prevention of local infections (Jorge et al., 2004).

However, several authors have cautioned that snakebite wounds should be carefully scrutinized (especially in Third World clinical facilities) because secondary infection may be a complication of some snakebites, particularly those that develop necrosis (Lam et al., 2010; Theakston et al., 1990). In a study of 310 snakebite victims who presented at Eshowe Hospital in Kwazulu-Natal, South Africa, <10% had necrotic wounds, and the author suggested that antibiotics be reserved for use only in these cases (Blaylock, 1999). Although relatively uncommon, cases of serious secondary infection have been documented; all from recognizably severe envenoming by front-fanged species (e.g., *A. hydrophila* infection that resulted in necrotizing fasciitis postenvenoming by *A. piscivorus*, Angel et al., 2002; mixed local infection 2 weeks postenvenoming by *B. jararaca*, Bucaretchi et al., 2010). Review of the available evidence (much of it from observational studies) emphasizes that antibiotics should only be used prophylactically in snakebites that feature, or have a known tendency for, necrosis. Otherwise, antibiotics should only be used when there is clinical evidence of infection, and in such a case should be started after specimens for culture (anaerobic and aerobic) and sensitivity testing have been obtained. Specific sensitivities of cultured organisms and regional antibiotic resistance patterns should guide the choice of antibiotics when these are deemed necessary. Antibiotics (empirical and specific) recommended for treating potential secondary infections associated with snakebites have included amoxicillin and clavulanic acid, or clindamycin for penicillin-allergic patients (Weinstein and Keyler, 2009); levofloxacin plus amoxicillin and clavulanic acid (Lam et al., 2010; Shek et al., 2009); and gentamycin with benzyl penicillin (Theakston et al., 1990).

In a prospective series of cases, Weed (1993) reported absence of infection in 68[28] patients bitten by nonvenomous snakes including *T. sirtalis*, *L. getula*, and pythoniids, and commented that although pathogenic bacteria are reported from the ophidian buccal cavity, nonvenomous bites do not usually require prophylactic antibiotics. As there is only a single well-documented non-front-fanged colubroid bite that included superficial necrotic effects (Knabe, 1939; see page 161), there is no evidence to support the use of antibiotics in the absence of clinically recognizable infection. The unnecessary and excessive use of prophylactic antibiotics (particularly for upper respiratory infections that are most often of viral etiology) has resulted in global antibiotic resistance among many common bacterial species. This very serious trend should be avoided whenever possible, including in cases of non-front-fanged snakebites that very rarely include significant secondary infection. Colubroid bites are very unlikely to develop necrosis due to the action of Duvernoy's secretion or venom components. However, the inappropriate and positively damaging use of tourniquets, wound incision, vacuum extraction, electric current, etc. for treatment of any snakebite may lead to serious secondary infection and necrosis.

4.6.2.16   Cautions and Contraindications

In general, the following **are to be avoided** in these cases:

*   **Do not** attempt to suture or surgically modify any bleeding wound, as this will likely result in massive hematoma and/or uncontrolled bleeding.
*   **Do not** give i.m. injections, such as updating tetanus immune status, until any coagulopathy or bleeding tendency has resolved; pressure should always be applied to the i.m. injection site. Note that tetanus is a risk in snakebite, albeit small, so tetanus immune status should be considered.
*   **Be aware** of the risk of ongoing and uncontrolled bleeding from any site of trauma, which includes any i.v. needle insertions. **Avoid**, unless no reasonable alternative exists, any i.v. sampling or canulation of the subclavian, jugular, or femoral vessels (e.g., insertion of central lines; if a central line is deemed essential, the femoral is the best option as hemostatic pressure can be applied as necessary). Due to the serious risks of uncontrollable hemorrhage, continuous monitoring via an intra-arterial line is **contraindicated** in any case of coagulopathic envenomation.
*   **Do not** permit patient intake of any supplements, botanical remedies, or naturopathic/homeopathic treatments (useless in management and may contain pro- or anticoagulant components, e.g., gingkosides of gingko biloba).
*   **Do not** provide antibiotics unless there is evidence of infection or necrotic tissue is evident, and/or there has been nonsterile interference with the wound.
*   **Carefully review** any medications routinely taken by the patient. Some medications [i.e., warfarin, some antidepressants (some mixed reuptake inhibitors such as venlafaxine and

[28] Weed (1993) included 72 patients in the study, but four patients had taken prophylactic antibiotics prior to presentation and therefore are not included in the brief assessment here.

duloxetine), aspirin and other NSAIDS (e.g., naproxen, ibuprofen, diclofenac, etc.), clopi-dogrel, etc.] may predispose to persistent bleeding or ecchymoses. Some medications may have to be discontinued or reduced to renal dosages during the course of venom disease.

- In the case of envenomation from a species for which specific commercial antivenom is available, **do not delay** attempts to procure one to two ampoules as this can be effective for up to 5–6 days postenvenoming.
- **Do not** underestimate the need for careful attention to the patient's constitutional require-ments. For example, hospital bedding should be inspected carefully for insufficient cush-ioning that may facilitate development of pressure-induced ecchymoses. In rural/field locations, patients must be insulated from biting insects and trauma from natural exposures to rough terrain, etc.
- In patients with uncontrolled hemostatic defects, **even the least trauma should be avoided**. Patients should remain on strict bed rest. Abdominal massage was sufficient to precipitate fatal retroperitoneal bleeding in one patient. Therefore, physical examination should be care-fully performed with the physician remaining cognizant of these significant risks.

4.6.2.17   Additional Considerations: The Possible Role of Hypersensitivity in the Effects of Colubrid Bites

Available data suggest that the vast majority of medically significant bites from non-front-fanged colubroid snakes are sustained while handling captive or field-collected specimens (Table 4.1). This suggests (and is often the case) that those bitten have had previous exposure to other snakes. This may include previous bites from non-venomous species, handling shed skins, performing captive husbandry, and so on. A smaller subgroup of patients may have a history of previous exposure to lyophi-lized venoms and/or prior bites from venomous species, and possible treatment with antivenom.

Type 1 IgE-mediated hypersensitivity is a recognized consequence of sensitiza-tion after such exposures (Madeiros et al., 2007; Malina et al., 2008; Reimers et al., 2000; Weinstein and Keyler, 2009). The multiple antigens shared among ophidian venoms, Duvernoy's secretions, and some other buccal secretions may play a con-tributory role in medically significant bites from colubroids (Weinstein and Keyler, 2009). Atopic tendencies may increase the severity of hypersensitivity reactions, but does not increase their incidence. After a protracted bite (the snake was forcibly removed after 2 min) on the right hand from a captive *P. patagoniensis*, a technician maintaining an institutional venomous animal collection (implying the possibility of previous exposure to venomous snakes and, possibly, venoms) experienced "con-stant itching" that preceded progressive edema that ultimately involved the arm and axilla (De Araújo and Dos Santos, 1997). Development of venom-specific IgE has been demonstrated in a patient with repeated exposure to ringhals (*Haemachatus haemachatus*) venom. The patient initially developed urticaria, but later experienced increasingly generalized atopy on exposure (Wadee and Rabson, 1987). Among eight patients with systemic effects from either *Vipera berus* (European viper or adder) or *Vipera aspis* (European asp, Asp viper) envenoming, seven had both posi-tive skin tests and IgE antibody against snake venoms, while testing was negative in two patients who exhibited only local reactions to snakebites (Reimers et al., 2000).

The authors emphasized an IgE-mediated mechanism as the likely cause of anaphylactic reactions following snakebites (Reimers et al., 2000).

Whether hypersensitivity develops from a snakebite or other provoking factor, mast cells are known to participate in the induction of hypersensitivity/inflammation through interaction of antigen with specific IgE bound to the high-affinity receptor for IgE (FcεRI; Tkaczyk et al., 2002). However, the possible contribution to this phenomenon of IgG subtypes cannot be excluded. For example, several investigators have identified the anaphylactic role of a subtype of IgG$_4$ (Bryant et al., 1975; Parish, 1970). Human mast cells and basophils contain high-affinity IgG receptors (FcγRI) that are activated and release pro-inflammatory mediators in immediate hypersensitivity reactions via IgG aggregation (Iwaki et al., 2005; Tkaczyk et al., 2002). Mediator release resulting from the activation of either FcεRI or FcγRI is reportedly indistinguishable (Okayama et al., 2001). Comparison of human and murine mast cell degranulation suggests that some of these responses may be species-specific (Tkaczyk et al., 2004). These findings support a complex relationship between the well-established hypersensitivity-antagonizing ("blocking") function of some IgG$_4$ isotypes (as are developed during desensitizing immunotherapy; Greenberger, 2002), and the pro-anaphylactic activation properties of others. Therefore, previous exposures to ophidian buccal secretion/venom antigens and antigens encountered as a consequence of exposure to snake products/shed skins may stimulate the development of complex sensitizing antibodies of γ and ε classes.

Type 1 hypersensitivity commonly presents with clinical manifestations that may be cutaneous (urticaria, pruritus), subcutaneous (angioedema), lymphatic (lymphangitis), GI and uterine (smooth muscle contraction), respiratory (bronchospasm), and cardiovascular (hypotension/shock, etc.). In the most frequent local disease, urticaria is common but not invariably present. Urticaria and angioedema may occur together or separately (Fauci et al., 2009). Thus, the absence of urticaria in a given case of suspected hypersensitivity should not preclude the diagnosis if supported by available evidence (see Section 4.2, *Thamnophis*; Table 4.1).

Uncomplicated local effects constitute the majority of symptoms/signs described in the relatively limited number of well-documented cases of medically significant non-front-fanged colubroid bites (Table 4.1; Section 4.1). It is unproven, but likely, that in some patients these effects (erythema, pruritus, edema, and blistering, etc.; Table 4.1) are a combination of Type 1 hypersensitivity, and the local effects of Duvernoy's secretion components (Weinstein and Keyler, 2009). Some cases may feature more extensive blistering, edema, and lymphangitis, and thus can resemble mild-to-moderate local envenoming from a crotaline viperid species (Weinstein and Keyler, 2009; however, see Plate 4.92A–F and p. 219). Unfortunately, to date there are no data regarding IgE or IgG levels in patients presenting with medically significant effects from non-front-fanged colubroid bites. Such information is very desirable and should be collected by performing the necessary serology whenever possible. Evidence of hypersensitivity in any patient should be managed with epinephrine, antihistamines, leukotriene receptor antagonists, fluid resuscitation, corticosteroids, and airway support as clinically indicated.

5 Summary and Conclusions

The taxonomically artificial ophidian assemblage, family Colubridae, is under dynamic revision. The previous uniform grouping of these snakes was phylogenetically incorrect and misleading as many are unrelated, and are gradually being reassigned to different families and subfamilies. An indeterminate number of non-front-fanged colubroid species produce secretions of varying toxicity from Duvernoy's gland; a low-pressure system that functions by supplying the secretion as needed, as in almost all studied to date there is no significant reservoir of secretion. None of these snakes has canaliculate fangs as in elapids, viperids, or atractaspidids. Some species have enlarged posterior or mid-maxillary teeth that may or may not be grooved associated with the Duvernoy's glands, others do not. Three-finger-fold neurotoxins, prothrombin activators, proteolytic fibrinogenases, and several other components have been characterized from a few taxa, but the secretion properties of the majority of these snakes remain poorly studied. Transcriptome and/or proteomic analyses of several non-front-fanged colubroid taxa have identified multiple classes of toxins, and other biologically active components shared with front-fanged species (Ching et al., 2006; Estrella et al, 2010; Fry et al., 2003, 2008; Weldon and Mackessy, 2010). Most of the characterized postsynaptic neurotoxins exhibit prey specificity (for birds, lizards, etc.). Several species produce highly toxic secretions that are medically important. These species (the Dispholidini, *D. typus*, *T. kirtlandii*, *T. capensis*, and the natricids, *R. tigrinus* and *R. subminiatus*) meet the criteria for the term "venomous" (Mebs, 2002; Russell, 1980), as they actively use their venom in prey capture and/or antipredator defense, as well as exhibit marked toxicity to other animal species. Prey capture/subjugation functions and toxicity have been poorly documented in most other species. Therefore, it is premature to use the term "venomous" for the secretion properties of many of these snakes, as their Duvernoy's glands and associated products have unproven or unverified roles. This is accentuated by the marked differences in functional morphology between glands of "true" venomous snakes (elapids, viperids, and atractaspidids) and those of other colubroids formerly termed colubrids (Greene, 1997; Jackson, 2003; Kardong, 1996; Taub, 1967; Weinstein and Kardong, 1994; Weinstein et al., 2010). Thus, the Duvernoy's secretions of a relatively small number of non-front-fanged colubroids have convincingly met the criteria defining the term "venom" (see p. 32).

Most Duvernoy's secretions studied to date have low toxicity, but several dispholidines and natricids (as noted earlier) produce venoms with marked lethal potency for prey species as well as humans. Characterization of avian or saurian prey-specific toxins present in some of these secretions (*B. dendrophila*, *B. irregularis*) supports their classification as "venoms." However, regardless of the need for a careful biological as well as pharmacological–biomedical definition and use of this term, the word "venom" carries a medical inference suggesting clinical importance. As has

"Venomous" Bites from Non-Venomous Snakes. DOI: 10.1016/B978-0-12-387732-1.00005-1

been discussed elsewhere (Kardong, 1996; Weinstein et al., 2010), it is unfortunate that oral secretions from squamate reptiles are most often defined in a medically/ pharmacologically biased context. Biological function—how the secretion is used— must contribute to the accurate and robust application of the term, "venom." It is necessary to again emphasize that the marked differences of venom delivery systems of elapids, viperids, and atractaspidids (high-pressure systems associated with canaliculate dentition) with the Duvernoy's gland system of non-front-fanged colubroids (low-pressure systems associated with noncanaliculate dentition) must be considered when assigning biological and clinical use of the term, "venom gland." Of course, the evolutionary development and derivation of venom delivery systems must be evaluated in their totality. However, critical analysis/synthesis of available evidence suggests that it is essential to avoid premature assignment of a broad, encompassing term (e.g., "venom," "venom gland"). This terminology inherently implies a dynamic process (evolution of oral glands of various functions, associated dentition, and recruitment/derivation of biologically active components of oral secretions) and should not be assigned to ophidian oral glands of unverified function (Duvernoy's gland) that undoubtedly are also the result of multiple evolutionary experiments, and preadaptation of multifunctional proteins, as well as many morphological modifications per selective needs. Therefore, these terms should be used with caution until biological function is verified/confirmed for a given species. For example, the premature use of the term "venom" for Duvernoy's secretions of taxa such as garter snakes (*Thamnophis* spp.) implies active use of their oral secretions in prey capture and, due to the frequently applied and popular interpretation of the term, also suggests medical importance. These impressions are misleading and unproven. As has been demonstrated here, these snakes have no significant medical importance, and active use of their secretions in prey capture/subjugation has not been verified. Therefore, it is likely that a more accurate term, such as "prey-specific venom," may be used as biological function becomes verified for additional species of non-front-fanged colubroids [e.g., as essentially verified for venom of *A.* (*Borikenophis*) *portoricensis*]. This could improve the accuracy of the term by including notation of use in prey capture and/or subjugation and simultaneously obviate the need to qualify the term by emphasizing a lack of medical importance.

Ophidian oral secretions may be defined as true venoms and promote rapid prey death, but many have additional roles such as producing quiescence/immobilization of prey (Rodriguez-Robles, 1992; Rodriguez-Robles and Leal, 1993), lubrication, digestion, poststrike trailing, defense, and others (Kardong, 2002). To date, a relatively small number of non-front-fanged colubroid genera have been found to produce Duvernoy's secretions of varying toxicity. This is largely due to limited investigation of the immobilization or subjugation qualities of these secretions (e.g., few studies have used potential prey items for testing) in addition to lethal potency studies. The relatively minimal attention to these secretions, in comparison to the many studies of front-fanged ophidian venoms, is not a result of disinterest on the part of venom researchers. Rather, this is due to technical difficulties (tedious collection of secretion, even with parasympathomimetic stimulation facilitating increased collected volumes; procurement of some species of snakes, etc.), perceived lack of medical importance, and very limited economic support for these investigations—an unfortunate reality partly derived from a rigid narrowmindedness on the part of many funding organizations that effectively limit the advancement of many "nonmainstream" research disciplines.

Published reports describing the effects of bites from some of these snakes have been hindered by: limited numbers of well-documented reports; a large amount of disseminated anecdotal information (occasionally perpetuated in the literature and on the Internet without verification); misidentification and/or unverified identity of snakes involved in reported cases; a common lack of qualified and critical clinical analysis and misinterpretation of reported/observed effects; frequent lack of thoroughly considered differential diagnoses for aberrant cases; and publication of many of these reports in nonclinically refereed journals or periodicals. Due to these flaws, critical assessment of a large proportion of these published cases reveals limited quality data available for risk analysis, and thus results in generally low evidence-based scores (Table 4.1).

Dispholidines or natricids that have inflicted life-threatening or fatal human envenoming all produce consumptive coagulopathy/DIC resulting in hemorrhagic diathesis. Unlike the medically significant effects of bites from most other non-front-fanged colubroids, the procoagulant and proteolytic/hemorrhagic toxins present in the venoms of these species exhibit clear functional correlation with the clinical effects observed in envenomed patients. Acute kidney injury figures in many of these cases and is often poorly responsive to diuretics and/or dialysis. There are commercial antivenoms available against venoms of two of these species (*D. typus* and *R. tigrinus*). However, it is fortunate that these life-threatening bites are relatively rare, as these antivenoms may be very difficult to obtain.

Management of envenomation from highly toxic species without antivenom, such as *Thelotornis* spp., consists of supportive measures. The use in management of heparin and antifibrinolytics is contraindicated by available evidence, but some unproven therapies (e.g., synthetic protease inhibitor, SPI) do not appear to exacerbate bleeding in Gram-negative endotoxemic coagulopathy and therefore may be used in selected cases of hazard level 1 colubrid envenoming. Replacement therapy with FFP, cryoprecipitate, and/or platelets is controversial but may be required according to clinical need. Patients envenomated by these species often exhibit anemia that requires treatment with repeated PRBC transfusions. The role in management of plasmapheresis or exchange transfusion is unclear. These procedures are unlikely to be of benefit. Although the respective pathological mechanisms/processes are distinctive, some coagulopathic envenomations by these species may share some similar pathophysiology and therefore some basic clinical management with that of Gram-negative endotoxemia.

Although bites from *Thelotornis* spp. are rare, effective antivenom against *T. capensis* is desirable. It might provide some protection against envenomation by congeners, and could be useful in a research context as well. However, development of such antivenom is extremely unlikely as it would be nonprofitable and bites are very infrequent. Aside from the hazard 1 species discussed previously, to date, there are no data supporting the commercial development of antivenoms against other colubrid species, although some authors have advocated this (e.g., Salomão et al., 2003), or suggested that such a "serum" could avoid the adverse effects of inappropriate provision of polyvalent antivenoms (e.g., anti-*Bothrops* spp.) for various colubrid bites (particularly *Philodryas* spp.; Correia et al., 2010). The risks of administering hypothetical antivenom in these cases would probably far outweigh any possible minimal benefit, as the vast majority of documented bites from many of these snakes feature insignificant or mild local effects. Commercial preparation of antivenom against species associated with frequent bites resulting in mild-to-moderate local effects in specific Third World regions (e.g., *Philodryas* spp. in Brazil) would be highly unlikely due to the unfavorable clinical risk/benefit profile and the complete lack of any commercial profit margin. Indeed, procurement of an adequate supply of safe, regionally specific antivenom against fully recognized medically important viperid and elapid species in Third World locales of great need is often a challenging, politically charged issue (Gutiérrez et al., 2006; Harrison et al., 2009; White, 2009; Williams et al., 2010). However, it is important to note that closer study and careful detailed reporting of clinical features of bites from these diverse colubroids should be included in the ambitious, and much needed, proposed global snakebite partnership/World Health Organization initiative.

As emphasized previously, the vast majority of these snakes inflict minor wounds without medically significant effects. Cases that do feature notable local effects are relatively uncommon and result from unclear etiology. Many people bitten by colubrid species have had prior contact with wild and/or captive snakes. This supports the concept that Type 1 hypersensitivity plays a part in their causation. These hypersensitivity reactions are due to classic IgE cross-linkage on mast cell and basophil receptors and, possibly, binding of a pro-anaphylactic subtype of IgG_4 to other mast cell-activating receptors. Medically significant local effects from many of these bites are probably due to the action of Duvernoy's secretion components such as proteolytic rhexic hemorrhagins and, in some individuals, hypersensitivity reactions.

There are only two well-documented cases of systemic effects after bites by *M. monspessulanus* (neurotoxicity) and *P. olfersii* (widespread ecchymoses). Therefore, although uncommon, these species must be considered capable of inflicting systemic envenomation. However, even though documented cases of bites by *B. irregularis* on Guam also have occasionally included systemic symptoms or signs suggesting systemic involvement, there are too few data to firmly establish the risk. This exemplifies the need for careful and cautious analysis of these cases along with precise documentation founded on evidence-based data. It also emphasizes the need for evaluation of these cases with due consideration of the verified identification and natural history of the ophidian species involved in a given case. Similarly, as CRISPS have been characterized from the Duvernoy's secretions of *H. angulatus* and *A. portoricensis*, as well as others, it is tempting to hypothesize a role for these in the occasional reports of wound paresthesia associated with bites from these taxa. However, it is important to avoid premature assignment of clinical risk based on limited biomedical data primarily derived from biochemical analysis of very restricted samples of Duvernoy's secretions or laboratory animal experiments. Concerns regarding these misinterpretations and their possible implications have been discussed elsewhere (Weinstein et al., 2010; and previous comments).

The diversity of this former assemblage of colubroids suggests that many biomedically important secretions, venoms, and their components will probably be discovered from further study of these snakes. Prey-specific toxins may have particular biomedical utility due to their often distinct specificities and selective lethal potencies. As more of these little-studied species increasingly enter the animal trade and private collections, assessment of their medical importance assumes additional significance. In recognizing 40 + species of non-front-fanged colubroids that reportedly produced medically significant bites, Warrell (1988) opined that an increasing number of species capable of envenomating humans would be gradually identified. This prediction is supported by some of the medically significant cases involving >100 taxa critically considered here. This emphasizes the need for increased study of these snakes that comprise the majority of extant ophidian species. Such study holds promise for contributions to the biomedical and clinical sciences, laboratory medicine, herpetology, and evolutionary biology.

Appendix A
Representative Unverified Cases of Medically Significant "Colubrid" Bites Posted on the Internet[1]

Case 1. Western Hognose Snake, *Heterodon nasicus*

Website

www.herpnet.net/bite/

Features of Case

Amateur hobbyist report describing a bite inflicted on the medial aspect of the right index finger (ascertained from photos accompanying the report) by an approximately 8-inch male long-term captive *H. n. nasicus*. Victim/author (male, age unknown) stated that the bite was a result of a "food response, not aggression," and that the snake "hung on like a little bulldog ... seemed to use its rear teeth almost exclusively, actively engaging the larger rear teeth." The snake reportedly "chewed" for 3–5 min and was eventually forcibly removed by immersion in cool tap water. Reported effects included bleeding, edema that began 2–3 h postbite and progressed, ultimately involving the forearm; digital stiffness; discharging wound; and the appearance of "small itchy blisters" and "tiny popped vessels." The victim reported that at 45 h postbite the edema extended to the elbow, while the hand edema began to decrease and blistering was noted at the base of the thumb. At 72 h, the edema reportedly was almost fully resolved. A "general reddish discoloration" was reported and deemed "not a rash." The victim stated that as the edema resolved, the hand was still tender, but reported that little "real pain" was experienced at any time during the described events.

---

[1] The cases included here are presented as representative samples of those posted at various websites. We have purposely declined inclusion of a comprehensive review of these cases as there is no objectively documented provenance, independent identification of snakes involved in the purported bite or recorded formal medical review of the victim. See section IV regarding the issues that seriously affect the utility of such cases.

Comments

As detailed in Section 4.5, although the victim/author attempted to provide a case account, the report is typically flawed due to a lack of formal medical review, subjectivity, and incorrect misinterpretation of factors influencing the outcome of the bite as well as the described symptoms/signs. It is noted that several features of the case are similar to some that have been formally reported (see Section 4.2; Weinstein & Keyler, 2009). Regardless, the case cannot be acceptably analyzed as it lacks the minimal standard of any appropriate clinical case report (Section 4.5). Evidence-based analyses of clinical cases must be held at an acceptable standard, whether the case involves a colubroid snakebite, myocardial infarction, diverticulitis, and so on. For instance, it is not possible to confidently analyze a case of haematuria posted on the Internet. Such a case requires formal medical history, examination, investigation, and documentation. The nature of any presentation must not change, lower, or in any way alter the standard expected in formal reporting of a clinical case. The identity of the snake in this case is not in question, as the victim posted photos of the specimen biting his finger. This should not encourage similar experimentation as the effects can, on occasion, be significant. Clearly, the victim allowed the snake to remain engaged on his finger in order to observe the effects of a protracted bite (Section 4.5). The victim's previous exposures, bites, and possible medical comorbidities are unknown. Obviously, at the least, the victim has had regular exposure to this snake for the period of ownership of the specimen (reportedly 8 years). In the USA, the medical history and, if applicable, documented details regarding previous snakebite incidents are personal medical data protected by Health Insurance Portability and Accountability Act (HIPAA)[2] statutes, and these constitute another reason (medicolegal) for the low evidence value of such cases posted on the Internet.

Case 2. Jackson's Black Tree Snake, *Thrasops jacksoni*

Websites

http://forums.kingsnake.com/view.php?id=1510152,1510152
http://www.reptileforums.co.uk/snake-pictures/124251-thrasops-jacksoni.html

Features of Case

Described by the victim/author (presumably male, age unknown), this case involved a bite inflicted by an approximately 48-inch captive *T. jacksoni*. Photos of the snake

[2]The HIPAA of 1996 provides security and privacy rules that establish US national standards for the protection of individually identifiable health information and security of electronically stored personal medical records. The implications of this Act also accentuate the need for competent medical evaluation and professional reporting of any clinical presentation, including medically significant snakebites. Such information publically posted on the Internet can be subject to misuse, whether purposely or unintentionally. See http://www.hhs.gov/ocr/privacy/ for further information regarding the medico-legal issues related to this Act.

were posted with the report, and although the snake responsible for the reported bite appears correctly identified, this was not officially verified. The victim was offering a mouse to the snake when the snake struck and, "... missed the proffered mouse entirely, slid up the tongs ..." and sank its teeth into the victim's left forefinger. The snake was allowed to "hang on" to the finger for "a couple of minutes" due to concerns of injuring the snake during forcible removal. The victim reported that the wound bled while the snake remained attached, and bleeding continued while attempts at removing the snake (by sliding a playing card between the jaws and finger) ensued. The attempt to remove the snake resulted in increased "chewing," and although the total time of attachment is unclear, the description obviously suggests a protracted bite. The victim stated, "Once I had finally got him off, I realized that I was going to feel some ill effects ..."

The reported effects included bleeding ("... a steady trickle of blood and plasma ...")/discharge from the wound for several days; pruritis of the hand/palm; stiffness of the affected finger as well as the adjacent digit and associated metacarpals; gradual development of edema involving the hand; and bruising at the bite site. The morning after the incident, the left hand was edematous to the wrist, and over the subsequent 48 h reportedly swelled "to about twice its original size." The victim also reported "quite severe pain" (approximately 1 week in duration) that he related to the edema, and that "lymph nodes in the left armpit were enfarcted (sic) and painful as hell." The bite wound became "black and blue" and the bitten finger reportedly remained "intensely painful, bloated, and unable to bend for weeks afterwards." The described effects followed a reported 10-day course, at which time the edema almost fully resolved and the wound was "invisible." There were no further effects or sequelae reported. The victim chose not to seek medical consultation (and retrospectively expressed regret regarding that decision), and the only treatment consisted of ingestion of an unknown dose of an unidentified antihistamine. He concluded that a "much larger specimen ... could conceivably cause a much more serious, even fatal, envenomation." He also compared the potential dangers of *T. jacksoni* to that of *D. typus* and noted the "handful of deaths recorded for *P. olfersii*" as an example of other "rearfangs" with lethal potential for humans.[3]

Comments

As in many Internet/popular periodical reports, the author/victim attempted to detail his experiences after receiving a bite from a captive snake, in this case, *T. jacksoni*. There is a scarcity of reports involving *Thrasops* spp., but this report cannot be accepted as a documented account due to issues involving absence of formal medical review and resulting description of physical exam, laboratory tests, and the like; subjectivity per victim as author; misinterpretation of signs/symptoms; and additional mitigating factors as noted in Section 4.5. As this case purportedly involved

---

[3]As detailed in section II, there are no acceptably documented or proven cases of human fatalities that have resulted from a *P. olfersii* bite. The only non-front-fanged colubroid species that have caused proven human fatalities belong to the genera, *Dispholidus*, *Thelotornis*, and *Rhabdophis*.

mild-to-moderate local effects—including a discharging wound—formal medical review, official verification, and documentation were clearly needed. The author recognized this and expressed regret for not seeking medical attention. In contrast with the assumptive assertions of some Internet contributors, to date there are no data supporting clinical similarity between medically significant bites from *D. typus* and *Thrasops* spp. There is only a single well-documented case of a medically significant bite from a *Thrasops* spp. (*T. flavigularis*, Table 4.1; Section 4.3), and it featured only local effects (Table 4.1; Section 4.3). Significant bites from *D. typus* and *Thelotornis* occasionally include moderate local effects, but these are most frequently followed by an unmistakable systemic disease featuring life-threatening consumptive coagulopathy/bleeding (Table 4.1; Section 4.3). However, as described in Section 4.3, there are data describing transcripts in *T. jacksoni* that may encode components (e.g., proteases, possibly disintegrins, procoagulants) similar to those of hazard level 1 dispholidines such as *D. typus* (Table 4.2). Therefore, any significant bite from a *Thrasops* spp. should be reviewed by a physician, the identity of the snake should be confirmed by an independent qualified person in a recognized institution, and the case (including laboratory test results) should be formally documented and subjected to qualified peer-review in an appropriate journal.

Case 3. Mangrove Snake, *Boiga dendrophila*

Websites

http://www.google.com/imgres?imgurl=http://i158.photobucket.com/albums/t85/stuartd_album/DSCF4588-1.jpg&imgrefurl=http://www.reptileforums.co.uk/forums/snakes/133156-snake-bite-picthread.html&usg=__FqhehFTy1wAoIUiHEOIKvq9QsbA=&h=768&w=1024&sz=823&hl=en&start=11&itbs=1&tbnid=PVwtOjduIMeDM:&tbnh=113&tbnw=150&prev=/images%3Fq%3Dboiga%2Bdendrophila%2Bbite%26hl%3Den%26client%3Dfirefoxa%26sa%3DN%26rls%3Dorg.mozilla:en-GB:official%26gbv%3D2%26ndsp%3D18%26tbs%3Disch:1
http://www.venomlist.com/forums/index.php?showtopic=21193

Features of Case

Victim posted a series of photos purporting to show the result of a bite inflicted on the right thumb by a 4-foot *B. dendrophila*. The victim stated that he was bitten while attempting to administer "medication" (details were unspecified) to the specimen via oral tube. The photos initially illustrate several bleeding punctures, and photos reportedly taken the next day feature erythema, edema (involving the thenar area as well as expanding to the dorsum and palmar aspects of the hand), ecchymoses, and sero-sanguinous discharge from a blister that formed in the presumed wound site. Described also were swollen glands in the right "armpit" accompanied by "almost unbearable" pain and "slight numbness on the right side of the face." The victim indicated that the major effects occurred hours after the incident. He also stated that *B. dendrophila* has, "… fairly potent venom known as a three-finger toxin consisting of the same neurotoxins that are present in cobra and mamba venom and the same hemotoxins as are present in viper venom. Fortunately, they lack an efficient delivery system and do not produce really significant amounts…."

Comments

As observed in the previous examples of Internet-posted cases, the numerous flaws and insufficiencies in these reports force their classification as only interesting anecdote (see Section 4.5). Although some tantalizingly offer subjective information regarding infrequently documented bites from several species (many, such as *B. dendrophila*, are common in private collections), the standard of clinical documentation must be held to the same professional and competent expectation as any other account of medically significant pathology. In fact, one could argue that the very contentious nature and misinterpretation of toxinological data common to these reports should require a *stringent* standard of objective documentation. For instance, the postsynaptically active three-finger neurotoxins characterized to date from Duvernoy's secretions of *B. dendrophila* and other non-front-fanged colubroids are strongly prey-specific (see Section 4.2). These probably play no role in any effects that result from bites of these snakes, and to date the medical effects of documented *B. dendrophila* bites are insignificant. As stated in Section 4.2, large specimens of all *Boiga* spp. should be handled with caution, especially in the setting of the handler having chronic illness or predisposing medical comorbidities. Additionally, it is important to note that the victim reported that he presented at an emergency room and that "they were totally at a loss as to what to do, I came away with anti-inflammatories and was told to take aspirin or paracetamol (acetaminophen) for the pain, which has eased off somewhat now without analgesia …" This also emphasizes the need for medical personnel to consult with an appropriately trained medical professional when confronted with an unfamiliar snakebite that caused significant local effects. In this, the case may also represent a lost opportunity to formally document some significant effects of a protracted bite from *B. dendrophila*.

Appendix B
Representative Lethal Potency Ranges and Yields of Duvernoy's Secretions and Venoms from Selected Non-Front-Fanged Colubroid Snakes

Species (Family, Subfamily)	Yield[a]		Range of Reported Murine LD$_{50}$ mg/kg (Route)[a]	Reference
	Liquid (μL)	Dry (mg)		
Alsophis [*Borikenophis*] *portoricensis* (Dipsadidae, Xenodontinae)	160[b]	5.9	2.1 mg/kg (i.p., murine) 3.8 mg/kg (i.p., anoline lizard)[c]	Weldon and Mackessy (2010)
Boiga [*Toxicodryas*] *blandingi* (Colubridae, Colubrinae)	147.5	1.6	2.85 (i.p.)–4.88 (i.p.)	Levinson et al. (1976); Weinstein and Smith (1993)
Boiga dendrophila (Colubridae, Colubrinae)	127.5	8.0	3.26 (i.p.)–4.85 (i.v.)	Sakai et al. (1984); Weinstein and Smith (1993)
Boiga irregularis (Colubridae, Colubrinae)	40–500[d]	0.642–19.2[d]	10.50 (i.p.)–80.00 (i.v.)[d]	Vest et al. (1991); Weinstein et al. (1991); Chiszar et al. (1992); Mackessy et al. (2006)
Spalerosophis diadema cliffordi (Colubridae, Colubrinae)	0.09	NR	2.75 (i.v.)	Rosenberg et al. (1985)

(*Continued*)

Species (Family, Subfamily)	Yield[a]		Range of Reported Murine LD_{50} mg/kg (Route)[a]	Reference
	Liquid (μL)	Dry (mg)		
Dispholidus typus (Colubridae, Colubrinae)	NR	0.5–8.0	0.06 (i.v.)–12.5 (s.c.)	Minton and Minton (1980); Weinstein and Smith (1993)
Thelotornis capensis (Colubridae, Colubrinae)	40	2.25	0.050 (i.p.)–1.24 (i.v.)	Christensen (1968); Weinstein and Smith (1993)
Rhabdophis tigrinus (Natricidae)	NR	8.5–20.5	0.265 (i.v.)–9.20 (s.c.)	Sakai et al. (1983)
Rhabdophis subminiatus (Natricidae)	10–15	NR	0.125 (i.v.)– 0.129 (i.v.)	Ferlan et al. (1983); Sakai et al. (1984)
Malpolon monspessulanus (Lamprophiidae, Psammophiinae)	0.44–5.2	NR	6.50 (i.v.)	Rosenberg et al. (1985)
Philodryas olfersii (Dipsadidae, Xenodontinae)	NR	NR	2.79 (i.p.)	Assakura et al. (1992)
Hydrodynastes gigas (Dipsadidae, Xenodontinae)	0–50	1.3 (single gland)	2.0 (i.p.)–9.4 (s.c.)	Glenn et al. (1992)
Heterodon nasicus (Dipsadidae, Heterodontinae)	24	NR	NR	Hill and Mackessy (2000)
Heterodon platirhinos (Dipsadidae, Heterodontinae)	1–5	0.050–0.200	NR	Young (1992)

(*Continued*)

Species (Family, Subfamily)	Yield[a]		Range of Reported Murine LD$_{50}$ mg/kg (Route)[a]	Reference
	Liquid (μL)	Dry (mg)		
Thamnophis elegans vagrans (Natricidae, Thamnophiinae)	0.71	0.057	13.85 (i.p.)	Vest (1981a,b)
Natrix tessellate (Natricidae)	0.16–0.76	NR	25.0 (i.v., MLD)	Rosenberg et al. (1985)
Cerberus rynchops (Homalopsidae)	10	NR	NR	Guinea et al. (1992)
Enhydris bocourti (Homalopsidae)	NR	NR	7.30 (i.v.)	Sakai et al. (1984)
Enhydris chinensis (Homalopsidae)	NR	NR	2.05 (i.v.)	Sakai et al. (1984)
Homalopsis buccata (Homalopsidae)	NR	NR	14.30 (i.v.)	Sakai et al. (1984)

Abbreviations: i.p., intraperitoneal; i.v., intravenous; s.c., subcutaneous; MLD, minimal lethal dose; NR, not reported.
[a]Aside from *R. tigrinus* yield, data obtained from macerated/dissected glands are excluded. Yields were obtained using microcapillary pipette extraction of living specimens ± sedation and/or parasympathomimetic stimulation (see text). Some of the quoted figures are average or mean of multiple determinations. For greater detail regarding yields and lethal potencies, see the text as well as Weinstein and Kardong (1994), and Mackessy (2002).
[b]Referenced data were published as an average of 30 extractions from six specimens.
[c]The mg/kg values are calculated from the published data (μg of "venom"/g lizard or mouse body weight).
[d]The ranges include intermediate values obtained from snakes of varying age and length. See the referenced studies for specific details.

Appendix C
Strategies of Management of Gram-Negative Septicemia: Are There Lessons to Be Learned for Managing Venom-Induced Coagulopathies?[1]

Although pathophysiologically distinctive, some general similarities between hazard level 1 colubrid envenoming and gram-negative septicemia can be identified. Septic patients with endotoxemia-induced consumptive coagulopathy/disseminated intravascular coagulation (DIC) often are treated with fresh-frozen plasma (FFP), cryoprecipitate, purified coagulation factors, platelets, protein C, and, occasionally, drotrecogin-α (Dempfle, 2004). Some investigators have highlighted differences between coagulopathic envenomations and DIC, questioning the appropriateness of the term for the venom-induced disease (Isbister, 2010). Isbister (2010) stated that the lack of evidence of systemic microthrombi, and end-organ failure in venom-induced coagulopathy, was indicative of an absence of DIC. In addition, he stressed the differences between the time course of venom-induced coagulopathy and the mechanism of initiation of coagulation activation, as thrombin generation in DIC is mediated by the tissue factor/factor VIIa pathway. It can be argued that the renal injury on hazard level 1 envenomation certainly may constitute end-organ damage and the pathways (e.g., "intrinsic" and "extrinsic" used as convenient terms of reference [see Figure 4.1]) can function simultaneously *in vivo* without precise detection.

A current Japanese expert consensus regarding potential pharmacotherapy for treatment of DIC generally recommends low-molecular weight heparin (LMWH), unfractionated heparin (UFH), antithrombin, and synthetic protease inhibitor (SPI; Wada et al., 2010). This consensus also asserted a provisional caution in regard to treatment of hemorrhagic diathesis in which LMWH, synthetic protease inhibitor (SPI), and antithrombin were recommended with recognition of a lack of quality evidence (Wada et al., 2010). However, this panel also declined recommendation of LMWH, UFH, and danaproid sodium for use in cases with life-threatening bleeding, while SPI is recommended in this scenario as it does not exacerbate bleeding (Wada et al., 2010). These authors also recognized replacement therapy (blood, FFP, platelets) as clinically indicated in life-threatening hemorrhagic diathesis. Their recommendations emphasized concerns regarding the frequent association of DIC with thrombosis (Wada et al., 2010). This is relevant to some serious hazard level 1 colubrid envenoming, as noted in some of the representative cases analyzed in this book (Table 4.1; Section 4.3). The extent of thrombosis in some of these cases can

[1] This appendix was solely authored by SAW.

be underappreciated. For example, streptokinase failed to dissolve postmortem clotted blood from a patient fatally envenomated by a *T. kirtlandii* (Mebs et al., 1978). The clinical pathology of the venom disease in the patient described by Mebs et al. (1978) suggests development of *purpura fulminans* from microvascular thrombosis. Therefore, this case featured some pathology in common with endotoxemia-induced DIC.

Interestingly, Wang et al. (2009) described a recombinant fibrinogenase derived from *Deinagkistrodon acutus* (Chinese snorkel-nosed viper or "hundred-pacer") venom that protected rabbits against lipopolysaccharide (LPS; endotoxin)-induced DIC. This recombinant also decreased renal fibrin deposition in the LPS-treated animals. It is not surprising that some venoms contain components that oppose the pharmacological effects of other venom toxins; some may even represent potential scaffolds for future therapeutics useful in the management of venom-induced DIC.

As noted by Dempfle (2004), no randomized trials have demonstrated evidence-supported therapies for consumptive coagulopathy. This author suggested recommendations similar to those of Wada et al. (2010), but reinforced the lack of proven clinical efficacy for most of these treatments. Therefore, recommendations for endotoxin-induced DIC present a guide that reflects some of the management strategies suggested by case studies of venom-induced consumptive coagulopathy/DIC. In summary, these are treatment of the specific cause of the coagulopathy (provision of antivenom if available); avoidance of unproven and possibly harmful therapies (heparin, vitamin K, antifibrinolytics, etc.); cautious provision of replacement therapy as clinically indicated and use, at the discretion of the physician, of therapeutics of unproven efficacy that have a low-risk profile (e.g., SPI).

Appendix D
Legal Considerations Regarding Private Ownership of Venomous Snakes (Including Hazard Level 1 "Colubrids"): An Opinionated Essay

Beginning in the mid-to-late 1980s, there was a notable explosion of interest in the private collection of living reptiles and amphibians. Since about 2001, approximately 2 million live reptiles are imported per annum in the United States alone. Of these, ≥25% are typically popular harmless species such as green iguanas (*Iguana iguana*), Central and South American boa constrictors (*Boa* spp.), and others (e.g., in 2001, around 2 million reptiles were imported of which about 500,000 were *I. iguana*).[1] This volume of importation, as well as exchange of captive-bred specimens, translates into hundreds of millions, possibly billions, of dollars (most published figures are inexact estimates). There are similarly large markets throughout Europe, Canada, and Japan. Due to the unprecedented, and relatively sudden, expansion of private ownership of reptiles and amphibians, an increasing number of species have become commercially available. Unfortunately, a proportion of amateur collectors often collect species of which they have little or no experience handling or maintaining. This lack of experience, and in some cases, overt carelessness/foolhardiness (free-handling, "self-immunization" with venoms, etc.), intersected with availability of dangerously venomous species occasionally results in serious morbidity or tragedy. An increasing number of "expos" or breeders' vendor shows, as well as Internet exchanges, provide open availability of many species to a broad expanse of interested prospective buyers. This relatively open access has some important positive aspects, as appropriately trained and/or informed hobbyists can obtain healthy captive-bred nonvenomous specimens to enhance their interest. Well-informed collection of captive-bred specimens also encourages further study as well as obviates collection pressures on wild populations. Many professional biologists (e.g., herpetologists, toxinologists, and other life scientists, including all of the authors) partly initiated and propagated their interests by maintaining a collection of living specimens. The responsible and reasonable trade in reptiles and amphibians also provides valuable specimens for research (including venom and Duvernoy's secretion research).

---

[1] http://www.worldwildlife.org/what/globalmarkets/wildlifetrade/faqs-reptile.html

However, these positives are increasingly negatively impacted by an irresponsible segment of amateurs as well as a growing lack of stringent self-monitored selectivity on the part of some breeders/vendors of potentially dangerous snake species in regard to the broad array of potential buyers. Many of these potential "customers" lack appropriate training, knowledge, and experience to keep species such as rhinoceros vipers (*Bitis nasicornis*), Gaboon vipers (e.g., the western Gaboon viper, *B. rhinoceros*), black mambas (*Dendroaspis polylepis*), eyelash tree or Schlegel's viper (*Bothriechis schlegeli*), or the hazard level 1 colubrid, *D. typus*, among many others. All of the aforementioned species (and many others) are either commonly offered for sale (e.g., *B. rhinoceros*, *B. schlegeli*), or periodically are available (*D. typus*, *D. polylepis*). Numerous genetic variants of various cobra species (e.g., leucistic, albino, "sunrise," of *Naja kaouthia*, and others) are commonly available via the Internet or select vendor shows (only a few expos allow the sale of venomous snakes). This circumstance is increasingly evidencing the proverb of "one rotten apple ...", as in the United States, for example, a mounting number of over-reaching state and local municipality regulations are becoming evident. Some of these laws negatively impact the responsible collection of popular nonthreatened/nonvenomous species. This is in response to a relatively small number of serious snakebites that occur among this amateur community. On the other hand, it must be noted that in many of these cases, the substantial expense (e.g., literally tens to hundreds of thousands of dollars) associated with management of a serious/life-threatening envenoming may be at least partly cost shifted to the local community. This is due to either a lack of insurance coverage or insufficient coverage of those envenomed under these circumstances, as many insurance providers will not absorb the totality of costs in these cases. Thus, some cases can incur significant cost shifted to the local community in which the envenomed patient resides. It is unclear if the health care initiative in the United States will change any of these implied complexities of costs incurred by such cases of envenoming by privately owned venomous snakes (it probably will not significantly relieve the incurred private costs).

Therefore, it is critical before statutory regulations are ultimately imposed and suffocate all access to many of these species (including numerous nonvenomous species), that vendors, breeders, commercial importers, and, most importantly, prospective collectors/hobbyists, exercise a notably increased rational introspection regarding captive maintenance of venomous species and those of unknown medical importance. Clearly, hazard level 1 colubrids (Table 4.2) must be considered equal to any venomous snake capable of inflicting a fatal envenoming. These species should only be legally maintained by professionals (e.g., in zoological parks and/or in research collections) or rarely by very experienced collectors. Stringent legal restrictions on these species are entirely justified, especially as antivenom is only available for *D. typus* and *R. tigrinus*, and these antivenoms are difficult to obtain. The vast majority of other colubrids (including many taxa readily available in the trade such as *H. gigas* and *B. dendrophila*) typically produce only mild local effects. Regardless, as noted in this book, these species may be capable of medically significant local effects, and some under unusual circumstances (e.g., large specimen, protracted bite associated with feeding behavior) may produce more severe morbidity that can result in extended convalescence. Other species, such as *P. olfersii* and *B. irregularis*, may be capable of inflicting bites that result in rare systemic effects in particularly susceptible victims (e.g., infants, children, the elderly, those with comorbidities or chronic illness, malnutrition, and/or substance dependency). Therefore, hazard levels 2 and 2/3 (Table 4.2) species must be handled with care and viewed with caution. Only increased responsibility and awareness of the need for appropriate training and individual limitations on the part of collectors and commercial/private suppliers will prevent the imposition of statutory regulations that will suffocate reasonable and *responsible* private access to many captive reptiles and amphibians.

Appendix E
List of Osteological Specimens
Examined at AMNH[1]

Taxa	Locality/Source	Museum Accession Number
Dispholidus typus	Durban, South Africa (FitzSimons)	75722
Thelotornis kirtlandii	Durban, South Africa (commercial dealer)	75091
Rhamnophis aethiopissa ituriensis	Niapu, Belgian Congo	12500
Thrasops jacksoni	Kampala, Uganda (Carnochan)	50572
Thrasops flavigularis	French Cameroon, Metet (Grissett)	R 50573
Rhabdophis tigrinus lateralis	Korea, "near Seoul" (Conant/Hanlon)	R 148037
Rhabdophis tigrinus lateralis	Korea, "near Seoul" (Conant/Hanlon)	R 148038
Macrelaps microlepidotus	Natal, Durban, South Africa	5897
Macrelaps microlepidotus	Natal, Mayville, South Africa	18227
Macropisthodon rudis	Fukien, Chungan Hsien (Pope)	34513
Tachymenis peruviana	Puno, Peru; San Antoine, Carabaya	5256
Boiga blandingi	Locality unavailable	84563
Boiga dendrophila	Locality unavailable	R 73608
Boiga irregularis	Northern Territory, Australia	114498
Philodryas baroni	Argentina	62831
Malpolon monspessulanus	Locality unavailable	75284
Heterodon platirhinos	Locality unavailable	63590
Heterodon platirhinos	Locality unavailable	75485
Heterodon nasicus	Locality unavailable	74842

(Continued)

[1] American Museum of Natural History, Department of Herpetology, New York, NY.

Taxa	Locality/Source	Museum Accession Number
Heterodon simus	South Carolina, USA	38165
Heterodon nasicus kennerlyi	Apache, Cochise Co, Arizona, USA (Bogert)	58234
Thamnophis sirtalis sirtalis	Locality unavailable	70096
Thamnophis elegans vagrans	Sandoval, New Mexico, USA (Applegarth)	R 148051
Oligodon cinereus	China, Hainan, Nodoa (Pope)	027899
Lycodon aulicus	Bombay, India (commercial dealer)	77025
Atractaspis irregularis	Niangara, Congo (Lang-Chapin)	12355
Corallus caninus	Locality unavailable	R 57788
Crotalus atrox	Locality unavailable	137173
Naja naja	North India	64418
Aipysurus laevis	Roebuck Bay, Western Australia (Spalding-Hosmer)	86176

Additional Recommended Reading

The vast majority of information about non-front-fanged colubroid snakes is dispersed among many different journals and periodicals. A large proportion of these is infrequently available or is difficult to obtain. As noted in Section 4.5, a significant number of these publications may be minimally referred. The Bibliography section lists many published materials that contribute information about non-front-fanged colubroids.

Aside from this book, no others deal exclusively, or extensively, with these snakes. Listed below are a few examples of recommended books that contain some information about non-front-fanged colubroids:

> Meier, J. and White, J. (Eds.), 1995. *CRC Handbook of Clinical Toxicology of Animal Venoms and Poisons*. CRC Press, Boca Raton, Florida. This book (co-edited by one of the authors [JW] of this book) is a thorough compendium of authoritatively written, detailed reviews of venomous animals, the toxinology of their venoms, and management of envenomations. Although it does not contain a specific section on non-front-fanged colubroids, information on some species is within several contributed sections.
>
> Mebs, D., 2002. *Venomous and Poisonous Animals*. CRC Press, Boca Raton, Florida. This attractive and well-written book contains detailed overviews of the biology and toxinology of venomous and poisonous species. It also includes a short section on non-front-fanged colubroids.
>
> Campbell, J.A. and Lamar, W.W. (Eds.), 2004. *The Venomous Reptiles of the Western Hemisphere*, 2 Vols. Cornell University Press, Ithaca, New York. This lavishly illustrated book contains a treasure trove of information about the ecology, biology, and toxinology of venomous reptiles of the Western Hemisphere. There is some substantive information about non-front-fanged colubroids (including a mini-review written by one of the authors [DAW] of this book) of reported medical risks associated with a number of "rear-fanged" taxa.
>
> Mackessy, S.P. (Ed.), 2010. *CRC Handbook of Reptile Venoms and Toxins*. Taylor and Francis, Boca Raton, Florida. This multi-authored text contains numerous well-written chapters on the biochemistry of venom components, the functional anatomy of venom delivery systems, and the clinical toxinology of medically important venomous snakes. It includes some detailed information on non-front-fanged colubroid Duvernoy's secretions/venoms, including an analysis of the comparative functional anatomy of Duvernoy's glands and "true" venom glands co-authored by one of the authors [SAW] of this book.

Aiding the Envenomated Patient and Further Information: Societies, Journals, Toxinology Courses, and Associated Contacts

Seeking Advice for Management of a Patient Bitten by a Non-Front-Fanged Colubroid Snake

A book like this one represents just one point in time. It cannot cover new knowledge and new treatments yet to come. Therefore, for a clinician faced with managing a case of non-front-fanged colubroid snakebite, it may sometimes be necessary to seek further expert advice. While there are individual consultants, covering their availability and contact details is impractical in a book, so it is better to seek advice through an organized expert service. In most parts of the world this function is fulfilled by a poisons' information center/service. Each country will have phone numbers for their service, which may change over time. If numbers in your country are not readily known, you may find contact details through the World Health Organization website (http://www.who.int/ipcs/poisons/centre/directory/en/).

Societies and Periodicals

A number of societies have involvement with various aspects of toxinology and envenoming, including occasional information about non-front-fanged colubroids. The International Society on Toxinology (IST) is the lead society at a global level covering both toxinology research and clinical toxinology. Details can be found on the Society's website (http://www.toxinology.org) and in their journal, *Toxicon*. The IST publishes original research and holds regular scientific meetings, both at a global level, and through regional sections of the Society (European Section, Asia-Pacific Section, Pan-American Section). A number of countries also have national or regional toxinology societies (e.g., the Brazilian Society of Toxinology, and the French Society on Toxinology). There are a number of national, regional, and global toxicology societies, most of which hold regular scientific meetings. Two well-known annual meetings of this type are the North American Congress of Clinical Toxicology (NACCT) and the Congress of the European Association of Poisons Centres and Clinical Toxicologists (EAPCCT), both of which frequently include presentations on aspects of snakebite. Some additional samplings of journals that specialize in toxinology are listed below. Contact/subscription information can be obtained via websearch:

Toxins—Open Access Journal
Egyptian Journal of Natural Toxins
Journal of Toxicology Toxin Reviews
Journal of Venomous Animals and Toxins including Tropical Diseases
Journal of Natural Toxins
Journal of Venom Research
Natural Toxins
Research Journal of Toxins.

There are also numerous local, national, regional, and international herpetological societies, some producing scientific journals of high repute that occasionally cover aspects of non-front-fanged colubroid snakes. A small representative sampling of well-established herpetological societies is listed below (their respective journals are in parentheses):

Society for Research on Amphibians and Reptiles in New Zealand Inc. (*SRARNZ notes*) www.victoria.ac.nz/srarnz/
American Society of Ichthyologists and Herpetologists (*Copeia*) www.asih.org

Australian Society of Herpetologists www.australiansocietyofherpetologists.org
British Herpetological Society (*The Herpetological Journal; The Herpetological Bulletin; The Natterjack*) http://www.thebhs.org
Herpetologists' League (*Herpetologica; Herpetological Monographs*) www.herpetologistsleague.org
Society for the Study of Amphibians and Reptiles (*Journal of Herpetology; Herpetological Review*) http://www.ssarherps.org

Contact information and subscription information for the following herpetological societies and/or their associated journals can be accessed through ZenScientist.com, or through Internet search:

Herpetological Association of Africa (*African Journal of Herpetology*)
Russian Journal of Herpetology
Phyllomedusa-Journal of Herpetology
Brazilian Society of Herpetology (*South American Journal of Herpetology*)
International Society for the History and Bibliography of Herpetology
Amphibian and Reptile Conservation
Applied Herpetology
Asiatic Herpetological Research
Australasian Journal of Herpetology
Herpetofauna
Herpetological Conservation and Biology
Japanese Journal of Herpetology.

The following organizations and toxicology societies may occasionally offer information and/or have subsections, as well as publish/present cases of non-front-fanged colubroid snakebites. Contact information can usually be easily obtained via websearch:

Viper Institute, University of Arizona
Animal Venom Research International
Center for Applied Toxinology.
Academy of Toxicological Sciences
American Academy of Clinical Toxicology
American Association of Poison Control Centers
American Board of Toxicology (ABT)
American Board of Forensic Toxicology (ABFT)
American Board of Veterinary Toxicology (ABVT)
American College of Medical Toxicology (ACMT)
American College of Toxicology
American Society for Pharmacology and Experimental Therapeutics-- Toxicology Division
Behavioral Toxicology Society
Canadian Network of Toxicology Centers (CNTC and RCCT)
European Society of Toxicologic Pathology (ESTP)
EuroTox
International Academy of Toxicologic Pathology
International Association of Therapeutic Drug Monitoring and Clinical Toxicology
International Neurotoxicology Association
International Society of Regulatory Toxicology and Pharmacology
International Union of Toxicology (IUTOX)

Italian Society of Toxicology
Japanese Society of Immunotoxicology
Society of Environmental Toxicology and Chemistry (SETAC)
Society of Forensic Toxicologists
Society of Toxicologic Pathology (STP)
Society of Toxicology of Canada (STC)
Society of Toxicology India (STOX)
Society of Toxicology (SOT)
Toxicology Education Foundation (TEF)
Turkish Society of Toxicology.

Some regional informatics-based organizations have substantial resources that may occasionally include publications or materials relevant to the study of non-front-fanged colubroids. One of these is the Center for North American Herpetology based in Lawrence, Kansas: http://www.cnah.org.

Another institution with relevant information and active research on non-front-fanged colubroids is the Instituto Butantan based in São Paulo, Brazil: http://www.butantan.gov.br.

Reptile hobbyist magazines may occasionally have features about different species of non-front-fanged colubroid snakes that are popular in private collections. Although these articles cannot be referenced in order to assess medically relevant information, some may offer interesting details about the basic biology and captive husbandry of some species. Some of these are listed below, and most have readily accessible websites:

United Kingdom

International Reptilian Magazine

United States/Canada

Iguana Times
Journal of the International Iguana Society
Reptiles Magazine

Europe

Reptilia—The European Herp Magazine
Terraria

France

La Tortue
Terrario Magazine

Italy

REPTImagazine

Several medical journals occasionally contain information relevant to the management of envenomation, although this uncommonly includes bites by non-front-fanged colubroids. The following list includes several representative examples, but is by no means exclusive:

Australian Medical Journal
American Family Physician
Lancet
Southern Medical Journal
South African Medical Journal
American Journal of Tropical Medicine and Hygiene
Wilderness and Environmental Medicine Journal
Brazilian Journal of Medical and Biological Research
Japan Medical Association Journal

Formal Training in Clinical Toxinology

Training in clinical toxinology, a subspecialty of clinical toxicology, is a relatively new phenomenon, as this highly specialized field of medicine moves toward formal recognition. The first and only comprehensive clinical toxinology course at an international level has been conducted since 1997 by the Toxinology Department, Women's & Children's Hospital, Adelaide, South Australia, in conjunction with the University of Adelaide. Details of upcoming courses may be found on the Clinical Toxinology Resources website (http://www.toxinology.com) or by contacting the Department. A few countries, such as Brazil, have local courses, while the Museum of Natural History, Paris, has a general toxinology course, not specific to clinical toxinology, but includes some clinical topics (for information contact: Muséum national d'Histoire naturelle, 57 rue Cuvier, CP 57, 75005, Paris). As a new initiative, the IST has adopted the establishment of clinical toxinology as a global medical field of expertise. It will likely take a number of years for this to become established and/or generally recognized.

A Call for Cases

Cases of non-front-fanged colubroid bites are actively sought for analysis, and even medically insignificant bites by little-known species may have value. Contributed cases containing carefully collected history and clinical data will be objectively analyzed, and some may be included in any possible future editions of this book or documented elsewhere as part of a collaborative effort. All contributors will be clearly acknowledged, and patient identity will be wholly and unconditionally protected. Please enquire and/or send case information to:

Scott A. Weinstein, PhD, MD, at: colubroidcase@gmail.com

Bibliography

Abbott, A.V., 2005. Diagnostic approach to palpitations. Am. Fam. Physician 71, 743–750.

Abercromby, A.F., 1910. The Snakes of Ceylon. Murray and Company, London, UK.

Acosta de Pérez, O., Leiva de Vila, L., Peichoto, M.E., Maruñak, S., Ruíz, R., Teibler, P., et al. 2003. Edematogenic and myotoxic activities of the Duvernoy's gland secretion of *Philodryas olfersii* from the north-east region of Argentina. Biocell 27, 363–370.

Ahasan, H.A., Mamna, A.A., Karim, S.R., Bakar, M.A., Gazi, E.A., Bala, C.S., 2004. Paralytic complications of puffer fish (tetrodotoxin) poisoning. Singapore Med. J. 45, 73–74.

Ahmed, I., Majeed, A., Powell, R., 2007. Heparin induced thrombocytopenia: diagnosis and management update. Postgrad. Med. J. 83, 575–582.

Aiken, S.P., Sellin, L.C., Schmidt, J.J., Weinstein, S.A., McArdle, J.J., 1992. A novel peptide toxin from *Trimeresurus wagleri* acts pre- and post-synaptically to block transmission at the rat neuromuscular junction. Pharm. Toxicol. 70, 459–462.

Aitchison, J.M., 1990. Boomslang bite-diagnosis and management. S. Afr. Med. J. 78, 39–42.

Akimoto, R., Watanabe, Y., Sakai, A., Kawamura, Y., Sawai, Y., 1991. A case of defibrination syndrome due to Japanese colubrid snake, yamakagashi (*Rhabdophis t. tigrinus*) bite, treated with antivenom. The Snake 23, 36–39.

Akubue, P.I., 1997. Poisons in Our Environment and Drug Overdose. A Guide for Health Professionals and the Lay Public. Snaaps Press, Enugu. pp. 77–82

Albolea, A.B.P., Salomão, M.D.G., Almeida-Santos, S.M., 2000. Why do non-poisonous snakes cause snakebites? Toxicon 38, 567–568.

Alburquerque, C.E., Ferrarezzi, H., 2004. A case of communal nesting in the Neotropical snake, *Sibynomorphus mikanii* (Serpentes, Colubridae). Phyllomedusa 3, 73–77.

Aleksankin, V.F., 1968. A case of acute drop in visual acuity of the right eye after snake bite. Oftalmol. Zh. 23, 58–60. (in Russian)

Alexander, G., Grothusen, J., Zepeda, H., Schwartzman, R.J., 1988. Gyroxin, a toxin from venom of *Crotalus durissus terrificus*, is a thrombin-like enzyme. Toxicon 26, 953–960.

Alfaro, M.E., Arnold, S.J., 2001. Molecular systematics and evolution of *Regina* and the thamnophiine snakes. Mol. Phylogenet. Evol. 21, 408–423.

American Psychiatric Association (2000). Diagnostic and Statistical Manual of Mental Disorders. Text Revision, fourth ed.. American Psychiatric Association, Washington, DC.

Amorós, C.L.B., 2004. *Liophis poecilogyrus* envenomation. Herp. Rev. 35, 69–70.

Anderson, P., 1965. The Reptiles of Missouri. University of Missouri Press, Columbia, MO. p. 330

Angel, M.F., Zhang, F., Jones, M., Henderson, J., Chapman, S.W., 2002. Necrotizing fasciitis of the upper extremity resulting from a water moccasin bite. South. Med. J. 95, 1090–1094.

Anton, T.G., 1994. Observation of predatory behavior in the regal ringneck snake (*Diadophis punctatus regalis*) under captive conditions. Bull. Chicago Herp. Soc. 29, 95.

Antunes, T.C., Yamashita, K.M., Barbaro, K.C., Saiki, M., Santoro, M.L., 2010. Comparative analysis of newborn and adult *Bothrops jararaca* snake venoms. Toxicon 56, 1443–1458.

Ariaratnam, C.A., Sheriff, M.H., Arambepola, C., Theakston, R.D., Warrell, D.A., 2009. Syndromic approach to treatment of snake bite in Sri Lanka based on results of a prospective national hospital-based survey of patients envenomed by identified snakes. Am. J. Trop. Med. Hyg. 81, 725–731.

Arthur, W., 2002. The emerging conceptual framework of evolutionary developmental biology. Nature 414, 757–764.

Arzola, J., Schenone, H., 1994. Dos nuevos casos de ofidismo en Chile. Boletin Chileno de Parasitologia 49, 69–70.

Assakura, M.T., Da Graca Salomão, M., Puorto, G., Mandelbaum, F.R., 1992. Hemorrhagic, fibrinogenolytic and edema-forming activities of the venom of the colubrid snake *Philodryas olfersii* (green snake). Toxicon 30, 427–438.

Atkinson, P.M., Bradlow, B.A., White, J.A., Greig, H.B.W., Gaillard, M., 1980. Clinical features of twig snake (*Thelotornis capensis*) envenomation. S. Afr. Med. J. 58, 1007–1010.

Atkinson, P.M., Rebello, M., Gaillard, M.C., Bradlow, B.A., 1981. The role of heparin therapy in *Dispholidus typus* envenomation: an experimental study. Thromb. Res. 23, 355–363.

Auffenberg, W., 1981. The Behavioural Ecology of the Komodo Monitor. University of Florida Press, Gainesville, FL.

Averill-Murray, R.C., 2006. Natural history of the western hognose snake (*Heterodon nasicus*) with notes on envenomation. Sonoran Herp. 19, 98–101.

Azuma, H., Sekizaki, S., Akizawa, T., Yasuhara, T., Nakajima, T., 1986. Activities of novel polyhydroxylated cardiotonic steroids purified from nuchal glands of the snake *Rhabdophis tigrinus*. J. Pharm. Pharmacol. 38, 388–390.

Bajaj, A., Bisseru, B., Powar, H.J., 1980. Snake bite. Med. J. Zambia 14, 109–112.

Ballard, V., Antonio, F.B., 2001. *Varanus griseus*. Toxicity. Herpetol. Rev. 32, 261.

Barun, A., Perry, G., Henderson, R.W., Powell, R., 2007. *Alsophis portoricensis anegadae* (Squamata: Colubridae): morphometric characteristics, activity patterns, and habitat use. Copeia 2007, 93–100.

Bechtel, H.B., 1999. In remembrance of Sherman Minton, Jr., 1919–1999. Herpetol. Rev 30, 202–204.

Beck, D.D., 2005. Biology of Gila Monsters and Beaded Lizards. University of California Press, Berkeley, CA.

Bedry, R., Hilbert, G., Goyffon, M., Laffort, P., Parrens, E., 1998. Is the saliva of the European whip snake (*Coluber viridiflavus*) neurotoxic? Toxicon 36, 1729–1730.

Beebe, W., 1946. Field notes on the snakes of Kartabo, British Guiana and Caripito, Venezuela. Zoologica: NY Zool. Soc. 41, 11–52.

Beiran, D., Currie, G., 1967. Snake bite due to *Thelotornis kirtlandii* (vine snake, bird snake or twig snake). Cent. Afr. J. Med. 13, 137.

Bibbs, C.S., Willis, F.B., Bratton, R.L., 2001. Iguana bites to the face. J. Am. Board Fam. Prac. 14, 152–154.

Bihorac, A., Schold, J.D., Hobson, C.E., 2010. Long-term mortality associated with acute kidney injury requiring dialysis. JAMA 303, 229.

Bizerra, A., Marques, O.A.V, Sazima, I., 2005. Reproduction and feeding of the colubrid snake *Tomodon dorsatus* in south-eastern Brazil. Amphibia-Reptilia 26, 33–38.

Blatchley, W.S., 1891. Notes on the batrachians and reptiles of Vigo County, Indiana. J. Cincinnati Soc. Nat. Hist. 14, 22–35.

Blaylock, R.S., 1960. A bite from a vine snake in Bulawayo. J. Herpetol. Assoc. Rhod. 12, 8–9.

Blaylock, R.S., 1982. Snakebites at Triangle Hospital, January 1975 to June 1981. Cent. Afr. Med. J. 28, 1–11.

Blaylock, R.S., 1983. Time of onset of clinical envenomation following snakebite. S. Afr. Med. J. 64, 357–360.

Blaylock, R.S., 1999. Antibiotic use and infection in snakebite victims. S. Afr. Med. J. 89, 874–876.

Blaylock, R.S., 2001. Normal oral bacterial flora from some southern African snakes. Onderstepoort J. Vet. Res. 68, 175–182.

Boeadi, J., Shine, R., Sugardigto, J., Amir, M., Sinaga, M.H., 1998. Biology of the commercially-harvested rat snake (*Ptyas mucosus*) and cobra (*Naja sputatrix*) in Central Java. Mertensiella 9, 99–104.

Bogert, C.M., 1943. Dentitional phenomena in cobras and other elapids with notes on adaptive modifications of the fangs. Bull. Am. Mus. Nat. Hist. 131, 285–360.

Bogert, C., Del Campo, R., 1956. The Gila monster and its allies. Bull. Am. Mus. Nat. Hist. 109, 1–238.

Bonaca, M.P., Steg, P.G., Feldman, L.J., Canales, J.F., Ferguson, J.J., Wallentin, L., et al. 2009. Antithrombotics in acute coronary syndromes. J. Am. Coll. Cardiol. 54, 969–984.

Boos, H.E.A., 2001. The Snakes of Trinidad and Tobago. Texas A&M University Press, College Station, TX.

Boquet, P., Saint Girons, H., 1972. Etude immunologique des glandes salivaires du vestibule-buccol de quelques Colubridae opisthoglyphes. Toxicon 10, 635–644.

Boulenger, G.A., 1896. Catalogue of the Snakes in the British Museum (Natural History). Volume III. Containing the Colubridae (Opisthoglyphae and Proteroglyphae), Amblycephalidae and Viperidae. British Museum (Natural History), London, UK.

Boulenger, G.A., 1913. The Snakes of Europe. Methuen and Company, London, UK.

Boulenger, E.G., 1915. On a colubrid snake (*Xenodon*) with a vertically moveable maxillary bone. Proc. Zool. Soc. Lond. 59, 83–85.

Bradlow, B.A., Atkinson, P.M., Gomperts, E.D., Gaillard, M.C., 1980. Studies on the coagulant effect of boomslang (*Dispholidus typus*) venom. Clin. Lab. Haemat. 2, 317–331.

Bragg, A.N., 1960. Is *Heterodon* venomous? Herpetologica 16, 121–123.

Branch, W.R., 1982. Venomous snakes of southern Africa, 3. Concluding part: Colubridae. The Snake 14, 1–17.

Branch, B., 1998. Bill Branch's Field Guide to the Snakes and Other Reptiles of Southern Africa. New Holland, London, UK.

Branch, W.R., McCartney, C.J., 1986. *Dispholidus typus* boomslang: envenomation. J. Herp. Assoc. Afr. 32, 34–35.

Broaders, M., Faro, C., Ryan, M.F., 1999. Partial purification of acetylcholine receptor binding components from the Duvernoy's secretions of Blanding's tree snake (*Boiga blandingi*) and the mangrove snake (*Boiga dendrophila*). J. Nat. Toxins 8, 155–166.

Broadley, D.G., 1957. Fatalities from the bites of *Dispholidus* and *Thelotornis* and personal case history. J. Herp. Assoc. Rhod. 1, 5.

Broadley, D.G., 1959. The herpetology of southern Rhodesia, Part I: Snakes. Bull. Mus. Comp. Zool. Harv. 120, 39–55.

Broadley, D.G., 1960. Case history of a boomslang (*Dispholidus*) bite. J. Herp. Assoc. Rhod. 11, 7–8.

Broadley, D.G., 1968. The venomous snakes of central and South Africa. In: Bucherl, W., Buckley, E.E., Deulofeu, V. (Eds.), Venomous Animals and Their Venoms (pp. 403–435). Academic Press, New York, NY.

Broadley, D.G., 1983. FitzSimons' Snakes of Southern Africa. Delta Books, Johannesburg, South Africa.

Broadley, D.G., Cock, E.V., 1975. Snakes of Rhodesia. Longman Rhodesia Ltd, Salisbury. 152 pp.

Broadley, D.G., Wallach, V., 2002. Review of the Dispholidini, with the description of a new genus and species from Tanzania (Serpentes, Colubridae). Bull. Nat. Hist. Mus. Lond. (Zool.) 68, 57–74.

Brown, B.C., 1939. The effect of *Coniophanes* poisoning in man. Copeia 2, 109.

Bryant, D.H., Burns, M.W., Lazarus, C., 1975. Identification of IgG antibody as a carrier of reaginic activity in asthmatic patients. J. Allergy Clin. Immunol. 56, 417–419.

Bucharetchi, F., de Capitani, E.M., Hyslop, S., Mello, S.M., Madureira, P.R., Zanardi, V., et al. 2010. Compartment syndrome after *Bothrops jararaca* snakebite: monitoring, treatment, and outcome. Clin. Toxicol. (Phila) 48, 57–60.

Buchtová, M., Handrigan, G.R., Tucker, A.S., Lozanoff, S., Town, L., Fu, K., et al. 2008. Initiation and patterning of the snake dentition are dependent on Sonic hedgehog signalling. Develop. Biol. 319, 132–145.

Bull, J.J., Jessop, T.S., Whiteley, M., 2010. Deathly drool: evolutionary and ecological basis basis of septic bacteria in Komodo dragon mouths. PLoS One 5, e11097. doi:10.1371/journal.pone.0011097.

Burger, W.I., 1975. A case of mild envenomation by the mangrove snake, *Boiga dendrophila*. The Snake 7, 99–100.

Burdmann, E.A., Woronik, V., Prado, E.B., Abdulkader, R.C., Saldanha, L.B., Barreto, O.C., et al. 1993. Snakebite-induced acute renal failure: an experimental model. Am. J. Trop. Med. Hyg. 48, 82–88.

Burgess, J.L., Dart, R.C., 1991. Snake venom coagulopathy: use and abuse of blood products in the treatment of pit viper envenomation. Ann. Emerg. Med. 20, 795–801.

Cable, D., McGehee, W., Wingert, W.A., Russell, F.E., 1984. Prolonged defibrination after a bite from a "nonvenomous" snake. JAMA 251, 925–926.

Cadle, J.E., 1987. Geographic distribution: problems in phylogeny and zoogeography. In: Seigel, R.A., Collins, J.T., Novak, S.S. (Eds.), Snakes: Ecology and Evolutionary Biology (pp. 77–105). Macmillan, New York, NY.

Cadle, J.E., 1988. Phylogenetic relationships among advanced snakes: a molecular perspective. Univ. California Publ. Zool. 119, 1–77.

Cadle, J.E., 2007. The snake genus *Sibynomorphus* (Colubridae: Dipsadidinae: Dipsadini) in Peru and Ecuador, with comments on the systematics of Dipsadini. Bull. Mus. Comp. Zool. 158, 183–284.

Cadle, J.E., Chuna, P.M., 1995. A new lizard of the genus *Macropholidus* (Teiidae) from a relictual humid forest of northwestern Peru, and notes on *Macropholidus ruthveni* Noble. Breviora 501, 1–39.

Campbell, J.A., 1998. Amphibians and Reptiles of Northern Guatemala, Yucatán and Belize. University of Oklahoma Press, Norman, OK.

Campbell, J.A., Lamar, W.W., 2004. The Venomous Reptiles of the Western Hemisphere, vols. I, II. Cornell University Press, Ithaca, NY. 1032 pp

Campden-Main, S.M., 1970. A Field Guide to the Snakes of South Vietnam. United States National Museum, Division of Reptiles and Amphibians, Smithsonian Institution, Washington, DC.

Capula, M., Filippi, E., Luiselli, L., Jesus, V.T., 1997. The ecology of the Western Whip snake, *Coluber viridiflavus* (Lacepede, 1789), in Mediterranean Central Italy. Herpetozoa 10, 65–79.

Cardoso, J.L., Fan, H.W., França, F.O., Jorge, M.T., Leite, R.P., Nishioka, S.A., et al. 1993. Randomized comparative trial of three antivenoms in the treatment of envenoming by lance-headed vipers (*Bothrops jararaca*) in São Paulo, Brazil. QJM 86, 315–325.

Caron, E.J., Manock, S.R., Maudlin, J., Koleski, J., Theakston, R.D.G., Warrell, D.A., et al. 2009. Apparent marked reduction in early antivenom reactions compared to historical controls: was it prophylaxis or method of administration? Toxicon 54, 779–783.

Centro de Informações Toxicológicas do Rio Grande do Sul, Importáncia médico-sanitária dos acidentes com cobra verde ou cobra cipó. Curare 2, 8.

Chan, Y., 2009. Differential diagnosis of dizziness. Curr. Opin. Otolaryngol. Head Neck Surg. 17, 200–203.

Chapman, D.S., 1968. The symptomatology, pathology and treatment of the bites of venomous snakes of central and southern Africa Bucherl, W. Buckley, E.E. Deulofeu, V. Venomous Animals and Their Venoms, vol. 1. Academic Press, New York, NY.

Ching, A.T., Rocha, M.M., Paes Leme, A.F., Pimenta, D.C., de Fatima, D., Furtado, M., et al. 2006. Some aspects of the venom proteome of the Colubridae snake *Philodryas olfersii* revealed from a Duvernoy's (venom) gland transcriptome. FEBS Lett. 580, 4417–4422 (Erratum in: FEBS Lett. 2006. 18:580: 5122-5123).

Chippaux, J.P., 1986. Les Serpents de la Guyane française. Editions de l'ORSTOM, Paris.

Chippaux, J.P., 1999. Les serpents d'Afrique occidentale et centrale. Éditions de l'IRD, Paris Collection Faune et Flore Tropicales 35, 1–278.

Chippaux, J.P., Boyer, L., 2010. The 3 + 3 dose escalation design is not appropriate for antivenom dose finding. Toxicon 55, 1408–1409. (and author reply pp. 1410–1411).

Chippaux, J.P., Williams, V., White, J., 1991. Snake venom variability: methods of study, results and interpretation. Toxicon 29, 1279–1304.

Chiszar, D., Weinstein, S.A., Smith, H.M., 1992. Liquid and dry venom yields from brown tree snakes, *Boiga irregularis* (Merrem). In: Strimple, P.D. (Ed.), Contributions in Herpetology (pp. 11–13). Greater Cincinnati Herpetological Society, Cincinnati, OH. 111 pp.

Chuang, T.Y., Lin, S.W., Chan, R.C., 1996. Guillain–Barré syndrome: an unusual complication after snake bite. Arch. Phys. Med. Rehabil. 77, 729–731.

Christensen, P.A., 1955. South African Snake Venoms and Antivenoms. South African Institute for Medical Research, Johannesburg, South Africa.

Christensen, P.A., 1968. The venoms of central and south African snakes. In: Bucherl, W., Buckley, E.E., Deulofeu, V. (Eds.), Venomous Animals and Their Venoms, vol. 1. Academic Press, New York, NY.

Chroni, E., Papapetropoulos, S., Argyriou, A.A., Papapetropoulos, T., 2005. A case of fatal progressive neuropathy. Delayed consequence of multiple bites of a non-venomous snake. Clin. Neurol. Neurosurg. 108, 45–47.

Clark, R.F., Selden, B.S., Furbee, B., 1993. The incidence of wound infection following *Crotalus* envenomation. Emerg. Med. 11, 583–586.

Clark, R.F., McKinney, P.E., Chase, P.B., Walter, F.G., 2002. Immediate and delayed allergic reactions to Crotalidae polyvalent immune Fab (ovine) antivenom. Ann. Emerg. Med. 39, 671–676.

Clarke, A.E., Fries, J.F., 1992. Health status instruments and physical examination techniques in clinical measurement methodologies. Curr. Opin. Rheumatol. 4, 145–152.

Clinch, C.R., Kahill, A., Klatt, L.A., Stewart, D., 2010. What is the best approach to benign paroxysmal positional vertigo in the elderly? J. Fam. Pract. 59, 295–297.

Coca, S.G., Yusuf, B., Schlipak, M.G., Garg, A.X., Parikh, C.R., 2009. Long-term risk of mortality and other adverse outcomes after acute kidney injury: a systematic review and meta-analysis. Am. J. Kidney Dis. 53, 961–973.

Cogger, H.G., 1983. Reptiles and Amphibians of Australia. Ralph Curtis Publishing, Sanibel, FL.

Conant, R., Collins, J.T., 1998. Reptiles and Amphibians of Eastern/Central North America, third ed.. Peterson Field Guides, Houghton Mifflin, New York, NY.

Cook, D.G., 1984. A case of envenomation by the neotropical colubrid snake, *Stenorrhina freminvillei*. Toxicon 22, 823–824.

Cooper, J.E., Reid, H.A., 1976. Ionides and snakebite. Trans. R. Soc. Trop. Med. Hyg. 70, 264–265.

Coopman, U., DeLeeuw, M., Cordonnier, J., Jacobs, W., 2009. Suicidal death after injection of a castor bean extract (*Ricinus communis*). Forensic Sci. Int. 189, e13–e20.

Cope, E.D., 1861. Catalogue of the Colubrids in the museum of the Academy of Natural Sciences of Philadelphia. Part 3. Proc. Acad. Nat. Sci. Philadelphia 12, 553–566.

Cope, E.D., 1892. A critical review of the characters and variations of the snakes of North America. Proc. U.S. Nat. Museum XIV, 589–694.

Cope, D., Bova, R., 2008. Steroids in otolaryngology. Laryngoscope 118, 1556–1560.

Corkill, N.L., 1932. Snakes and Snake Bite in Iraq. Bailliere Tindall & Cox, London, UK.

Correia, J.M., de Lima Santana Neto, P., Sardou Sabino Pinho, M., Afrânio da Silva, J., Lucineide Porto Amorim, M., Arturo Costa Escobar, J., 2010. Poisoning due to Philodryas olfersii (Lichtenstein, 1823) attended at Restauração Hospital in Recife, State of Pernambuco, Brazil: case report. Rev. Socied. Brasil. Med. Trop. 43, 336–338.

Cox, M.J., 1991. The Snakes of Thailand and Their Husbandry. Krieger Publishing, Malabar, FL.

Cox, M.J., Van Dijk, P.P., Nabhitabhata, J., Thirakhupt, K., 1998. A Photographic Guide to Snakes and Other Reptiles of Peninsular Malaysia, Singapore and Thailand. Ralph Curtis Publishing, Sanibel, FL. p. 144

Crimmins, M.L., 1937. A case of Oxybelis poisoning in man. Copeia 1937, 233.

Cupo, P., Azevedo-Marques, M.M., de Menezes, J.B., Hering, S.E., 1991. Immediate hypersensitivity reactions after intravenous use of antivenin sera: prognostic value of intradermal sensitivity tests. Rev. Inst. Med. Trop. Sao Paulo 33, 115–122.

Curcio, F.F., Piacentini, V.D.Q., Fernandes, D.S., 2009. On the status of the snake genera Erythrolamprus Boie, Liophis Wagler and Lygophis Fitzinger (Serpentes, Xenodontinae). Zootaxa 2173, 66–68.

Dabo, A., Diawara, S.I., Dicko, A., Katilé, A., Diallo, A., Doumbo, O., 2002. Evaluation and treatment of snake bites in Bancoumana village in Mali. Bull. Soc. Pathol. Exot. 95, 160–162.

D'Abreu, E.A., 1931. Effect of a bite from Schneider's water snake, Hypsyrhina enhydris. J. Bombay Nat. Hist. Soc. 22, 203.

D'Cruze, N.C., 2008. Envenomation by the Malagasy colubrid snake, Langaha madagascariensis. J. Venom. Anim. Toxins incl. Trop. Dis. 14, 546–551.

Daley, B.J., Alexander, A.M., 2010. Snakebite. http://emedicine.medscape.com/article/168828-overview.

Daniel, J.C., 1983. The Book of Indian Reptiles. Bombay Natural History Society, Bombay, India.

Date, A., Pulimood, R., Jacob, C.K., Kirubakaran, M.G., Shastry, J.C., 1986. Haemolytic-uraemic syndrome complicating snake bite. Nephron 42, 89–90.

Da Rocha, M.M.T., Furtado, M.F.D., 2007. Análise das atividades biológicas dos venenos de Philodryas olfersii [Lichtenstein] e P. patagoniensis [Girard] [Serpentes, Colubridae]. Revista Brasil. Zool. 24, 410–418.

Da Silva, N.J., Aird, S.D., Seebart, C., Kaiser, I.I., 1989. A gyroxin analog from the venom of the bushmaster (Lachesis muta muta). Toxicon 27, 763–771.

DeLoughery, T.G., 2005. Critical care clotting catastrophies. Crit. Care Clin. 21, 531–562.

De Medeiros, C.R., Barbaro, K.C., Lira, M.S., França, F.O.S., Zaher, V.L., Kokron, C.M., et al. 2007. Predictors of Bothrops jararaca venom allergy in snake handlers and snake venom handlers. Toxicon 51, 672–680.

Dempfle, C.E., 2004. Coagulopathy of sepsis. Thromb. Haemost. 91, 213–224.

Deraniyagala, P.E.P., 1955. A Coloured Atlas of Some Vertebrates from Ceylon, Serpentoid Reptilia, vol. 3. Government Press, Ceylon.

Dessauer, H.C., Cadle, J.E., Lawson, R., 1987. Patterns of snake evolution suggested by their proteins. Fieldiana: Zool. N. A. 34, 1–34.

Deufel, A., Cundall, D., 2003. Feeding in Atractaspis (Serpentes: Atractaspididae): a study in conflicting functional constraints. Zoology 106, 43–61.

Devitt, T.J., LaDuc, T.J., McGuire, J.A., 2008. The Trimorphodon biscutatus (Squamata: Colubridae) species complex revisited: a multivariate statistical analysis of geographic variation. Copeia 2008, 370–387.

De Araújo, M.E., dos Santos, A.C., 1997. Cases of human envenoming caused by *Philodryas olfersii* and *Philodryas patagoniensis* (Serpentes: Colubridae). Rev. Soc. Bras. Med. Trop. 30, 517–519.

De Carvalho, M.A., Nogueira, F.N., 1998. Snakes from the urban area of Cuiaba, Mato Grosso: ecological aspects and associated snakebites. Cad. Saude. Publ. 14, 753–763.

De Haro, L., Pommier, P., 2003. Envenomation: a real risk of keeping exotic house pets. Vet. Hum. Toxicol. 45, 214–216.

De Lema, T., 2007. Descrição de acidente ofídico com *Phalotris trilineatus* (Serpente-Colubridae) no Brasil. Caderno de Pesquisa, serie Biolog 19, 6–16.

De Lisle, H.F., 1984. *Boiga cyanea* (Green Cat-eye Snake): envenomation. Herpetol. Rev. 15, 112.

De Madeiros, C.R., Hess, P.L., Nicoleti, A.F., Sueiro, L.R., Duarte, M.R., de Almeida-Santos, S.M., et al. 2010. Bites by the colubrid snake *Philodryas patagoniensis*: a clinical and epidemiological study of 297 cases. Toxicon 56, 1018–1024.

de Oliveira, L., Jared, C., da Costa Prudente, A.L., Zaher, H., Antoniazzi, M.M., 2007. Oral glands in dipsadine "goo-eater" snakes: morphology and histochemistry of the infralabial glands in *Atractus reticulatus*, *Dipsas indica*, and *Sibynomorphus mikanii*. Toxicon 51, 898–913.

De Perez, O.A., de Vila, L.L., Peichoto, M.E., Maruñak, S., Ruiz, R., Teibler, P., et al. 2003. Edematogenic and myotoxic activities of the Duvernoy's gland secretion of *Philodryas olfersii* from the north-east region of Argentina. Biocell 27, 363–370.

De Quieroz, A., Lawson, R., Lemos-Espinal, J.A., 2002. Phylogenetic relationships of North American garter snakes (*Thamnophis*) based on four mitochondrial genes: how much DNA sequence is enough? Mol. Phylogenet. Evol. 22, 315–329.

De Silva, A., 1976a. The pattern of snake bite in Sri Lanka. The Snake 8, 43–51.

De Silva, A., 1976b. Venomous snakes of Sri Lanka. The Snake 8, 31–42.

De Silva, A., 1990a. Colour Guide to the Snakes of Sri Lanka. R&A Publishing, Avon, UK.

De Silva, A., 1990b. Venomous snakes, their bites and treatment in Sri Lanka. In: Gopalakrishnakone, P., Chou, L.M. (Eds.), Snakes of Medical Importance (Asia Pacific Region) (pp. 479–556). Venom and Toxin Research Group, National University of Singapore.

De Silva, A., Aloysius, D.J., 1983. Moderately and mildly venomous snakes of Sri Lanka. Ceylon Med. J. 28, 118–127.

Diaz, F., Navarrete, L.F., Pefaur, J., Rodriguez-Acosta, A., 2004. Envenomation by neotropical opisthoglyphous colubrid, *Thamnodynastes cf. pallidus* Linné, 1758 (Serpentes: Colubridae) in Venezuela. Rev. Inst. Med. Trop. Sao Paulo 46, 287–290.

Ditmars, R.L., 1896. The snakes found within fifty miles of New York City. Proc. Linn. Soc. N.Y. 8, 9–24.

Ditmars, R.L., 1912. Feeding habits of serpents. Zoologica 1, 204.

Ditmars, R.L., 1948. A Field Book of North American Snakes. Doubleday and Company, Garden City, NY.

Domergue, C.A., 1989. Un serpent venimeux de Madagascar. Observation de deux cas de morsure par Madagascarophis (*Colubridé opisthoglyphe*). Arch. Inst. Pasteur Madagascar 56, 299–311.

Domergue, C.H.A., Richaud, J., 1971. Hemolytic activity of the secretions of Duvernoy's gland in *Lioheterodon* (Colubridae, Aglypha). Arch. Inst. Pasteur Madagascar 40, 145–148.

Donoso-Barros, R., 1966. Reptiles de Chile. University of Chile, Santiago. 458 pp.

Dos Santos-Costa, M.C., Outeiral, A.B., D'Agostini, F.M., Cappellari, L.H., 2000. Envenomation by the neotropical colubrid *Boiruna maculata* (Boulenger, 1896): a case report. Rev. Inst. Med. Trop. Sao Paulo 42, 283–286.

Dos Santos-Costa, M.C., Di-Bernadino, M., 2001. Human envenomation by an aglyphous colubrid snake *Liophis miliaris* (Linnaeus, 1758). Cuadernos Herpetogica 14, 153–154. (dated 2000).

Dowling, H.G., Highton, R., Maha, G.C., Maxson, L.R., 1983. Biochemical evaluation of colubrid snake phylogeny. J. Zool. 201, 309–329.

Dowling, H.G., Hass, C.A., Hedges, S.B., Highton, R., 1996. Snake relationships revealed by slow-evolving proteins: a preliminary survey. J. Zool. 240, 1–28.

Duarte, M.R., Puorto, G., Franco, F.L., 1995. A biological survey of the pit viper, *Bothrops insularis* Amaral (Serpentes, Viperidae): an endemic and threatened offshore snake of southeastern Brazil. Stud. Neotrop. Fauna Environ. 30, 1–13.

Duddu, V., Isaac, M.K., Chatuvedi, S.K., 2006. Somatization, somatosensory amplification, attribution styles and illness behavior: a review. Int. Rev. Psychiatry 18, 25–33.

Duméril, A.M.C., Bibron, G., Duméril, A.H.A., 1854. Erpétologie Générale ou Histoire Naturelle Complète des Reptiles, Tome Septième. Deuxième Partie, Comprenant l'histoire des Serpents Venimeux. Librairie Encyclopédique de Roret, Paris, France. pp. 781–1536.

Du Toit, D.M., 1980. Boomslang (*Dispholidus typus*) bite. A case report and a review of diagnosis and management. S. Afr. Med. J. 57, 507–510.

Ebell, M.H., Siwek, J., Weiss, B.D., Woolf, S.H., Susman, J., Ewigman, B., et al. 2004. Strength of Recommendation Taxonomy (SORT): a patient-centered approach to grading evidence in the medical literature. Am. Fam. Physician 69, 548–556.

Edgren, R.A., 1955. The natural history of the hog-nosed snakes, genus *Heterodon*: a review. Herpetologica 11, 105–117.

Ekenbäck, K., Hulting, J., Persson, H., Wernell, I., 1985. Unusual neurological symptoms in a case of severe crotalid envenomation. J. Toxicol. Clin. Toxicol. 23, 357–364.

Endo, W., Amend, M., Fleck, L.C., 2007. *Oxybelis fulgidus* (green vine snake) prey. Herpetol. Rev. 38, 209.

Epley, J.M., 1992. The canalith repositioning procedure for treatment of benign paroxysmal positional vertigo. Otolaryngol. Head Neck Surg. 107, 399–404.

Ergul, Y., Ekici, B., Tastan, Y., Sezer, T., Uysal, S., 2006. Vestibular neuritis caused by enteroviral infection. Pediatr. Neurol. 34, 45–46.

Ernst, C.H., Barbour, R.W., 1989. Snakes of Eastern North America. George Mason University Press, Fairfax, VA.

Ernst, C.H., Ernst, E.M., 2003. Snakes of the United States and Canada. Smithsonian Books, Washington, DC.

Estrella, A., Sánchez, E.E., Galán, J.A., Tao, W.A., Guerrero, B., Navarrete, L.F., et al. 2010. Characterization of toxins from the broad-banded water snake *Helicops angulatus* (Linnaeus, 1758): isolation of a cysteine-rich secretory protein, Helicopsin. Arch. Toxicol doi: 10.1007/s00204-010-0597-6.

Fauci, A., Braunwald, E., Kasper, D., Hauser, S., Longo, D., Jameson, J., et al. 2009. Harrison's Manual of Medicine. McGraw-Hill Professional, New York, NY.

Ferlan, I., Ferlan, A., King, T., Russell, F.E., 1983. Preliminary studies on the venom of the colubrid snake *Rhabdophis subminiatus* (red-necked keelback). Toxicon 21, 570–574.

Ferquel, E., de Haro, L., Jan, V., Guillemin, I., Jourdain, S., Teynié, A., et al. 2007. Reappraisal of *Vipera aspis* venom neurotoxicity. Plos One 2, e1194.

Finley, R.B., Chiszar, D., Smith, H.M., 1994. Field observations of salivary digestion of rodent tissue by the wandering garter snake, *Thamnophis elegans vagrans*. Bull. Chicago Herp. Soc. 29, 5–6.

Fitzinger, L.J., 1833. *Elaphe parreyssii*—Parreyss's *Elaphe*. In: Wagler, J. (Ed.), Descriptiones et Icones Amphibiorum: 3. JG Cotta, München, Germany

FitzSimons, F.W., 1909. On the toxic action of the bite of the boomslang or South African tree-snake (*Dispholidus typus*). Ann. Mag. Nat. Hist. 3 (8), 271–278.

FitzSimons, F.W., 1912. The Snakes of Southern Africa: Their Venom and Treatment of Snake Bite. TM Miller, Cape Town, South Africa.

FitzSimons, F.W., 1919. The Snakes of Southern Africa. TM Miller, Cape Town, South Africa.

FitzSimons, V.F.M., 1962. Snakes of Southern Africa. Purnell & Sons, Johannesburg, South Africa.

FitzSimons, D.C., Smith, H.M., 1958. Another rear-fanged South African snake lethal to humans. Herpetologica 14, 198–202.

Fowler, I.R., Salomão, M.D.G., 1994. Activity patterns in the colubrid snake genus *Philodryas* and their relationship to reproduction and snakebite. Bull. Chicago Herp. Soc. 29, 229–232.

Fowlie, J.A., 1965. The Snakes of Arizona. Azul Quinta Press, Fallbrook, CA.

Franco, F.L., Fernandes, D.S., Bentin, B.M., 2007. A new species of *Hydrodynastes* Fitzinger, 1843 from central Brazil (Serpentes: Colubridae: Xenodontinae). Zootaxa 1613, 57–65.

Frembgen, J., 1966. The folklore of geckos: ethnographic data from South and West Asia. Asian Folklore Stud. April 1996.

Fritts, T.H., McCoid, M.J., 1999. The threat to humans from snakebite by snakes of the genus *Boiga* based on data from Guam and other areas. In: Rodda, G.H., Sawai, Y., Chiszar, D., Hiroshi, T. (Eds.), Problem Snake Management. Cornell University Press, Ithaca, NY

Fritts, T.H., McCoid, M.J., Haddock, R.L., 1990. Risks to infants on Guam from bites of the brown tree snake (*Boiga irregularis*). Am. J. Trop. Med. 42, 607–611.

Fritts, T.H., McCoid, M.J., Haddock, R.L., 1994. Symptoms and circumstances associated with bites by the brown tree snake (Colubridae: *Boiga irregularis*) on Guam. J. Herpetol. 28, 27–33.

Fry, B.G., Lumsden, N.G., Wuster, W., Wickramaratan, J.C., Hodgson, W.C., Kini, R.M., 2003. Isolation of neurotoxin (alpha-colubritoxin) from a nonvenomous colubrid: evidence for early origin of venomous snakes. J. Mol. Evol. 57, 446–452.

Fry, B.G., Vidal, N., Norman, J.A., Vonk, F.J., Scheib, H., Ramjan, R., et al. 2006. Early evolution of the venom system in lizards and snakes. Nature 439, 509–632.

Fry, B.G., Scheib, H., van der Weerd, L., Young, B., McNaughtan, J, Ryan Ramjan, S.F., et al. 2008. Evolution of an arsenal. Structural and functional diversification of the venom system in the advanced snakes (Caenophidia). Mol. Cell. Proteomics 7, 215–246.

Fry, B.G., Vidal, N., van der Weerd, L., Kochva, E., Renjifo, C., 2009a. Evolution and diversification of the Toxicofera reptile venom system. J. Proteomics 72, 127–136.

Fry, B.G., Wroe, S., Teeuwisse, W., van Osch, M.J., Moreno, K., Ingle, J., et al. 2009b. A central role for venom in predation by *Varanus komodoensis* (Komodo dragon) and the extinct giant *Varanus* (*Megalania*) *priscus*. Proc. Natl. Acad. Sci. U.S.A. 106, 8969–8974.

Fukushima, H., 1986. Clinical aspects of bite by Yamakagashi, *Rhabdophis tigrinus*. J. Kagoshima Soc. Inter. Med. 18, 60–85.

Gacek, R.R., 2008. Evidence for a viral neuropathy in recurrent vertigo. ORL J. Otorhinolaryngol. Relat. Spec. 70, 6–14.

Gans, C., 1978. Reptilian venoms: some evolutionary considerations. In: Gans, C., Gans, K.A. (Eds.), Biology of the Reptilia (pp. 1–39). Academic Press, New York, NY.

García-Gubern, C., Bello, R., Rivera, V., Rocafort, A., Colon-Rolon, L., Acosta-Tapia, H., 2010. Is the Puerto Rican racer, *Alsophis portoricensis*, really harmless? A case report series. Wilderness Environ. Med. 21, 353–356.

Gardner-Thorpe, C., 1967. Snakebite poisoning. Br. Med. J. 26, 558.

Garg, A., Sujatha, S., Garg, J., Srinivas Acharya, N., Parija, S.C., 2009. Wound infections secondary to snakebite. J. Infect. Dev. Ctries 3, 221–223.

Gay, T., 1978. Notes on the green keel-back snake (*Macropisthodon plumbicolor*). J. Bombay Nat. Hist. Soc. 75, 854–859.

Geddes, J., Thomas, J.E.P., 1985. Boomslang bite—a case report. Cent. Afr. J. Med. 31, 109–112.

Geffeney, S.L., Fujimoto, E., Brodie III, E.D., Brodie Jr., E.D., Ruben, P.C., 2005. Evolutionary diversification of TTX-resistant sodium channels in predator–prey interaction. Nature 434, 759–763.

Gehlbach, F.R., 1974. Evolutionary relations of southwestern ringneck snakes (*Diadophis puntatus*). Herpetologica 30, 140–148.

Gell, P.G.H., Coombs, R.R.A. (Eds.),, 1963. Clinical Aspects of Immunology (first ed.). Blackwell, Oxford, UK

George, A., Tharakan, V.T., Solez, K., 1987. Viper bite poisoning in India: a review with special reference to renal complications. Ren. Fail. 10, 91–99.

Gerber, J.D., Adendorff, H.P., 1980. Boomslang (*Dispholidus typus*) bite: case report. South Afr. Med. J. 57, 710–711.

Gillissen, A., Theakston, R.D., Barth, J., May, B., Krieg, M., Warrell, D.A., 1994. Neurotoxicity, haemostatic disturbances and haemolytic anaemia after a bite by a Tunisian saw-scaled or carpet viper (*Echis "pyramidum"*-complex): failure of antivenom treatment. Toxicon 32, 937–944.

Giraudo, A.R., Arzamendia, V., Cacciali, P., 2006. Geographic variation and taxonomic status of the southernmost populations of *Liophis miliaris* (Linnaeus, 1758) (Serpentes, Colubridae). Herpetol. J. 16, 213–220.

Glenn, J.L., Straight, R.C., Wolfe, M.C., Hardy, D.L., 1983. Geographical variation in Mojave rattlesnake (*Crotalus scutulatus scutulatus*) venom properties. Toxicon 21, 119–130.

Göçmen, B., Yildiz, M.Z., 2006. Snakes and their relations with humans. Kibris Bilim (Cyprus Science) 2, 28–31. (in Turkish)

Göçmen, B., Werner, Y.L., Elbeyli, B., 2008. Cannibalism in *Dolicophis jugularis* (Serpentes: Colubridae): more than random? Curr. Herpetol. 27, 1–7.

Goetz, C.G., 2007. Textbook of Clinical Neurology. Saunders, New York, NY.

Goldstein, E.J.C., Citron, D.M., Gonzalez, H., Russell, F.E., Finegold, S.M., 1979. Bacteriology of rattlesnake venom and implications for therapy. J. Infect. Dis. 140, 818–821.

Goldstein, E.J.C, Agyare, E.O., Vagvolgyi, A.E., Halpern, M., 1981. Aerobic bacterial oral flora of garter snakes: development of normal flora and pathogenic potential for snakes and humans. J. Clin. Microbiol. 13, 954–956.

Gomes, V.M., Carvalho, A.O., Da Cunha, M., Keller, M.N., Bloch Jr., C., Deolindo, P., et al. 2005. Purification and characterization of a novel peptide with antifungal activity from *Bothrops jararaca* venom. Toxicon 45, 817–827.

Gomez, H.F., Davis, M., Phillips, S., McKinney, P., Brent, J., 1994. Human envenomation from a wandering garter snake. Ann. Emerg. Med. 23, 1119–1122.

Gomperts, E.D., Demetriou, D., 1977. Laboratory studies and clinical features in a case of boomslang envenomation. S. Afr. Med. J. 51, 173–175.

Gonçalves, L.R.C., Yamanouye, N., Nun z-Burgos, G.B., Furtado, M.F.D., Britto, L.R.G., Nicolau, J., 1997. Detection of calcium-binding proteins in venom and Duvernoy's glands of South American snakes and their secretions. Comp. Biochem. Physiol. 118C, 207–211.

Gonzáles, D., 1979. Bissverletzungen durch *Malpolon monspessulanus*. Salamandra 15, 266–268.

Gonzáles, D., 1982. Epidemiological and clinical aspects of certain venomous animals of Spain. Toxicon 20, 925–928.

Goodman, J.D., 1985. Two record size Blanding's tree snakes from Uganda. East Afr. Nat. Hist. Bull. Nairobi 1985, 56–57.

Gopalakrishnakone, P., Chou, L.M., 1990. Snakes of Medical Importance (Asia-Pacific Region). Venom and Toxin Research Group: National University of Singapore, Singapore.

Gorzula, S., 1982. *Leptodeira annulata ashmeadii* envenomation. Herpetol. Rev. 13, 47.

Gould, S.J., 2002. The Structure of Evolutionary Theory. Belknap Press, Cambridge, MA.

Gould, S.J., Vrba, S., 1982. Exaptation–a missing term in the science of form. Paleobiology 8, 4–15.

Grasset, E., Schaafsma, A.W., 1940. Antigenic characteristics of "boomslang" (*Dispholidus typus*) venom and preparation of a specific antivenene by means of formalized venom. S. Afr. Med. J. 14, 484–489.

Greenberger, P.A., 2002. Immunotherapy update: mechanism of action. Allergy Asthma Proc. 23, 373–376.

Greene, H.W., 1989. Ecological, evolutionary and conservation implications of feeding biology in old world cat-eyed snakes genus *Boiga* (Colubridae). Proc. Calif. Acad. Sci. 46, 193–207.

Greene, H.W., 1997. Snakes: The Evolution of Mystery in Nature. University of California Press, Berkeley, CA.

Gregory, P.T., Macartney, J.M., Rivard, D.H., 1980. Small mammal predation and prey handling by the garter snake, *Thamnophis elegans*. Herpetologica 36, 87–93.

Grogan, W.L., 1974. Effects of accidental envenomation from the saliva of the Eastern hognose snake, *Heterodon platyrhinos*. Herpetologica 30, 248–249.

Groves, F., 1973. Reproduction and venom in Blanding's tree snake *Boiga blandingi*. International Zoo Yearbook 13, 106–108.

Guillemin, I., Bouchier, C., Garrigues, T., Wisner, A., Choumet, V., 2003. Sequences and structural organization of phospholipase A_2 genes from *Vipera aspis aspis*, *V. aspis zinnekeri*, and *Vipera berus berus* venom. Identification of a new viper population based on ammodytin I1 heterogeneity. Eur. J. Biochem. 270, 2697–2706.

Guillin, M.C., Bezeand, A., Ménaché, D., 1978. The mechanism of activation of human prothrombin by an activator isolated from *Dispholidus typus* venom. Biochem. Biophys. Acta 537, 160–165.

Guinea, M.L., McMorrow, L., Peerzada, N., 1992. Yield and molecular weight of the Duvernoy's gland secretions of the dog-faced watersnake, *Cerberus rynchops* (Serpentes: Colubridae: Homalopsinae). Toxicon 30: 516 (abstract).

Gupta, A., Rhodes, G.J., Berg, D.T., Gerlitz, B., Molitoris, B.A., Grinnellf, B.W., 2007. Activated protein C ameliorates LPS-induced kidney injury and downregulates renal INOS and angiotensin 2. Am. J. Physiol. Renal Physiol. 293, F245–F254.

Gutiérrez, J.M., Mahmood, S., 2002. Bites and envenomations by colubrid snakes in Mexico and Central America. J. Toxicol. Toxin Rev. 21, 105–112.

Gutiérrez, J.M., Avilac, C., Camacho, Z., Lomonte, B., 1990. Ontogenic changes in venom of the snake *Lachesis muta stenophrys* (Bushmaster) from Costa Rica. Toxicon 28, 419–426.

Gutiérrez, J.M., Theakston, R.D.G., Warrell, D.A., 2006. Confronting the neglected problem of snake bite envenoming: the need for a global partnership. PloS Med. 3 (6), e150. doi:10.1371/journal.pmed.0030150.

Gygax, P., 1971. Entwicklung, Bau und Funktion der Giftdrüse (Duvernoy's gland) von *Natrix tessellata*. Acta Trop. Zool. 28, 225–274.

Haagner, G.V., Smit, R., 1987. Case history of boomslang (*Dispholidus typus*) envenomation in the eastern Transvaal, South Africa. Brit. Herp. Soc. Bull. 21, 43–45.

Haas, G., 1931. Dber die Morphologie der Kiefermuskulatur und die Schadelmechanik einiger Schlangen. Zool. Jahrb. 54, 332–416.

Habib, A.G., 2003. Tetanus complicating snake bite in Northern Nigeria: clinical presentation and public health implications. Acta Trop. 85, 87–91.

Hardy, L.M., McDiarmid, R.W., 1969. The amphibians and reptiles of Sinaloa, Mexico. Mus. Nat. Hist 18, 39–252.

Harris, J.B., Faiz, M.A., Rahman, M.R., Jalil, M.M., Ahsan, M.F., Theakston, R.D., et al. 2010. Snake bite in Chittagong Division, Bangladesh: a study of bitten patients who developed no signs of systemic envenoming. Trans. R. Soc. Trop. Med. Hyg. 104, 320–327.

Harrison, R.A., Hargreaves, A., Wagstaff, S.C., Faragher, B., Lalloo, D.G., 2009. Snake envenoming: a disease of poverty. PLoS Negl. Trop. Dis. 3, e569.

Hartman, P.A., Marques, O.A.V., 2005. Diet and habitat use of two sympatric species of *Philodryas* (Colubridae), in south Brazil. Amphibia-Reptilia 26, 25–31.

Hass, C.A., Maxson, L.R., Hedges, S.B., 2001. Relationships and divergence times of West Indian amphibians and reptiles: insights from albumin immunology. In: Woods, C.A., Sergile, F.E. (Eds.), Biogeography of the WestIndies: Patterns and Perspectives (pp. 157–174). CRC Press, Boca Raton, FL.

Hati, A.K., Mondal, M., De, M.K., Mukherjee, H., Hati, R.N., 1992. Epidemiology of snake bite in the district of Burdwan, West Bengal. J. Indian Med. Assoc. 90, 145–147.

Hay, O.P., 1892. The Batrachians and Reptiles of the State of Indiana. William B. Burford, Indianapolis, IN.

Hayes, W.K., Hayes, F.E., 1985. Human envenomation from the bite of the eastern garter-snake, *Thamnophis s. sirtalis* (Serpentes: Colubridae). Toxicon 23, 719–721.

Hayes, W.K., Lávin-Murcio, P., Kardong, K.V., 1993. Delivery of Duvernoy's secretion into prey by the brown tree snake, *Boiga irregularis* (Serpentes: Colubridae). Toxicon 31, 881–887.

Heatwole, H., Banuchi, I.B., 1966. Envenomation by the colubrid snake, *Alsophis portoricensis*. Herpetologica 22, 132–134.

Heatwole, H., Cogger, H.G., 1993. Family Hydrophiidae. In: Glasby, C.J., Ross, G.J.B., Beesley, P.L. (Eds.), Fauna of Australia, Chapter 36, vol. 2A, Amphibia and Reptilia. Australian Government Publishing Service, Canberra, ACT, pp. 310–318.

Hedges, S.B., Couloux, A., Vidal, N., 2009. Molecular phylogeny, classification, and biogeography of West Indian racer snakes of the Tribe Alsophiini (Squamata, Dipsadidae, Xenodontinae). Zootaxa 2067, 1–28.

Hegeman, G., 1961. Enzymatic constitution of *Alsophis* saliva and its biological implications. Breviora 134, 1–8.

Heise, P.J., Maxson, L.R., Dowling, H.G., Hedges, S.B., 1995. Higher-level snake phylogeny inferred from mitochondrial DNA sequences of 12S rRNA and 16S rRNA genes. Mol. Biol. Evol. 12, 259–265.

Hejnar, P., Bardon, J., Sauer, P., Kolár, M., 2007. *Stenotrophomonas maltophilia* as a part of normal oral bacterial flora in captive snakes and its susceptibility to antibiotics. Vet. Microbiol. 121, 357–362.

Hermann, J. 1804. Observationes Zoologicae quibus novae complures aliaeque animalium species, describuntur et illustrantur (opus posthumum) edidit Fridericus Ludovicus Hammer, Paris.

Hernández-Ríos, A., Luna-Alcantara, H.S., García-Padilla, E., 2011. *Leptodeira septentrionalis polysticta* (Central American cat-eyed snake). Diet. Herpetol. Rev. 42, 100.

Herrel, A., O'Reilly, J.C., 2006. Ontogenetic scaling of bite force in lizards and turtles. Physiol. Biochem. Zool. 79, 31–42.

Hiestand, P.C., Hiestand, R.R., 1979. *Dispholidus typus* (boomslang) snake venom: purification and properties of the coagulant principle. Toxicon 17, 489–498.

Hill, R.E., Mackessy, S.P., 1997. Venom yields from several species of colubrid snakes and differential effects of ketamine. Toxicon 35, 671–678.

Hill, R.E., Mackessy, S.P., 2000. Characterization of venom (Duvernoy's secretion) from twelve species of colubrid snakes and partial sequence of four venom proteins. Toxicon 38, 1663–1687.

Hoffmann, J.J.M.L., Vijgen, M., Smeets, R.E.H., Melman, P.G., 1992. Haemostatic effects *in vivo* after snakebite by the red-necked keelback (*Rhabdophis subminiatus*). Blood Coagul. Fibrinolysis 3, 461–464.

Hoole, M., Goddard, A., 2007. Boomslang envenomation in 2 dogs in Kwazulu-Natal, South Africa. J. S. Afr. Vet. Assoc. 78, 49–51.

Hoso, M., Asami, T., Hori, M., 2007. Right-handed snakes: convergent evolution of asymmetry for functional specialization. Biol. Lett. 3, 169–172.

Hsieh, S., Babel, F.E., 1999. *Serratia marcescens* cellulitis following an iguana bite. Clin. Infect. Dis. 28, 1181–1182.

Hutchinson, D.A., Mori, A., Savitzky, A.H., Burghardt, G.M., Wu, X., Meinwald, J., et al. 2007. Dietary sequestration of defensive steroids in nuchal glands of the Asian snake, *Rhabdophis tigrinus*. Proc. Natl. Acad. Sci. U.S.A. 104, 2265–2270.

Ineich, I., Goyffon, M., Dang, V., 2006. Qu'est-ce qu'un serpent dangereux pour l'homme? Un cas d'envenimation par un colubridae aglyphe opisthodonte du Cameroun, *Thrasops flavigularis* (Hallowell, 1852). Bull. Soc. Zool. Fr. 131, 135–145.

Isbister, G.K., 2010. Snakebite doesn't cause disseminated intravascular coagulation: coagulopathy and thrombotic microangiopathy in snake envenoming. Semin. Thromb. Hemost. 36, 444–451.

Isbister, G.K., Williams, V., Brown, S.G., White, J., Currie, B.J., Australian Snakebite Project Investigators, 2006. Clinically applicable laboratory end-points for treating snakebite coagulopathy. Pathology 38, 568–572.

Isbister, G.K., Little, M., Cull, G., McCoubrie, D., Lawton, P., Szabo, F., et al. 2007. Thrombotic microangiopathy from Australian brown snake (*Pseudonaja*) envenoming. Intern. Med. J. 37, 523–528.

Isbister, G.K., Brown, S.G., MacDonald, E., White, J., Currie, B.J., Australian Snakebite Project Investigators, 2008. Current use of Australian snake antivenoms and frequency of immediate type hypersensitivity reactions and anaphylaxis. Med. J. Aust. 188, 473–476.

Isbister, G.K., Dufull, S.B., Brown, S.G., Australian Snakebite Project Investigators, 2009. Failure of antivenom to improve recovery in Australian snakebite coagulopathy. QJM 102, 563–568.

Isemonger, R.M., 1955. Snakes and Snake Catching in Southern Africa. Howard Timmins, Cape Town, South Africa.

Ishunin, G. 1950. Reports of A.S. Uzbec, SSR 1950, 6.

Ismail, A.K., Weinstein, S.A., Auliya, M., Sabardin, D.M., Herbosa, T.J., Saiboon, I.M., et al. 2010. A bite by the twin-barred tree snake, *Chrysopelea pelias* (Linnaeus, 1758). Clin. Toxicol. 48, 222–226.

Iwaki, S., Tkaczyk, C., Metcalfe, D.D., Gilfillan, A.M., 2005. Roles of adaptor molecules in mast cell activation. Chem. Immunol. Allergy 87, 43–58.

Jackson, K., 2002. How tubular venom-conducting fangs are formed. J. Morphol. 252, 292–297.

Jackson, K., 2003. The evolution of venom-delivery systems in snakes. Zool. J. Linn. Soc. 137, 337–354.

Jackson, K., 2007. The evolution of venom-conducting fangs: insights from developmental biology. Toxicon 49, 975–981.

Jackson, K., Fritts, T.H., 1995. Evidence from tooth surface morphology for posterior maxillary origin of the proteroglyph fang. Amphibia-Reptilia 16, 273–288.

Jackson, K., Fritts, T.H., 2004. Dentitional specialisations for durophagy in the Common Wolf snake, *Lycodon aulicus capucinus*. Amphibia-Reptilia 25, 247–254.

Jacobson, E., 2007. Infectious Diseases and Pathology of Reptiles. CRC Press, Boca Raton, FL.

Jan, V., Maroun, R.C., Robbe-Vincent, A., De Haro, L., Choumet, V., 2002. Toxicity evolution of *Vipera aspis aspis* venom: identification and molecular modeling of a novel phospholipase A_2 heterodimer neurotoxin. FEBS Lett. 527, 263–268.

Jang, I.K., Hursting, M.J., 2005. When heparins promote thrombosis. Review of heparin-induced thrombocytopenia. Circulation 111, 2671–2683.

Jansen, D.W., Foehring, R.C., 1983. The mechanism of venom secretion from Duvernoy's gland of the snake *Thamnophis sirtalis*. J. Morphol. 175, 271–277.

Jansen, D.W., 1987. The myonecrotic effect of Duvernoy's gland secretion of the snake *Thamnophis elegans vagrans*. J. Herpetol. 21, 81–83.

Jaume, M.L., 1983. Notas sobre mordeduras tóxicas de serpientes (Reptilia, Serpentes, Colubridae). Rev. Cubana Med. Trop. 35, 224–230.

Jaume, M.L., Garrido, O.H., 1980. Notes on *Alsophis cantherigerus* Bibron (Reptilia-Serpentes, Colubridae) bites in Cuba. Rev. Cubana Med. Trop. 32, 145–148.

Jelinek, G.A., Smith, A., Lynch, D., Calenza, A., Irving, I., Michalopoulos, N., et al. 2005. The effect of adjunctive fresh frozen plasma administration on coagulation parameters and survival in a canine model of antivenom-treated brown snake envenoming. Anaesth. Intensive Care 33, 36–40.

Jenner, J.V., Dowling, H.G., 1985. Taxonomy of American xenodontine snakes: the tribe Pseudoboini. Hepetologica 41, 161–172.

Jessop, T.S., Madsen, T., Sumner, J., Rudiharto, H., Phillips, J.A., Ciofi, C., 2006. Maximum body size among insular Komodo dragon populations covaries with large prey densities. OIKOS 112, 422–429.

Johanbocke, M.M., 1974. Effects of a bite from *Conophis lineatus* (Squamata: Colubridae). Bull. Philadel. Herp. Soc. 22, 39.

Johansson, S.G., Bieber, T., Dahl, R., Friedmann, P.S., Lanier, B.Q., Lockey, R.F., et al. 2004. Revised nomenclature for allergy for global use: report of the Nomenclature Review Committee of the World Allergy Organization, October 2003. J. Allergy Clin. Immunol. 113, 832–836.

Johnson, J.D., 1988. Comments on the report of envenomation by the colubrid snake, *Stenorrhina freminvillei*. Toxicon 26, 519–521.

Jorge, M.T., Malaque, C., Ribeiro, L.A., Fan, H.W., Cardoso, J.L., Nishioka, S.A., et al. 2004. Failure of chloramphenicol prophylaxis to reduce the frequency of abscess formation as a complication of envenoming by *Bothrops* snakes in Brazil: a double-blind randomized controlled trial. Trans. R. Soc. Trop. Med. Hyg. 98, 529–534.

Joseph, J.S., Chung, M.C., Mirtschin, P.J., Kini, R.M., 2002. Effect of snake venom procoagulants on snake plasma: implications for the coagulation cascade of snakes. Toxicon 40, 175–183.

Joshua, A.M., Celermajer, D.S., Stockler, M.R., 2005. Beauty is in the eye of the examiner: reaching agreement about physical signs and their value. Intern. Med. J. 35, 178–187.

Kamiguti, A.S., Theakston, R.D., Sherman, N., Fox, J.W., 2000. Mass spectrophotometric evidence for P-III/P-IV metalloproteinases in the venom of the boomslang (*Dispholidus typus*). Toxicon 38, 1613–1620.

Kang, T.S., Vrabec, J.T., Giddings, N., Terris, D.J., 2002. Facial nerve grading systems (1985–2002): beyond the House-Brackmann scale. Otol Neurotol. 23, 767–771.

Kapus, E.J., 1964. Anatomical evidence for *Heterodon* being poisonous. Herpetologica 20, 137–138.

Kardong, K.V., 1979. "Protovipers" and the evolution of snake fangs. Evolution 33, 433–443.

Kardong, K.V., 1980a. Evolutionary patterns in advanced snakes. Am. Zool. 20, 269–282.

Kardong, K.V., 1980b. Jaw musculature of the West Indian snake *Alsophis catherigerus brooksi* (Colubridae, Reptilia). Breviora 463, 1–26.

Kardong, K.V., 1982. The evolution of the venom apparatus in snakes from colubrids to viperids and elapids. Mem. Inst. Butantan 46, 105–118.

Kardong, K.V., 1996. Snake toxins and venoms: an evolutionary perspective. Herpetologica 52, 36–46.

Kardong, K.V., 2002. Colubrid snakes and Duvernoy's "venom" glands. J. Toxicol. Toxin Rev. 21, 1–15.

Kardong, K.V. 2009. Colubrid venoms: pharmacology vs biological role. Presentation at Venom Week 2009, June 2009, Alburquerque, New Mexico.

Kardong, K.V., Luchtel, D.L., 1986. Ultrastructure of Duvernoy's gland from the wandering garter snake, *Thamnophis elegans vagrans* (Serpentes, Colubridae). J. Morphol. 188, 1–13.

Kardong, K.V., Lavin-Murcio, P.A., 1993. Venom delivery of snakes as high-pressure and low-pressure systems. Copeia 1993, 650–654.

Karns, D.R., 2001. Sherman A. Minton, Jr. 1919–1999. Copeia 2001, 891–894.

Kärppä, M., 2009. Acute polyradiculitis—from prickling to intensive care. Duodecim 125, 1615–1621.

Karatas, M., 2008. Central vertigo and dizziness: epidemiology, differential diagnosis and common causes. Neurologist 14, 355–364.

Kasturiratne, A., Wickremasinghe, A.R., de Silva, N., Gunawardena, N.K., Pathmeswaran, A., Premaratna, R., et al. 2008. The global burden of snakebite: a literature analysis and modelling based on regional estimates of envenoming and deaths. PLoS Med. 5, e218.

Kawamoto, F., Kumada, N., 1989. A case report of eye-injury caused by cervical gland venom of a snake, *Rhabdophis tigrinus* (Boie). Japan. J. Sanit. Zool. 40, 211–212.

Kawamura, Y., Sakai, A., Sawai, Y., 1986. Studies on the pathogenesis of envenomation of the Japanese colubrid, yamakagashi, *Rhabdophis tigrinus* (Boie). 3. Preparation of anti-yamakagashi antivenom. The Snake 18, 1–5.

Kawamura, Y., Sawai, Y., Toriba, M., Hokama, Y., Sakai, A., Kouda, T., et al. 1988. Study on the preparation of anti-yamakagashi (*Rhabdophis tigrinus*) rabbit and goat antivenom. The Snake 20, 4–8.

Keenlyside, R.A., Schonberger, L.B., Bregman, D.J., Bolyal, J.Z., 1980. Fatal Gulláin–Barre syndrome after the national influenza immunization program. Neurology 30, 929–933.

Kelly, C.M., Barker, N.P., Villet, M.H., Broadley, D.G., Branch, W.R., 2008. The snake family Psammophiidae (Reptilia: Serpentes): phylogenetics and species delimitation in the African sand snakes (*Psammophis* Boie, 1825) and allied genera. Mol. Phylogenet. Evol. 47, 1045–1060.

Kelsey, J., Ehrlich, M., Henderson, S.O., 1997. Exotic reptile bites. Am. J. Emerg. Med. 15, 536–537.

Kennedy, H.L., Whitlock, J.A., Sprague, M.K., Kennedy, L.J., Buckingham, T.A., Goldberg, R.J., 1985. Long-term follow-up of asymptomatic healthy subjects with frequent and complex ventricular ectopy. N. Engl. J. Med. 312, 193–197.

Kerber, K.A., 2009. Vertigo and dizziness in the emergency department. Emerg. Med. Clin. North Am. 27, 39–50.

Kerrigan, K.R., Mertz, B.L., Nelson, S.J., Dye, J.D., 1997. Antibiotic prophylaxis for pit viper envenomation: a prospective, controlled trial. World J. Surg. 21, 369–372. (discussion pp. 372–373).

Keyler, D.E., 2008. Envenomation by the lowland viper (*Proatheris superciliaris*): severe case profile documentation. Toxicon 52, 836–841.

Kijjirak, R., et al. 1998. Interesting case conference (in Thai) "Ngu laysab khodeng gat" (red-necked keel-back bite). Chula J. Int. Med. 11, 268–272.

Kikuchi, H., Takamura, T., Ishii, M., Ichihara, T., Kawamura, Y., Sawai, Y., 1987. Study on the effectiveness of the yamakagashi (*Rhabdophis tigrinus*) antivenom. The Snake 19, 95–98.

Kirmayer, L.J., Young, A., Robbins, J.M., 1994. Symptom attribution in cultural perspective. Can. J. Psychiatry 39, 584–595.

Klauber, L.M., 1928. The *Trimorphodon* (lyre snake) of California, with notes on the species of the adjacent areas. Trans. San Diego Soc. Nat. Hist. 5, 183–194.

Knabe, K., 1939. Schlangenbiss eines Kamerunnegers durch grüne Baumschlange (*Dipholidus typus*). Arch. Schiffs-u. Tropenhyg. 43, 173–174.

Kochva, E., 1965. The development of the venom gland in the opisthoglyph snake, *Telescopus fallax*, with remarks on *Thamnophis sirtalis* (Colubridae, Reptilia). Copeia 1965, 147–154.

Kochva, E., 1978. Oral glands of the Reptilia. In: Gans, C., Gans, K.A. (Eds.), Biology of the Reptilia, vol. 8. Academic Press, New York, NY, pp. 43–161.

Kochva, E., 1987. The origin of snakes and evolution of the venom apparatus. Toxicon 25, 65–106.

Kochva, E., 1998. Venomous snakes of Israel: ecology and snakebite. Public Health Rev. 26, 209–232.

Kochva, E., Oron, U., Ovadia, M., Simon, T., Bdolah, A., 1980. Venom glands, venom synthesis, venom secretion and evolution. In: Eaker, D., Wadstrom, T. (Eds.), Natural Toxins (pp. 3–12). Pergamon Press, Oxford, UK.

Komori, K., Konishi, M., Maruta, Y., Toriba, M., Sakai, A., Matsuda, A., et al. 2006. Characterization of a novel metalloproteinase in Duvernoy's gland of *Rhabdophis tigrinus tigrinus*. J. Toxicol. Sci. 31, 157–168.

Kono, H., Sawai, Y., 1975. Systemic poisoning from the bite of *Rhabdophis tigrinus*. The Snake 7, 38–39.

Kornalik, F., Táborská, E., 1978. Procoagulant and defibrinating potency of the venom gland extract from *Thelotornis kirtlandii*. Thromb. Res. 12, 991–1001.

Kornalik, F., Táborská, E., Mebs, D., 1978. Pharmacological and biochemical properties of a venom gland extract from the snake, *Thelotornis kirtlandii*. Toxicon 16, 535–542.

Kraus, F., Brown, W.M., 1998. Phylogenetic relationships of colubroid snakes based on mitochondrial DNA sequences. Zool. J. Linn. Soc. 62, 421–442.

Kroll, J.C., 1976. Feeding adaptations of hognose snakes. Southwest Naturalist 20, 537–557.

Kuch, U., Jesberger, U., 1993. Human envenomation from the bite of the South American colubrid snake species *Philodryas baroni* Berg, 1895. The Snake 25, 63–65.

Kuch, U., 1999. Notes on two cases of envenomation by the South American colubrid snakes *Philodryas olfersii latirostris* Cope, 1862, and *Philodryas chamissonis* (Wiegmann, 1834) (Squamata: Serpentes: Colubridae). Herpetozoa 12, 11–16.

Kuch, U., Müller, J., Mödden, C., Mebs, D., 2006. Snake fangs from the Lower Miocene of Germany: evolutionary stability of perfect weapons. Naturwissenschaften 92, 84–87.

Kumlutas, Y., Mehmet, O., Tunc, M.R., Kaska, Y., Ozdemir, A., Dusen, S., 2004. On species of the Western Taurus Range, Turkey. Nat. Croat. 13, 19–33.

Kurnik, D., Haviv, Y., Kochva, E., 1999. A snake bite by the burrowing asp, *Atractaspis engaddensis*. Toxicon 37, 223–227.

Lakier, J.B., Fritz, V.U., 1969. Consumptive coagulopathy caused by a boomslang bite. S. Afr. Med. J. 43, 1052–1055.

Lam, K.K., Crow, P., Leung, N.K.H., Shek, K.C., Fung, H.T., Ades, G., et al. 2010. A cross-sectional survey of snake oral bacterial flora from Hong Kong, SAR, China. Emerg. Med. J. 28, 107–114.

Lampert, K.P., Schartl, M., 2010. A little bit is better than nothing: the incomplete partheno-genesis of salamanders, frogs and fish. BMC Biol. 8, 78.

Langen, M.J., Spawls, S., 2010. Amphibians and Reptiles of Ethiopia and Eritrea. Edition Chimaira, Frankfurt, Germany.

Latifi, M., 1991. Latifi's Snakes of Iran. Society for the Study of Amphibians and Reptiles, Oxford, OH.

Lawson, R., Slowinski, J.B., Crother, B.I., Burbrink, F.T., 2005. Phylogeny of the Colubroidea (Serpentes): new evidence from mitochondrial and nuclear genes. Mol. Phylogenet. Evol. 37, 581–601.

Lazkowski-Jones, L., 2009. A case of envenomation from a non-venomous snake? Wilderness Environ. Med. 2009 (Summer), 18–19.

Leal, M., Thomas, R., 1994. Notes on the feeding behaviour and caudal luring by juvenile *Alosphis portoricensis* (Serpentes: Colubridae). J. Herpetol. 28, 126–128.

Leder, D., 1990. Clinical interpretation: the hermeneutics of medicine. Theor. Med. 11, 9–24.

Lee, J.C., 1996. The Amphibians and Reptiles of the Yucatan Peninsula. Comstock/Cornell University Press, Ithaca, NY.

Lee, H., Kim, B.K., Park, H.J., Koo, J.W., Kim, J.S., 2009. Prodromal dizziness in vestibu-lar neuritis: frequency and clinical implication. J. Neurol. Neurosurg. Psychiatry 80, 355–356.

Lee, C.H., Jones, D.K., Ahern, C., Sarhan, M.F., Ruben, P.C., 2011. Biophysical costs associated with tetrodotoxin resistance in the sodium channel pore of the garter snake, *Thamnophis sirtalis*. J. Comp. Physiol. A. Neuroethol. Sens. Neural Behav. Physiol. 197, 33–43.

Leisewitz, A.L., Blaylock, R.S., Kettner, F., Goodhead, A., Goddard, A., Schoeman, J.P., 2004. The diagnosis and management of snakebite in dogs—a southern African perspective. J. S. Afr. Vet. Assoc. 75, 7–13.

Leite, P.T., Kaefer, I.L., Cechin, S.Z., 2009. Diet of *Philodryas olfersii* (Sepentes, Colubridae) during hydroelectric dam flooding in southern Brazil. North-Western J. Zool. 5, 53–60.

Lemoine, K., Salqueiro, L.M., Rodríguez-Acosta, A., Acosta, J.A., 2004a. Neurotoxic, hemor-rhagic, and proteolytic activities of Duvernoy's gland secretion from Venezuelan opistho-glyphous snakes in mice. Vet. Hum. Toxicol. 46, 10–14.

Lemoine, K., Girón, M.E., Aguilar, I., Navarette, L.F., Rodríguez-Acosta, A., 2004b. Proteolytic, hemorrhagic, and neurotoxic activities caused by *Leptodeira annulata ashmeadii* (Serpentes: Colubridae) Duvernoy's gland secretion. Wilderness Environ. Med. 15, 82–89.

León, G., Segura, A., Herrera, M., Otero, R., França, F.O., Barbaro, K.C., et al. 2008. Human heterophilic antibodies against equine immunoglobulins: assessment of their role in the early adverse reactions to antivenom administration. Trans. R. Soc. Trop. Med. Hyg. 102, 1115–1119.

Levine, E.G., Manilov, A., McAllister, S.C., Heymann, W.R., 2003. Iguana bite-induced hypersensitivity reaction. Arch. Dermatol. 139, 1658–1659.

Levinson, S.R., Evans, M.H., Groves, F., 1976. A neurotoxic component of the venom from Blanding's tree snake (*Boiga blandingi*). Toxicon 14, 307–312.

Leynaud, G.C., Bucher, E.H., 1999. La fauna de serpientes del Chaco Sudamericano: diversidad, distribución geografica y estado de conservación. Acad. Nacion. Ciencias Misc. 98, 1–46.

Li, Q.B., Huang, G.W., Kinjoh, K., Nakamura, M., Kosugi, T., 2001. Hematological studies on DIC-like findings observed in patients with snakebite in south China. Toxicon 39, 943–948.

Linder, R., 2006. Alan W. Bernheimer. Microbe (obituary section) June 2006.

Liner, E.A., 1960. A new subspecies of false coral snake (*Pliocercus elapoides*) from San Luis Potosi, Mexico. Southwest Naturalist 5, 217–220.

Liner, E.A., 1994. Scientific and common names for the amphibians and reptiles of Mexico in English and Spanish. SSAR Herpetol. Circular 23, 113. pp

Longmore, M., Wilkinson, I., Török, E., 2001. Oxford Handbook of Medicine, fifth ed.. Oxford University Press, Oxford, UK.

LoVecchio, F., Klemens, J., Welch, S., Rodriguez, R., 2002. Antibiotics after rattlesnake envenomation. J. Emerg. Med. 23, 327–328.

Lowe, C.H, Schwalbe, C.R., Johnson, T.B., 1986. The Venomous Reptiles of Arizona. Arizona Game and Fish Department, Phoenix, AZ. 115 pp

Lumsden, N.G., Fry, B.G., Manjunatha Kini, R., Hodgson, W.C., 2004. In vitro neuromuscular activity of colubrid venoms: clinical and evolutionary implications. Toxicon 43, 819–827.

Lumsden, N.G., Fry, B.G., Ventura, S., Kini, R.M., Hodgson, W.C., 2005. Pharmacological characterisation of a neurotoxin from the venom of Boiga dendrophila (mangrove catsnake). Toxicon 45, 329–334.

Lumsden, N.G., Ventura, S., Dauer, R., Hodgson, W.C., 2005. A biochemical and pharmacological examination of Rhamphiophus oxyrhynchus (Rufous beaked snake) venom. Toxicon 45, 219–231.

Macedo, E., Abdulkader, R., Castro, I., Sobrinho, A.C.C., Yu, L., Vieira Jr., J.M., 2006. Lack of protection of N-acetylcysteine (NAC) in acute renal failure related to elective aortic aneurysm repair—a randomized controlled trial. Nephrol. Dial. Transplant. 21, 1863–1869.

MacCabe, R.J., 2009. Desert nomads. A study of health and disease of the Turkana people of North Western Kenya. Irish Carmalites, Dublin, Ireland.

MacKay, N., Ferguson, J.C., Ashe, J., Bagshawe, A., Forrester, A.T.T., McNicol, G.P., 1969. The venom of the boomslang (Dispholidus typus): in vivo and in vitro studies. Thromb. Diasth. Hemorrhag. 21, 234–244.

Mackessy, S.P., 1988. Venom ontogeny in the pacific rattlesnakes Crotalus viridis helleri and C. v. oreganus. Copeia 1988, 92–101.

Mackessy, S.P., 2002. Biochemistry and pharmacology of colubrid venoms. J. Toxicol. Toxin Rev. 21, 43–83.

Mackessy, S.P., Baxter, L.M., 2006. Bioweapons synthesis and storage: the venom gland of front-fanged snakes. Zool. Anz. 245, 147–159.

Mackessy, S.P., Sixberry, N.M., Heyborne, W.H., Fritts, T., 2006. Venom of the Brown Treesnake, Boiga irregularis: ontogenetic shifts and taxa-specific toxicity. Toxicon 47, 537–548.

Magalhaes, A., Da Fonseca, B.C., Diniz, C.R., Gilroy, J., Richardson, M., 1993. The complete amino acid sequence of a thrombin-like enzyme/gyroxin analogue from the venom of the bushmaster snake (Lachesis muta muta). FEBS Lett. 329, 116–120.

Mahasandana, S., Rungruxsirivorn, Y., Chantarangkul, V., 1980. Clinical manifestations of bleeding following Russell's viper and green pit viper bites in adults. Southeast Asian J. Trop. Med. Public Health 11, 285–293.

Malasit, P., Warrell, D.A., Chanthavanich, P., Viravan, C., Mongkolsapaya, J., Singhthong, B., et al. 1986. Prediction, prevention and mechanism of early (anaphylactic) antivenom reactions in victims of snakebites. Br. Med. J. (Clin. Res. Ed.) 292, 17–20.

Malhotra, A., Thorpe, R.S., 2004. A phylogeny of four mitochondrial gene regions suggests a revised taxonomy for Asian pitvipers (Trimeresurus and Ovophis). Mol. Phylogenet. Evol. 32, 83–100.

Malik, G.M., 1995. Snake bites in adults from the Asir region of southern Saudi Arabia. Am. J. Trop. Med. Hyg. 52, 314–317.

Malina, T., Krecsák, L., Korsós, Z., Takács, Z., 2008. Snakebites in Hungary—Epidemiological and clinical aspects over the past 36 years. Toxicon 51, 943–951.

Malnate, E.V., 1960. Systematic division and evolution of the colubrid snake genus Natrix, with comments on the subfamily Natricinae. Proc. Acad. Nat. Sci. Philadelphia 112, 41–71.

Mamonov, G., 1977. Case report of envenomation by the mountain racer, *Coluber ravergieri* in USSR. The Snake 9, 27–28.

Mandal, S., Bhattacharyya, D., 2007. Ability of a small, basic protein isolated from Russell's viper venom (*Daboia russelli russelli*) to induce renal tubular necrosis in mice. Toxicon 50, 236–250.

Mandell, F., Bates, J., Mittleman, M.B., Loy, J.W., 1980. Major coagulopathy and "nonpoisonous" snake bites. Pediatrics 65, 314–317.

Manning, B., Galbo, M., Klapman, G., 1999. First report of a symptomatic South American false water cobra envenomation. J. Toxicol. Clin. Toxicol. 37, 613.

Marais, J., 1985. Snake Versus Man: A Guide to Dangerous and Common Harmless Snakes of Southern Africa. Macmillan, Johannesburg, South Africa.

Marino, P.L., 2009. The Little ICU Book of Facts and Formulas. Lippincott, Williams and Wilkins, Philadelphia, PA.

Marsh, N., Williams, V., 2005. Practical applications of snake venom toxins in haemostasis. Toxicon 45, 1171–1181.

Martins, N., 1916. Das opistoglyphas brasileiras e seu veneno. Colet. Trab. Inst. Butantan 1916, 427–496.

Martens, E.J., de Jonge, P., Na, B., Cohen, B.E., Lett, H., Whooley, M.A., 2010. Scared to death? Generalized anxiety disorder and cardiovascular events in patients with stable coronary artery disease: The Heart and Soul Study. Arch. Gen. Psychiatry 67, 750–758.

Marunäk, S.L., Acosta, O.C., Leiva, L.C., Ruiz, R.M., Aguirre, M.V., Teibler, P., 2004. Mice plasma fibrinogen consumption by thrombin-like enzyme present in rattlesnake venom from the north-east region of Argentina. Medicina (B. Aires) 64, 509–517.

Matell, G., Nyman, D., Werner, B., Wilhelmsson, S., 1973. Consumption coagulopathy caused by a boomslang bite: a case report. Thromb. Res. 3, 173–182.

Mather, H.M., Mayne, S., McMonagle, T.M., 1978. Severe envenomation from "harmless" pet snake. Br. Med. J. 1, 1324–1325.

Matsuda, R., Narai, S., Iizuka, M., 1990. A case of defibrination syndrome due to snake (*Rhabdophis tigrinus*) bite. Tottori Med. J. 18, 182–187.

McAlister, W.H., 1963. Evidence of mild toxicity in the saliva of the hognose snake (*Heterodon*). Herpetologica 19, 132–137.

McArdle, J.J., Lentz, T.L., Witzemann, V., Schwarz, H., Weinstein, S.A., Schmidt, J.J., 1999. Waglerin I selectively blocks the epsilon form of the muscle nicotinic acetylcholine receptor. J. Pharm. Exp. Ther. 289, 543–550.

McCue, M.D., 2005. Enzyme activities and biological functions of snake venoms. Appl. Herpetol. 2, 109–123.

McCue, M.D., 2007. Prey envenomation does not improve digestive performance in Western diamondback rattlesnakes (*Crotalus atrox*). J. Exp. Zool. A Ecol. Genet. Physiol. 307A, 568–577.

McDiarmid, R.W., Campbell, J.A., Touré, T.A., 1999. Snake Species of the World, vol. 1. Herpetologists' League, Lawrence, KS.

McDowell, S.B., 1986. The architecture of the corner of the mouth of colubroid snakes. J. Morphol. 20, 353–407.

McKinstry, D.M., 1978. Evidence of toxic saliva in some colubrid snakes of the United States. Toxicon 16, 523–534.

McKinstry, D.M., 1983. Morphologic evidence of toxic saliva in colubrid snakes: a checklist of world genera. Herp. Rev. 14, 12–15.

McNally, S.L., Reitz, C.J., 1987. Victims of snakebite: a 5-year study at Shongwe Hospital, Kangwane, 1978–1982. S. Afr. Med. J. 72, 855–860.

McPhee, S.J., Papadakis, M., 2009. Current Medical Diagnosis and Treatment 2009 (Lange Current Series). McGraw-Hill Professional, New York, NY.

Means, D.B., 2010. Ophidism by the green palm snake. Wilderness Environ. Med. 21, 46–49.

Mebs, D., 1968. Analysis of *Leptodeira annulata* venom. Herpetologica 24, 338–339.

Mebs, D., 1978. Pharmacology of reptile venoms. In: Gans, C., Gans, K.A. (Eds.), Biology of the Reptilia, vol. 8. Academic Press, New York, NY

Mebs, D., 2002. Venomous and Poisonous Animals. CRC Press, Boca Raton, FL.

Mebs, D., Scharrer, I., Stille, W., Hauk, H., 1978. A fatal case of snake bite due to *Thelotornis kirtlandii* Toxins: Animal, Plant and Microbial: Proceedings of the Fifth International Symposium. Pergamon Press, Oxford, UK. pp. 477–479.

Mebs, D., Parr, D., Graben, N., Hassel, U., 1987. Severe envenomation after a bite from *Rhabdophis subminiatus*. Toxicon 25, 372.

Mebs, D., Holada, K., Kornalik, F., Simák, J., Vanková, H., Müller, D., et al. 1998. Severe coagulopathy after a bite of a green bush viper (*Atheris squamiger*): case report and biochemical analysis of the venom. Toxicon 36, 1333–1340.

Meier, J., 1981. The fangs of *Dispholidus typus* Smith and *Thelotornis kirtlandii* Smith (Serpentes: Colubridae). Rev. Suisse Zool. 88, 897–902.

Merhtens, J.M., 1987. Living Snakes of the World. Sterling Publishing, New York, NY.

Merin, D.S., Bush, S.P., 2000. Severe hand injury following a green iguana bite. Wilderness Environ. Med. 11, 225–226.

Michaud, E.J., Dixon, J.R., 1989. Prey items of 20 species of the neotropical snake genus. *Liophis*. Herpetol. Rev. 20, 39–41.

Miguti, G.I., Dube, M., 1998. Severe envenomation by a "pet" vine snake. Cent. Afr. J. Med. 44, 232–234.

Minton, S.A., 1964. A contribution to the herpetology of West Pakistan. Bull. Am. Mus. Nat. Hist. 134, 29–184. p. 73.

Minton, S.A., 1974. Venom Diseases. Thomas Publishing, Springfield, IL.

Minton, S.A., 1976. A list of colubrid envenomations. Kentucky Herp. 7, 4.

Minton, S.A., 1979. Beware: non-poisonous snakes. Clin. Toxicol. 15, 259–265.

Minton, S.A., 1986. Venomous bites by "nonvenomous" snakes. Wilderness Environ. Med. 3, 6–7.

Minton, S.A., 1990. Venomous bites by non-venomous snakes: an annotated bibliography of colubrid envenomation. J. Wilderness Med. 1, 119–127.

Minton, S.A., 1996. Are there are any nonvenomous snakes? An update on colubrid envenoming. Adv. Herpetocult. 1, 127–134.

Minton, S.A., 2001. Life, Love and Reptiles: An Autobiography of Sherman A. Minton, MD. Krieger, Malabar, FL.

Minton, S.A., Dunson, W.A., 1978. Observations on the Palawan mangrove snake, *Boiga dendrophila multicincta* (Reptilia, Serpentes, Colubridae). J. Herpetol. 12, 107–108.

Minton, S.A., Mebs, D., 1978. Four cases of bites by colubrids (Reptilia: Serpentes: Colubridae). Salamandra 14, 41–43.

Minton, S.A., Minton, M.R., 1969. Venomous Reptiles, first ed.. Scribners, New York, NY.

Minton, S.A., Minton, M.R., 1980. Venomous Reptiles, second ed.. Scribners, New York, NY.

Minton, S.A., Weinstein, S.A., 1984. Protease activity and lethal toxicity of venoms from some little-known rattlesnakes. Toxicon 22, 828–830.

Minton, S.A., Weinstein, S.A., 1986. Geographic and ontogenetic variation in venom of the Western diamondback rattlesnake (*Crotalus atrox*). Toxicon 24, 71–80.

Minton, S.A., Weinstein, S.A., 1987. Colubrid snake venoms: immunologic relationships, electrophoretic patterns. Copeia 1987, 993–1000.

Mitchell, J.S., Heckert, A.B., Sues, H.D., 2010. Grooves to tubes: evolution of the venom delivery system in a Late Triassic "reptile". Naturwissenschaften 97, 1117–1121.

Mittleman, M.B., Goris, R.C., 1974. Envenomation from the bite of the Japanese colubrid snake, *Rhabdophis tigrinus* (Boie). Herpetologica 2, 113–119.

Mittleman, M.B., Goris, R.C., 1978. Death caused by the bite of the Japanese colubrid snake, *Rhabdophis tigrinus* (Boie) (Reptilia, Serpentes, Colubridae). J. Herpetol. 12, 109–111.

Mole, R.R., 1924. The Trinidad snakes. Proc. Gen. Meet. Sci. Bus. Zool. Soc. 1924, 234–278.

Monk, A.R., 1991. A case of mild envenomation from a mangrove snake bite. Litt. Serp. 11, 21–23.

Montgomery, J.M., Gillespie, D., Sastrawan, P., Fredeking, T.M., Stewart, G.L., 2002. Aerobic salivary bacteria in wild and captive Komodo dragons. J. Wildl. Dis. 38, 545–551.

Monzel, M., Wüster, W., 2008. Neotropische Grubenottern—Evolution, Biogeographie und Ökologie. Draco 8 (33), 4–27.

Moran, N.F., Newman, W.J., Theakston, R.D., Warrell, D.A., Wilkinson, D., 1998. High incidence of early anaphylactoid reaction to SAIMR polyvalent snake antivenom. Trans. R. Soc. Trop. Med. Hyg. 92, 69–70.

Mori, A., Burghardt, G.M., 2000. Does prey matter? Geographic variation in antipredator responses of hatchlings of a Japanese natricine snake (*Rhabdophis tigrinus*). J. Comp. Psychol. 114, 408–413.

Mori, A., Burghardt, G.M., 2008. Comparative experimental tests of natricine antipredator displays, with special reference to the apparently unique displays in the Asian genus, *Rhabdophis*. J. Ethol. 26, 61–68.

Mori, A, Mizuta, T., 2006. Envenomation by the Madagascan colubrid snake, *Ithycyphus miniatus*. J. Venom. Anim. Toxins incl. Trop. Dis. (online ISSN 1678-9199).

Mori, K., Hisa, S., Suzuki, S., Sugai, K., Sakai, H., Kiruchi, T., et al. 1983. A case of severe defibrination syndrome due to snake (*Rhabdophis tigrinus*) bite. Jap. J. Haematol. 24, 256–262.

Morita, T., Matsumoto, H., Iwanaga, S., Sakai, A., 1988. A prothrombin activator found in *Rahbdophis tigrinus* (Yamakagashi snake) venom. In: Pirkle, H., Markland, F.S. (Eds.), Hemostasis and Animal Venoms. Marcel Dekker, New York, NY, pp. 55–66.

Morocco, A.P., Hendrickson, R.G., Haddock, R.L., 2006. Envenomation by the brown tree snake (*Boiga irregularis*) on Guam. Clin. Toxicol. 44, 643. (abstract)

Morris, M., 1985. Envenomation from the bite of *Heterodon nasicus* (Serpentes: Colubridae). Herpetologica 41, 361–363.

Morrison, J.J., Pearn, J.H., Covacevich, J., Nixon, J., 1983. Can Australians identify snakes? Med. J. Aust. 2, 66–70.

Muguti, G.I., Dube, M., 1998. Severe envenomation by a "pet" vine snake. Cent. Afr. J. Med. 44, 232–234.

Mulcahy, D.G., 2008. Phylogeography and species boundaries of the western North American night snake (*Hypsiglena torquata*): revisiting the subspecies concept. Mol. Phylogenet. Evol. 46, 1095–1115.

Myers, C.W., 1965. Biology of the ringneck snake, *Diadophis punctatus*, in Florida. Bull. Florida State Mus. 10, 43–90.

Myers, C.W., Daly, J.W., Malkin, B., 1978. A dangerously toxic new frog (*Phyllobates*) used by Emberá Indians of western Colombia, with discussion of blowgun fabrication and dart poisoning. Bull. Am. Mus. Nat. Hist. 161, 309–365.

Myint-Lwin, Tin-Nu-Swe, Myint-Aye-Mu, Than-Than, Thein-Than, Tun-Pe, Heparin therapy in Russell's viper bite victims with impending dic (a controlled trial). Southeast Asian J. Trop. Med. Public Health 20, 271–277.

Nagy, Z.T., Lawson, R., Joger, U., Wink, M., 2004. Molecular systematics of racers, whipsnakes and relatives (Reptilia: Colubridae) using mitochondrial and nuclear markers. J. Zool. Syst. Evol. Res. 42, 223–233.

Nagy, Z.T., Schmidtler, J.F., Joger, U., Wink, M., 2004. Systematik der Zwergnattern (Reptilia: Colubridae: Eirenis) und verwandter Gruppen anhand von DNA-Sequenzen und morphologischen Daten. Salamandra 39, 149–168.

Nagy, Z.T., Glaw, F., Andreone, F., Wink, M., Vences, M., 2007. Species boundaries in Malagasy snakes of the genus *Madagascarophis* (Serpentes: Colubridae *sensu lato*) assessed by nuclear and mitochondrial markers. Org. Divers. Evol. 7, 241–251.

Nahas, L., Kamiguchi, A.S., Hoge, A.R., Goris, R., 1976. Characterization of the coagulant activity of the venom of aglyphous (*Rhabdophis tigrinus*) snake. In: Ohsaka, A. (Ed.), Animal, Plant and Microbial Toxins (pp. 159–170). Plenum Press, New York, NY.

Nair, D.G., Fry, B.G., Alewood, P., Kumar, P.P., Kini, R.M., 2007. Antimicrobial activity of omwaprin, a new member of the waprin family of snake venom proteins. Biochem. J. 402, 93–104.

Nakayama, Y., Furuya, S., Yamada, T., Hirakawa, Y., Fosaka, F., 1973. The treatment by artificial dialysis of a snakebite patient with an intravascular coagulation syndrome. Jap. J. Nephrol. 4, 269. (Note: in Japanese; features of the case translated and published in English by Mittleman and Goris, 1978).

Narayan, S.M., Kazi, D., Krummen, D.E., Rappel, W.J., 2008. Repolarization and activation restitution near human pulmonary veins and atrial fibrillation initiation: a mechanism for the initiation of atrial fibrillation by premature beats. J. Am. Coll. Cardiol. 52, 1222–1230.

Neill, W.T., 1949. Two cases of snake bite in New Guinea. Copeia 3, 228–229.

Neill, W.T., 1954. Evidence of venom in snakes of the genera *Alsophis* and *Rhadinaea*. Copeia 8, 59–60.

Neira, P.O., Jofré, L.M., Oschilewski, D.L., Subercaseaux, B.S., Munöz, N.S., 2007. Mordedura por *Philodryas chamissonis*. Presentación de un caso y revisión de la literature. Rev. Chil. Infectol. 24, 236–241.

Newman, C.J., 1985. Notes on the bite of the Montpellier snake. The Vipera 1, 35–39.

Nichols, A., 1986. Envenomation by a blue-striped garter snake, *Thamnophis sirtalis similis*. Herp. Rev. 17, 6.

Nicholson, E., 1874. Indian Snakes. An Elemenatry Treatise on Ophiology with a Descriptive Catalogue of the Snakes Found in India and the Adjoining Countries, second ed.. Higginbotham and Company, Madras, India.

Nicolson, I.C., Ashby, P.A., Johnson, N.D., Versey, J., Slater, L., 1974. Boomslang bite with haemorrhage and activation of complement by the alternate pathway. Clin. Exp. Immun. 16, 295–300.

Nickerson, M.A., Henderson, R.W., 1976. A case of envenomation by the South American colubrid, *Philodryas olfersii*. Herpetologica 32, 197–198.

Nishioka, S., Silveira, P.V.P., 1994. *Philodryas patagoniensis* bite and local envenoming. Rev. Inst. Med. Trop. São Paulo 36, 279–281.

Nomura, T., Nagata, T., Kawamura, Y., Sawai, Y., 1989. A case of severe yamakagashi (*Rhabdophis tigrinus*) bite treated by antivenom. The Snake 21, 85–86.

Napolitano, L.M., Warkentin, T.E., Almahameed, A., Nasraway, S.A., 2006. Heparin-induced thrombocytopenia in the critical care setting: diagnosis and management. Crit. Care Med. 34, 2898–2911.

Odeleye, A.A., Presley, A.E., Passwater, M.E., Mintz, P.D., 2004. Report of two cases: Rattlesnake venom-induced thrombocytopenia. Ann. Clin. Lab. Sci. 34, 467–470.

O'Donnell, R.P., Staniland, K., Mason, R.T., 2007. Experimental evidence that oral secretions of northwestern ring-necked snakes (*Diadophis punctatus occidentalis*) are toxic to their prey. Toxicon 50, 810–815.

Ogawa, H., Sawai, Y., 1986. A fatal bite of the yamakagashi (*Rhabdophis tigrinus*). The Snake 18, 53–54.

Okayama, Y., Hagaman, D.D., Woolhiser, M., Metcalfe, D.D., 2001. Further characterization of FcgammaRII and FcgammaRIII expression by cultured human mast cells. Int. Arch. Allergy Immunol. 124, 155–157.

Omogbai, E.K.I., Nworgu, Z.A.M., Imhafidon, M.A., Ikpeme, A.A., Ojo, D.O., Nwako, C.N., 2003. Snake bites in Nigeria: a study of the prevalence and treatment in Benin City. Trop. J. Pharmaceut. Res. 1, 39–44.

OmPraba, G., Chapeaurouge, A., Doley, R., Devi, K.R., Padmanaban, P., Venkatraman, C., et al. 2010. Identification of a novel family of snake venom proteins veficolins from *Cerberus rhynchops* using a venom gland transcriptomics and proteomics approach. J. Proteome Res. 9, 1882–1893.

Orcés, G., 1948. Notas sobre los ofidios venosos del Ecuador. Revista Filosofia Letras (Quito) 3, 231–250.

Orduna, T.A., Martino, O.A.L., Bernachea, P., Maulen, S., 1994. Ophidism produced by snakebite of the genus *Philodryas*. Prensa. Méd. Argentina 81, 636–638.

Orlov, B.N., Gelashvili, D.B., Ibrahimov, A.K., 1990. Venomous Animals and Plants of USSR. Vysshaya Shkola, Moscow. pp. 107–112.

O'Shea, M., 1996. A Guide to the Snakes of Papua New Guinea. Independent Publishing, Port Moresby, Papua New Guinea.

Otto, J., Blaylock, R., 2003. Vine snake (*Thelotornis capensis*) bite in a dog. J. S. Afr. Vet. Assoc. 74, 27–28.

Ovadia, M., 1984. Embryonic development of Duvernoy's gland in the snake, *Natrix tessellata* (Colubridae). Copeia 1984, 516–521.

Padial, J.M., 2006. Commented distributional list of the reptiles of Mauritania (West Africa). Graellsia 62, 159–178.

Pahlajani, D.B., Iya, V., Tahiliani, R., Shah, V.K., Khokhani, R.C., 1987. Sinus node dysfunction following cobra bite. Indian Heart J. 39, 48–49.

Parnes, L.S., McClure, J.A., 1991. Posterior semicircular canal occlusion in the normal hearing ear. Otolaryngol. Head Neck Surg. 104, 52–57.

Parish, W.E., 1970. Short-term anaphylactic antibodies in human sera. Lancet 2, 591.

Parrish, H.M., 1967. Pitfalls in treating pit viper bites. Med. Times 95, 809–815.

Parrish, H.M., Maclaurin, A.W., Tuttle, R.L., 1956. North American pit vipers: bacterial flora of the mouth and venom glands. Va. Med. Mon. 83, 383–385.

Paul, V., Pudoor, A., Earali, J., John, B., Anil Kumar, C.S., Anthony, T., 2007. Trial of low molecular weight heparin in the treatment of viper bites. J. Assoc. Physicians India 55, 338–342.

Pawlak, J., Mackessy, S.P., Fry, B.G., Bhatia, M., Mourier, G., Fruchart-Gaillard, C., et al. 2006. Denmotoxin, a three-finger toxin from the colubrid snake, *Boiga dendrophila* (Mangrove catsnake) with bird-specific activity. J. Biol. Chem. 281, 29030–29041.

Pawlak, J., Mackessy, S.P., Sixberry, N.M., Stura, E.A., Le Du, M.H., Menez, R, et al. 2009. Irditoxin, a novel covalently linked heterodimeric three-finger toxin with high taxon-specific neurotoxicity. FASEB J. 23, 534–545.

Peichoto, M.E., Leiva, L.C., Guaimás Moya, L.E., Rey, L., Acosta, O., 2005. Duvernoy's gland secretion of *Philodryas patagoniensis* from the northeast of Argentina: its effects on blood coagulation. Toxicon 45, 527–534.

Peichoto, M.E., Teibler, P., Ruiz, R., Leiva, L., Acosta, O., 2006. Systemic pathological alterations caused by *Philodryas patagoniensis* colubrid snake venom in rats. Toxicon 48, 520–528.

Peichoto, M.E., Cespedez, J.A., Pascual, J.A., 2007a. Report of a bite by the South American colubrid snake *Philodryas olfersii latirostris* (Squamata: Colubridae). Acta Herp. 2, 11–15.

Peichoto, M.E., Teibler, P., Mackessy, S.P., Leiva, L., Acosta, O., Gonçalves, L.R., et al. 2007b. Purification and characterization of patagonfibrase, a metalloproteinase showing alpha-fibrinogenolytic and hemorrhagic activities, from *Philodryas patagoniensis* snake venom. Biochim. Biophys. Acta. 1770, 810–819.

Peichoto, M.E., Mackessy, S.P., Teibler, P., Tavares, F.L., Burckhardt, P.L., Breno, M.C., et al. 2009. Purification and characterization of a cysteine-rich secretory protein from *Philodryas patagoniensis* snake venom. Comp. Biochem. Physiol. C Toxicol. Pharmacol. 150, 79–84.

Pérez, A.V., Saravia, P., Rucavado, A, Sant'Ana, C.D., Soares, A.M., Gutiérrez, J.M., 2007. Local and systemic pathophysiological alterations induced by a serine proteinase from the venom of the snake *Bothrops jararacussu*. Toxicon 49, 1063–1069.

Pérez, A.V., Rucavado, A., Sanz, L., Calvete, J.J., Gutiérrez, J.M., 2008. Isolation and characterization of a serine proteinase with thrombin-like activity from the venom of the snake *Bothrops asper*. Braz. J. Med. Biol. Res. 41, 12–17.

Perry, G., 1988. Mild toxic effects resulting from the bites of Jan's desert racer, *Coluber rhodorachis*, and Moila's snake, *Malpolon moilensis* (Ophidia: Colubridae). Toxicon 26, 523–524.

Peters, J.A., Orejas-Miranda, B.R., 1970. Catalogue of Neotropical Squamata. Part I. Snakes. Bull. U.S. Nat. Mus., 347. Washington, DC

Phillips, S., Rose, B., Kulig, K., Brent, J., 1997. Envenomation from the bite of the Western hognose snake. J. Toxicol. Clin. Toxicol. 35, 532.

Phisalix, M., 1922. Animaux Venimeux et Venins, vol. 2. Masson et Cie, Paris, France.

Pineda Lizano, W., 2010. *Oxybelis fulgidus* (green vinesnake). Foraging behavior. Herpetol. Rev. 41, 369–370.

Pinho, F.M., Zanetta, D.M., Burdmann, E.A., 2005. Acute renal failure after *Crotalus durissus* snakebite: a prospective survey on 100 patients. Kidney Int. 67, 659–667.

Pinou, T., Vicario, S., Marschner, M., Caccone, A., 2004. Relict snakes of North America and their relationships within Caenophidia, using likelihood-based Bayesian methods on mitochondrial sequences. Mol. Phylogenet. Evol. 32, 563–574.

Pinto, R.R., Fernandes, R., 2004. Reproductive biology and diet of *Liophis poecilogyrus poecilogyrus* (Serpentes, Colubridae) from southeastern Brazil. Phyllomedusa 3, 9–14.

Pinto, R.N., Jorge da Silva, N., Aird, S.D., 1991. Human envenomation by the South American opisthglyph, *Clelia clelia plumbea* (Wied). Toxicon 29, 1512–1516.

Pitman, C.R.S., 1974. A Guide to the Snakes of Uganda. Wheldon & Wesley, London, UK.

Pizzatto, L., 2005. Body size, reproductive biology and abundance of the rare pseudoboini snakes genera *Clelia* and *Boiruna* (Serpentes, Colubridae). Phyllomedusa 4, 111–122.

Poey, D.F., 1873. Mordedura de un jubo. El Genio Cient. La Habana 1, 94–98.

Pommier, P., de Haro, L., 2007. Envenomation by Montpellier snake (*Malpolon monspessulanus*) with cranial nerve disturbances. Toxicon 50, 868–869.

Pope, C.H., 1947. Amphibians and Reptiles of the Chicago Area. Chicago Museum of Natural History, Chicago, IL.

Pope, C.H., 1958. Fatal bite of captive African rear-fanged snake (*Dispholidus*). Copeia 4, 280–282.

Porath, A., Gilon, D., Schulchynska-Castel, H., Shalev, O., Keynan, A., Benbassat, J., 1992. Risk indicators after envenomation in humans by *Echis coloratus* (mid-east saw scaled viper). Toxicon 30, 25–32.

Pozio, E., 1988. Venomous snake bites in Italy: epidemiological and clinical aspects. Trop. Med. Parasitol. 39, 62–66.

Prado-Franceschi, J., Hyslop, S., Cogo, J.C., Andrade, A.L., Assakura, M., Cruz-Hofling, M.A., et al. 1996. The effects of Duvernoy's gland secretion from the xenodontine colubrid *Philodryas olfersii* on striated muscle and the neuromuscular junction: partial characterization of a neuromuscular fraction. Toxicon 34, 459–466.

Prozialeck, W.C., Edwards, J.R., 2007. Cell adhesion molecules in chemically-induced renal injury. Pharmacol. Ther. 114, 74–93.

Pyron, R.A., Burbrink, F.T., Colli, G.R., Nieto Montes de Oca, A., Vitt, L.J., Kuczynski, C.A., Wiens, J.J., 2011. The phylogeny of advanced snakes (Colubroidea), with discovery of a new subfamily and comparison of support methods for likelihood trees. Mol. Phylogenet. Evol. 58, 329–342.

Quelch, J.J., 1893. Venom in harmless snakes. J. Linn. Soc. Zool. 17, 30–31.

Quintela, F.M., 2010. *Liophis poecilogyrus sublineatus* (Serpentes: Dipsadidae) bite and symptoms of envenomation. Herpetol. Notes 3, 309–311.

Rao, V.S., Joseph, J.S., Kini, R.M., 2003. Group D prothrombin activators from snake venom are structural homologues of mammalian blood coagulation factor Xa. Biochem. J. 369, 635–642.

Ramachandran, S., Ganaikabahu, B., Pushparajan, K., Wijesekera, J., 1995. Electroencephalographic abnormalities in patients with snake bites. Am. J. Trop. Med. Hyg. 52, 25–28.

Ratcliffe, P.J., Pukrittayakamee, S., Ledingham, J.G., Warrell, D.A., 1989. Direct nephrotoxicity of Russel's viper venom demonstrated in the isolated perfused rat kidney. Am. J. Trop. Med. Hyg. 40, 312–319.

Ray, J.M., Wilson, B., Griffith-Rodriquez, E.J., Ross, H.L., 2011. *Sibon argus* (blotched snail sucker). Diet. Herpetol. Rev. 42, 102–103.

Reid, H.A., 1964. Cobra bites. Br. Med. J. 2, 540–545.

Reid, H.A., 1967. Snakebite poisoning. Br. Med. J. 5, 367.

Reid, H.A., 1980. Antivenom reactions and efficacy. Lancet 1 (8176), 1024–1025.

Reid, H.A., Thean, P.C., Chan, K.E., Baharom, A.R., 1963. Clinical effects of bites by Malayan pit viper (*Ancistrodon rhodostoma*). Lancet 1, 617–621.

Reimers, A.R., Weber, M., Müller, U.R., 2000. Are anaphylactic reactions to snake bites immunoglobulin E-mediated? Clin. Exp. Allergy 30, 276–282.

Reinhardt, J., Lütken, C.F., 1862. Bidrag tii det vestindiske Öriges og navnligen tii de danskvestindiske Oers Herpetologie. Vidensk. Meddel. Naturhist. For. Kjöbenhavn, 153–291.

Reinstein, L., Pargament, J.M., Goodman, J.S., 1982. Peripheral neuropathy after multiple tetanus toxoid injections. Arch. Phys. Med. Rehabil. 63, 332–334.

Reitz, C.J., 1989. Boomslang bite—time of onset of clinical envenomation. S. Afr. Med. J. 76, 39–40.

Ribeiro, J., 1989. Fatalidade Histórica da Ilha de Ceilão. Publicações Alfa, Lisboa, Portugal.

Ribeiro, L.A., Puorto, G., Jorge, M.T., 1999. Bites by the colubrid snake, *Philodryas olfersii*: a clinical and epidemiological study of 43 cases. Toxicon 37, 943–948.

Robbins, J.M., Kirmayer, L.J., 1991. Attributions of common somatic symptoms. Psychol. Med. 21, 1029–1045.

Robertson, S.S.D., Delpierre, G.R., 1969. Studies on African snake venoms-IV. Some enzymatic studies in the venom of the boomslang, *Dispholidus typus*. Toxicon 7, 189–194.

Rochelle, M., Kardong, K.V., 1993. Constriction versus envenomation in prey capture by the brown tree snake, *Boiga irregularis* (Squamata: Colubridae). Herpetologica 49, 297–300.

Rodríguez-Acosta, A., Girón, M.E., Aguilar, I., Fuentes, O., 1997. A case of envenomation by a "non-venomous" snake (*Philodryas viridissimus*) and a comparison between this snake's Duvernoy's gland secretion and northern South American rattlesnake's venoms. Arch. Venezol. Med. Trop. 1, 29032.

Rodriguez-Robles, J.A., 1992. Notes on the feeding behavior of the Puerto Rican racer, *Alsophis portoricensis* (Serpentes: Colubridae). J. Herpetol. 26, 100–102.

Rodriguez-Robles, J.A., Leal, M., 1993. Feeding envenomation by *Arrhyton exiguum* (Serpentes: Colubridae). J. Herpetol. 27, 107–109.

Rodriguez-Robles, J.A., Thomas, R., 1992. Venom function in the Puerto Rican racer, *Alsophis portoricensis* (Serpentes: Colubridae). Copeia 1992, 62–68.

Romer, A.S., 1956. Osteology of the Reptiles. University of Chicago Press, Chicago, IL. 793 pp

Rosenberg, H.I., 1992. An improved method for collecting secretion from Duvernoy's gland of colubrid snakes. Copeia 1992, 244–246.

Rosenberg, H.I., Bdolah, A., Kochva, E., 1985. Lethal factors and enzymes in the secretion from Duvernoy's gland of three colubrid snakes. J. Exp. Zool. 233, 5–14.

Rosenberg, H.I., Kinamon, S., Kochva, E., Bdolah, H., 1992. The secretion of Duvernoy's gland of *Malpolon monspessulanus* induced hemorrhage in the lungs of mice. Toxicon 30, 920–924.

Rossman, D.A., 1961. A Taxonomic Study of the Sauritus Group of the Gartersnakes, Genus *Thamnophis* Fitzinger. University of Florida, PhD Dissertation.

Rossman, D.A., Ford, N.B., Seigel, R.A., 1996. The Garter Snakes: Evolution and Ecology. University of Oklahoma Press, Norman, OK. Animal Natural History Series, 332 pp.

Russell, F.E., 1980. Snake Venom Poisoning. Lippincott, New York, NY.

Ruthven, A.G. 1908. Variations and Genetic Relationships of the Garter Snakes. Smithsonian Institution, U.S. Museum Bulletin, p. 61.

Saddler, M., Paul, B., 1988. Vine snake envenomation. Cent. Afr. J. Med. 1988, 31–33.

Saha, B.K., Hati, A.K., 1998. A comparative study on some epidemiological aspects of non-poisonous and poisonous snake bite cases. The Snake 28, 59–61.

Sakai, A., 2007. Clinical feature of envenomation by the snake, Yamakagashi (*Rhabdophis tigrinus*). Chudoku Kenkyu 20, 235–243.

Sakai, A., Hatsuse, M., 1995. Pathogenesis of envenomation by the Japanese snake (*Rhabdophis tigrinus*) and the effect of antivenom. Toxicon 33, 275–276.

Sakai, A., Honma, M., Sawai, Y., 1983. Studies on the pathogenesis of envenomation of the Japanese colubrid snake, yamakagashi, *Rhabdophis tigrinus tigrinus*.1. Study on the toxicity of the venom. The Snake 15, 7–13.

Sakai, A., Honma, M., Sawai., Y., 1984. Study on the toxicity of venoms extracted from Duvernoy's gland of certain Asian colubrid snakes. The Snake 16, 16–20.

Sakai, A., Hatsuse, M., Sawai, Y., 1990. Study on the pathogenesis of envenomation by the Japanese colubrid snake, yamakagashi, *Rhabdophis tigrinus tigrinus*. 4. Hematological and histological studies. The Snake 22, 11–19.

Sakamoto, T., 1932. A severe case of "yamakagashi" (*Natrix tigrina*) snakebite with self-limited hemorrhaging. Gurentsugebito 6, 116–120. (in Japanese).

Salomão, M.D.G., Laporta-Ferreira, I.L., 1994. The role of secretions from the supralabial, infralabial, and Duvernoy's glands of the slug-eating snake, *Sibynomorphus mikanii* (Colubridae: Dipsadinae) in the immobilization of molluscan prey. J. Herpetol. 28, 369–371.

Salomão, M.D.G., Albolea, A.B.P, Santos, S.M.A., 2003. Colubrid snakebite: a public health problem in Brazil. Herpetol. Rev. 34, 307–312.

Salazar, A.M., Aguilar, I., Guerrero, B., Girón, M.E., Lucena, S., Sánchez, E.E., et al. 2008. Intraspecies differences in hemostatic venom activities of the South American rattlesnakes, *Crotalus durissus cumanensis*, as revealed by a range of protease inhibitors. Blood Coagul. Fibrinolysis 19, 525–530.

Satora, L., 2004. Bites by the grass snake *Natrix natrix*. Vet. Human Toxicol. 46, 334.

Savitzky, A.H., 1980. The role of venom-delivery strategies in snake evolution. Evolution 34, 1194–1204.

Savitzky, A.H., 1981. Hinged teeth in snakes: an adaptation for swallowing hard-bodied prey. Science 212, 346–349.

Savitzky, A.H., 1983. Coadapted character complexes among snakes: fossoriality, piscivory, and durophagy. Am. Zool. 23, 397–409.

Sawai, Y., Sakai, A., Honma, M., 1985. Studies on the pathogenesis of envenomation due to *Rhabdophis tigrinus tigrinus* (Boie) a colubrid. Toxicon 23, 607.

Scartozzoni, R.R., Marques, O.A.V., 2004. Sexual dimorphism, reproductive cycle, and fecundity of the water snake *Ptychophis flavovirgatus* (Serpentes, Colubridae). Phyllomedusa 3, 69–71.

Schätti, B., Monsch, P., 2004. Systematics and phylogenetic relationships of Whip snakes (*Hierophis* Fitzinger) and *Zamenis andreana* Werner 1917 (Reptilia: Squamata: Colubrinae). Rev. Suisse Zool. 111, 239–256.

Schätti, B., Wilson, L.D., 1986. Coluber Linnaeus. Holarctic racers. Catalog. Am. Amphibians Reptiles 399, 1–4.

Schenone, H., Reyes, H., 1965. Animales ponzoñosos de Chile. Boletin Chileno Parasitol. 20, 104–108.

Schlegel, H., 1828. Untersuchung der Speicheldrusen bei den Schlangen mit gefurchten Zahnen, im Vergleich mit denen der Giftlosen und Giftigen. Nova Acta Acad. Caes. Leopoldino-Carolinae Nat. Curiosorum vol. 14

Schmid, E.U., 1966. Snake bite. S. Afr. Med. J. 40, 766–770.

Schmidt, K.P., 1939. Reptiles and amphibians from Southwestern Asia. Publ. Field Mus. Nat. Hist., Zool. Ser. 24, 49–92.

Schmidt, K.P., Inger, R.F., 1966. Living Reptiles of the World. (third edition). Doubleday & Co., New York, New York.

Schneck, J., 1878. Is the bite of the *Heterodon* or spreading adder, venomous? Chicago Med. J. Exam. 37, 585–587.

Schneemann, M., Cathomas, R., Laidlaw, S.T., El Nahas, A.M., Theakston, R.D.G., Warrell, D.A., 2004. Life-threatening envenoming by the Saharan horned viper (*Cerastes cerastes*) causing micro-angiopathic haemolysis, coagulopathy and acute renal failure: clinical cases and review. QJM 97, 717–727.

Schouten, E.S., van de Pol, A.C., Schouten, A.N.J., Turner, N.M., Jansen, N.J.G., Bollen, C.W., 2009. The effect of aprotinin, tranexamic acid, and aminocaproic acid on blood loss and use of blood products in major pediatric surgery: a meta-analysis. Pediatr. Crit. Care Med 10, 182–190.

Schuknecht, H.F., 1969. Cupulolithiasis. Arch. Otolaryngol. 90, 765–778.

Schwartz, A., Henderson, R.W., 1991. The Reptiles and Amphibians of the West Indies: Descriptions, Distributions, and Natural History. University of Florida Press, Gainesville, FL.

Secor, S.M., Lane, J.S., Whang, E.E., Ashley, S.W., Diamond, J., 2002. Luminal nutrient signals for intestinal adaptation in pythons. Am. J. Physiol. Gastrointest. Liver Physiol. 283, G1298–G1309.

Seib, R.L., 1980. Human envenomation from the bite of an aglyphous false coral snake, *Pliocercus elapoides* (Serpentes: Colubridae). Toxicon 18, 399–401.

Senter, P., 1998. A bite from the rear-fanged colubrid, *Psammophis phillipsi*. Herpetol. Rev. 29, 216–217.

Seow, E., Kuperan, P, Goh, S.K., Gopalakrishnakone, P., 2000. Morbidity after a bite from a "non-venomous" pet snake. Singapore Med. J. 41, 34–35.

Shaw, C.E., Campbell, S., 1974. Snakes of the American West. Alfred A. Knopf, New York, NY. 328 pp

Shek, K.C., Tsui, K.L., Lam, K.K., Crow, P., Ng, K.H., Ades, G., et al. 2009. Oral bacterial flora of the Chinese cobra (*Naja atra*) and bamboo pit viper (*Trimeresurus albolabris*) in Hong Kong SAR, China. Hong Kong Med. J. 15, 183–190.

Shine, R., Schwaner, T., 1985. Prey constriction by venomous snakes: a review, and new data on Australian species. Copeia 1985, 1067–1071.

Shine, R., Branch, W.R., Harlow, P.S., Webb, J.K., Shine, T., 2006. Biology of burrowing asps (Atractaspididae) from Southern Africa. Copeia 2006, 103–115.

Shuster, T.A., Silliman, W.R., Coats, R.D., Mureebe, L., Silver, D., 2003. Heparin-induced thrombocytopenia: twenty-nine years later. J. Vasc. Surg. 38, 1316–1322.

Silveira, P.V., Nishioka, S.D.A., 1992. Non-venomous snake bite and snake bite without envenoming in a Brazilian teaching hospital. Analysis of 91 cases. Rev. Inst. Med. Trop. São Paulo 34, 499–503.

Silver-Júnior, M. 1956. O ofidismo no Brasil. Ministério da Saúde, Serviço Nacional de Educação Sanitária, Rio de Janeiro, Brazil.

Simbotwe, M.P., 1982. Epidemiology and clinical study of snakebite in Kasempa District of northwestern Zambia. The Snake 14, 101–104.

Simpson Jr., R.J., Cascio, W.E., Schreiner, P.J., Crow, R.S., Rautaharju, P.M., Heiss, G., 2002. Prevalence of premature ventricular contractions in a population of African American and white men and women: the Atherosclerosis Risk in Communities (ARIC) study. Am. Heart J. 143, 535–540.

Sindern, E., Schröder, J.M., Krismann, M., Malin, J.P., 2001. Inflammatory polyradiculoneuropathy with spinal cord involvement and lethal outcome after hepatitis B vaccination. J. Neurol. Sci. 186, 81–85.

Slaughter, T.F., Greenberg, C.S., 1997. Antifibrinolytic drugs and perioperative hemostasis. Am. J. Hematol. 56, 32–36.

Slotta, K., Fraenkel-Conrat, H., 1938. Two active proteins from rattlesnake venom. Nature 142, 213.

Smeets, R.E., Melman, P.G., Hoffmann, J.J., Mulder, A.W., 1991. Severe coagulopathy after a bite from a "harmless" snake (*Rhabdophis subminiatus*). J. Inter. Med. 230, 351–354.

Smith, M.A., 1935. The Fauna of British India. Reptiles and Amphibians. Taylor & Francis, London, UK.

Smith, M.A., 1938. The nucho-dorsal glands of snakes. Proc. Zool. Soc. (Series B), 575–583.

Smith, M.A., 1943. The Fauna of British India, Ceylon and Burma, Including the Whole of the Indo-Chinese Sub-Region. Reptilia and Amphibia. 3 (Serpentes). Taylor & Francis, London, UK.

Smith, M.A., Bellairs, A., 1947. Head glands of snakes. J. Linn. Soc. Lond. Zool. 41, 353–368.

Smith, H.M., Brodie, E.D., 1982. A Guide to Field Identification of Reptiles of North America. Golden Press, New York, NY.

Soderberg, P.S., 1971. Striking behavior in the common green whip snake (*Ahaetulla nasutus*). J. Bombay Nat. Hist. Soc. 68, 839.

Sopiev, O., Makeev, B.M., Kudryavtsev, S.B., Makarov, A.N., 1987. A case of intoxication by a bite of the gray monitor (*Varanus griseus*). Izv. Akad. Nauk Turkm. SSR. Ser. Biol. Nauk 87, 78.

Spawls, S., 1979. Sun, Sand and Snakes. William Morrow and Company, New York, NY.

Spawls, S., Howell, K., Drewes, R., Ashe, J., 2002. A Field Guide to the Reptiles of East Africa. Kenya, Tanzania, Uganda, Rwanda and Burundi. Natural World Press, San Diego, CA.

Spies, S.K., Malherbe, L.F., Pepier, W.J., 1962. Boomslangbyt met afibrinogemie. S. Afr. Med. J. 36, 834–838.

Sra, J., Zaidi, S.T., Krum, D., Georgakopoulos, N., Ahmad, A., Akhtar, M., 2001. Correlation of spontaneous and induced premature atrial complexes initiating atrial fibrillation in humans: electrophysiologic parameters for guiding therapy. J. Cardiovasc. Electrophysiol. 12, 1347–1352.

Starace, F., 1998. Guide des Serpents et Amphisbènes de Guyane. Ibis Rouge Editions, Guadeloupe, Guyane.

Stebbins, R.C., 1985. A Field Guide to the Western Reptile and Amphibians. Houghton Mifflin Company, Boston, MA.

Stejneger, L., 1893. The poisonous snakes of North America. Ann. Report US Nat. Mus. 1893, 337–487.

Stevens, K., 2000. Brief notes on the captive care of the false water cobra (Cyclagras gigas, Dumeril, Bibron and Dumeril 1854). The Herptile 25, 94–97.

Stewart, M.M., 2000. Historical perspectives: Madge and Sherman Minton. Copeia 2000, 304–309.

Stiles, B.G., Sexton, F.W., Weinstein, S.A., 1991. Antibacterial effects of different snake venoms: purification and characterization of antibacterial proteins from Pseudechis australis (Australian king brown or mulga snake) venom. Toxicon 29, 1129–1141.

Suankratay, C., Wilde, H., Nunthapisud, P., Khantipong, M., 2002. Tetanus after white-lipped green pit viper bite. Wilderness Environ. Med. 13, 256–261.

Subaraj, R., 2008. A personal account of envenomation by a blue-necked keelback, Macropisthodon rhodomelas (Boie) (Reptilia: Squamata: Natricidae). Nature Singapore 1, 109–111.

Sutherland, S.K., Tibballs, J., 2001. Australian Animal Toxins. Oxford University Press, Oxford, UK.

Svensson, P., Rosenberg, J., Ostergren, J., Karlson-Stiber., C., 1993. Do ACE inhibitors potentiate snake venom? Severe and prolonged hypotension caused by adder bite. Lakartidningen 90, 2653–2654.

Sweeney, R.C.H., 1971. Snakes of Nyasaland. Asher & Company, Amsterdam.

Szczerbak, N.N., 2003. Guide to the Reptiles of the Eastern Palearctic. Krieger, Malabar, FL. 260 pp.

Tantanun, S., 1957. The venom of the Malayan pit viper and its complications. J. Med. Assoc. Thai. 40, 175–191.

Taub, A.M., 1966. Ophidian cephalic glands. J. Morphol. 118, 529–542.

Taub, A.M., 1967. Comparative histological studies on Duvernoy's gland of colubrid snakes. Bull. Am. Mus. Nat. Hist. 138, 1–50.

Taylor, E.H., 1922. The Snakes of the Philippine Islands. Department of Agriculture and Natural Resources, Bureau of Science, Manila, Philippines.

Taylor, E.H., Smith, H.M., 1938. Miscellaneous notes on Mexican snakes. Univ. Kansas Sci. Bull. 25, 239–258.

Theakston, R.D.G., Reid, H.A., Romer, J.D., 1979. Biological properties of the red-neck reelback snake (Rhabdophis subminiatus). Toxicon 17 (Suppl. 1), 190.

Theakston, R.D., Phillips, R.E., Looareesuwan, S., Echevarria, P, Makin, T., Warrell, D.A., 1990. Bacteriological studies of the venom and mouth cavities of wild Malayan pit vipers (Calloselasma rhodostoma) in southern Thailand. Trans. R. Soc. Trop. Med. Hyg. 84, 875–879.

Thein-Than, Tin-Tun, Hla-Pe, Philips, R.E., Myint-Lwin, Tin-Nu-Swe, Development of renal function abnormalities following bites by Russell's vipers (Daboia russelli siamensis) in Myanmar. Trans. R. Soc. Trop. Med. Hyg. 85, 404–409.

Thesiger, W., 1964. The Marsh Arabs. Longmans, London, UK. pp. 114–115.

Tkaczyk, C., Okayama, Y., Woolhiser, M.R., Hagaman, D.D., Gilfillan, A.M., Metcalfe, D.D., 2002. Activation of human mast cells through the high affinity IgG receptor. Mol. Immunol. 38, 1289–1293.

Tkaczyk, C., Okayama, Y., Metcalfe, D.D., Gilfillan, A.M., 2004. Fcgamma receptors on mast cells: activatory and inhibitory regulation of mediator release. Int. Arch. Allergy Immunol. 133, 305–315.

Trestrail, J.H., 1982. The "underground zoo"—the problem of exotic venomous snakes in private possession in the United States. Vet. Hum. Toxicol. 24, 144–149.

Toriba, M., Sawai, Y., 1990. Venomous snakes of medical importance in Japan. In: Gopalakrishnakone, P., Chou, L.M. (Eds.), Snakes of Medical Importance (Asia Pacific Region) (pp. 323–347). Venom and Toxin Research Group, National University of Singapore, Singapore.

Thomas, R.G., Pough, F.H., 1979. The effect of rattlesnake venom on digestion of prey. Toxicon 17, 221–228.

Thomas, R., Prieto-Hernandez, J.A., 1985. The use of venom by the Puerto Rican snake, *Alsophis portoricensis*. Decimo Simposio de Recursos Naturales 1985, 13–22.

Tiedemann, F., Grillitsch, H., 1999. Ergänzungen zu den Katalogen der Typusexemplare der Herpetologischen Sammlung des Naturhistorischen Museums in Wien. Herpetolozoa 12, 147–156.

Trapp, B., 2007. Amphibien und Reptilien des Griechischen Festlandes. Ntv Natur Und Tier-Verlag, Berlin, Germany.

Trevor, A.J., Katzung, B.G., Masters, S., 2008. Katzung and Trevor's Pharmacology. Examination and Board Review, eighth ed.. McGraw-Hill/Lange Medical, New York, NY.

Underwood, G., 2002. On the rictal structures of some snakes. Herpetologica 58, 1–17.

Underwood, G., Kochva, E., 1993. On the affinities of the burrowing asps, *Atractaspis* Serpentes: Atractaspidae. Zool. J. Linn. Soc. 107, 3–64.

Utiger, U., Schätti, B., Helfenberger, N., 2005. The oriental colubrine genus *Coelognathus* Fitzinger, 1843 and classification of old and New World racers and ratsnakes (Reptilia, Squamata, Colubridae, Colubrinae). Russ. J. Herpetol. 12, 39–60.

Valenta, J., Stach, Z., Fricova, D., Zak, J., Balik, M., 2008. Envenoming by the viperid snake, *Proatheris superciliaris*: a case report. Toxicon 52, 392–394.

Vallon, V., Osswald, H., 2009. Adenosine receptors and the kidney. Handbook Exp. Pharmacol. 2009, 443–470.

Valls-Moraes, F., De Lema, T., 1997. Envenomation by *Phalotris trilineatus* in Rio Grande Do Sul State, Brazil: a case report. J. Venom. Anim. Toxins 3, 1.

Vaughan, S.T., Lobetti, R.G., 1995. Boomslang envenomation in a dog. S. Afr. Vet. Assoc. 66, 265–267.

Vaz-Ferreira, R., Covelo de Zolessi, L., Archával, F., 1970. Oviposicion y desarrollo de ofidios y lacertilios em hormigueros de Acromyrmex. Physis XXIX 79, 431–459.

Vellard, J., 1955. Propriétés venimeuses de "*Tachimenis peruviana*". Wiegm. Fol. Biol. And. 1, 1–14.

Vest, D.K., 1981a. Envenomation following the bite of the wandering garter snake, *Thamnophis elegans vagrans*. Clin. Toxicol. 18, 573–579.

Vest, D.K., 1981b. The toxic secretion of the wandering garter snake, *Thamnophis elegans vagrans*. Toxicon 19, 831–839.

Vest, D.K., 1988. Some effects and properties of Duvernoy's gland secretion from *Hypsiglena torquata texana* (Texas night snake). Toxicon 26, 417–419.

Vest, D.K., Mackessy, S.P., Kardong, K.V., 1991. The unique Duvernoy's secretion of the brown tree snake (*Boiga irregularis*). Toxicon 29, 532–535.

Vetter, R.S., 2009. Arachnids misidentified as brown recluse spiders by medical personnel and other authorities in North America. Toxicon 54, 545–547.

Vidal, N., Kindl, S.G., Wong, A., Hedges, S.B., 2000. Phylogenetic relationships of xenodontine snakes inferred from 12S and 16S ribosomal RNA sequences. Mol. Phylogenet. Evol. 14, 389–402.

Vidal, N., Delmas, A.-S., David, P., Cruaud Couloux, A., Hedges, S.B., 2007. The phylogeny and classification of caenophidian snakes inferred from seven nuclear protein-coding genes. C. R. Biol. 330, 182–187.

Vidal, N., Branch, W.R., Pauwels, O.S.G., Hedges, S.B., Broadley, D.G., Wink, M., et al. 2008. Dissecting the major African snake radiation: a molecular phylogeny of the Lamprohiidae Fitzinger (Serpentes, Caenophidia). Zootaxa 1945, 51–66.

Vidal, N., Dewynter, M, Gower, D.J., 2010. Dissecting the major snake radiation: a molecular phylogeny of the Dipsadidae Bonaparte (Serpentes, Caenophidia). C. R. Biol. 333, 48–55.

Villa, J., 1969. Notes on *Conophis nevermanni*, an addition to the Nicaraguan herpetofauna. J. Herpetol. 3, 169–171.

Viravan, C., Looareesuwan, S., Kosakarn, W., Wuthiekanun, V., McCarthy, C.J., Stimson, A.F., et al. 1992. A national hospital-based survey of snakes responsible for bites in Thailand. Trans. R. Soc. Trop. Med. Hyg. 86, 100–106.

Visser, J., Chapman, D.S., 1978. Snakes and Snakebite—Venomous Snakes and Management of Snakebite in Southern Africa. Purnell & Sons, Cape Town, South Africa.

Vitt, L.J., 1983. Ecology of an anuran-eating guild of terrestrial tropical snakes. Herpetologica 39, 52–66.

Vitt, L.J., Caldwell, J.P., 2008. Herpetology: An Introductory Biology of Amphibians and Reptiles, third ed.. Academic Press, Burlington, MA.

Vogel, G., David, P., 2006. On the taxonomy of the *Xenochrophis piscator* complex (Serpentes, Natricidae). In: Vences, M., Köhler, J., Ziegler, T., Böhme, W. (Eds.), Herpetologia Bonnensis II. Proceedings of the 13th Congress of the Societas Europaea Herpetologica (pp. 241–246).

Vogel, G., David, P., Lutz, M., Rooijen, J.V., Vidal, N., 2007. Revision of the *Tropidolaemus wagleri*-complex (Serpentes: Viperidae: Crotalinae). I. Definition of included taxa and redescription of *Tropidolaemus wagleri* (Boie, 1827). Zootaxa 1644, 1–40.

Vonk, F.J., Admiraal, J.F., Jackson, K., Reshef, R, de Bakker, M.A., Vanderschoot, K., et al. 2008. Evolutionary origin and development of snake fangs. Nature 454, 630–633.

Wada, H., Asakura, H., Okamoto, K., Iba, T., Uchiyama, T., Kawasugi, K., et al. 2010. Expert consensus for the treatment of disseminated intravascular coagulation in Japan. Thromb. Res. 125, 6–11.

Wadee, A.A., Rabson, A.R., 1987. Development of specific IgE antibodies after repeated exposure to snake venom. J. Allergy Clin. Immunol. 80, 695–698.

Wagner, P., Townsend, E., Barej, M., Rödder, D., Spawls, S., 2009. First record of human envenomation by *Atractaspis congica* Peters, 1877 (Squamata: Atractaspididae). Toxicon 54, 368–372.

Wakamatsu, T., Kawamura, Y., Sawai, Y., 1986. A successful trial of yamakagashi antivenom. The Snake 18, 4–5.

Wald, R., Quinn, R.R., Luo, J., Li, P., Scales, D.C., Mamdani, M.M., et al. 2009. Chronic dialysis and death among among survivors of acute kidney injury requiring dialysis. JAMA 302, 1179–1185.

Wall, F., 1913. The Poisonous Terrestrial Snakes of Our British Indian Dominions (Including Ceylon) and How to Recognize Them with Symptoms of Snake Poisoning and Treatment. Bombay Natural History Society, Bombay, India.

Wall, F., 1921. Ophidia Taprobanica or The Snakes of Ceylon. Cottle Government Printer, Colombo, Ceylon.

Walley, H.D., 2002. An incident of envenomation from *Heterodon nasicus*. Bull. Chicago Herp. Soc. 37, 31.

Walls, J., 1991. Caution: look alikes. The *Rhabdophis–Amphiesma* problem. Trop. Fish Hobbyist 39, 138–141.

Wan, L., Bellomo, R., Di Giantomasso, D., Ronco, C., 2003. The pathogenesis of septic acute renal failure. Curr. Opin. Crit. Care 9, 496–502.

Wang, R., Cai, J., Huang, Y., Xu, D., Sang, H., Yan, G., 2009. Novel recombinant fibrinogenase of *Agkistrodon acutus* venom protects against LPS-induced DIC. Thromb. Res. 123, 919–924.

Wapnick, S., Levin, L., Broadley, D.G., 1972. A study of snake bites admitted to a hospital in Rhodesia. Cent. Afr. J. Med. 18, 137–141.

Warkentin, T.E., 1999. Heparin-induced thrombocytopenia: a ten-year retrospective. Ann. Rev. Med. 50, 129–147.

Warrell, D.A., 1979. Clinical snake bite problems in the Nigerian savanna region. Technische Hochschule Darmstadt. Schriftenreihe Wissenschaft u-Technik 14, 31–60.

Warrell, D.A., 1988. Injuries, envenoming, poisoning and allergic reactions caused by animals (second ed.) In: Weatherall, D.J., Ledingham, J.G.G., Warrell, D.A. (Eds.), Oxford Textbook of Medicine, vol. 1. Oxford University Press, Oxford, UK pp. 6.66–6.85.

Warrell, D.A., 1995. Clinical toxicology of snakebite in Asia. In: Meier, J., White, J. (Eds.), CRC Handbook of Clinical Toxicology of Animal Venoms and Poisons (pp. 493–594). CRC Press, Boca Raton, FL.

Warrell, D.A., 1995. Clinical toxicology of snakebite in Africa and the Middle East/Arabian Peninsula. In: Meier, J., White, J. (Eds.), CRC Handbook of Clinical Toxicology of Animal Venoms and Poisons (pp. 433–492). CRC Press, Boca Raton, FL.

Warrell, D.A., 2004. Snakebites in Central and South America: epidemiology, clinical features, and clinical management. In: Campbell, J.A., Lamar, W.W. (Eds.), The Venomous Reptiles of the Western Hemisphere, vol. II. Cornell University Press, Ithaca, NY.

Warrell, D.A., 2005. Snake bites in Europe, Africa, Asia and Oceania. In: White, J. (Ed.), Clinical Toxinology Short Course Handbook (pp. 259–285). University of Adelaide, Faculty of Health Sciences, Adelaide, South Australia.

Warrell, D.A., 2009. Management of exotic snakebites. QJM 102, 593–601.

Warrell, D.A., Ormerod, L.D., Davidson, N.M., 1976. Bites by the night adder (*Causus maculatus*) and burrowing vipers (genus *Atractaspis*) in Nigeria. Am. J. Trop. Med. Hyg. 25, 517–524.

Warrell, D.A., Pope, H.M., Prentice, C.R.M., 1976. Disseminated intravascular coagulation caused by the carpet viper (*Echis carinatus*): trial of heparin. Br. J. Haematol. 33, 335–342.

Weed, H.G., 1993. Nonvenomous snakebite in Massachusetts: prophylactic antibiotics are unnecessary. Ann. Emerg. Med. 22, 220–224.

Weinstein, S.A., 2003. In Memoriam: Professor Sherman Anthony Minton (24/2/19–15/2/99). Toxicon 41, 733–735.

Weinstein, S.A., Kardong, K.V., 1994. Properties of Duvernoy's secretions from opisthoglyphous and aglyphous colubrid snakes. Toxicon 32, 1161–1185.

Weinstein, S.A., Keyler, D.E., 2009. Local envenoming by the Western hognose snake, *Heterodon nasicus*: a case report and review of medically significant *Heterodon* bites. Toxicon 54, 354–360.

Weinstein, S.A., Smith, L.A., 1990. Preliminary fractionation of tiger rattlesnake (*Crotalus tigris*) venom. Toxicon 28, 1447–1455.

Weinstein, S.A., Smith, L.A., 1993. Chromatographic profiles and properties of Duvernoy's secretions from some boigine and dispholidine colubrids. Herpetologica 49, 78–94.

Weinstein, S.A., Minton, S.A., Wilde, C.E., 1985. Distribution among ophidian venoms of a toxin isolated from venom of the Mojave rattlesnake, Crotalus scutulatus scutulatus. Toxicon 23, 825–844.

Weinstein, S.A., Schmidt, J.J., Bernheimer, A.W., Smith, L.A., 1991. Characterization and amino acid sequences of two lethal peptides from venom of Wagler's pit viper, Trimeresurus wagleri. Toxicon 29, 227–236.

Weinstein, S.A., DeWitt, C.F., Smith, L.A., 1992. Variation in venom-neutralization capacities of serum from snakes of the colubrid genus Lampropeltis. J. Herpetol. 26, 452–461.

Weinstein, S.A., Stiles, B.G., McCoid, M.J., Smith, L.A., Kardong, K.V., 1993. Variation and lethal potencies and acetylcholine receptor binding activity of Duvernoy's secretions from the brown tree snake, Boiga irregularis. J. Nat. Toxins 2, 187–198.

Weinstein, S.A., Dart, R.C., Staples, A., White, J., 2009. Envenomations: an overview of clinical toxinology for the primary care physician. Am. Fam. Physician 80, 793–802.

Weinstein, S.A., Smith, T., Kardong, K.V., 2010. Reptile venom glands: form, function and future. In: Mackessy, S.P. (Ed.), CRC Handbook of Reptile Venoms and Toxins (pp. 63–90). Taylor & Francis, Boca Raton, FL.

Weldon, C.L., Mackessy, S.P., 2010. Biological and proteomic analysis of venom from the Puerto Rican racer (Alsophis portoricensis: Dipsadidae). Toxicon 55, 558–569.

Wellington, K., Wagstaff, A.J., 2003. Transexamic acid: a review of its use in the management of menorrhagia. Drugs 63, 1417–1433.

Whitaker, R., 1968. The dog-faced watersnake (Cerberus rhynchops) in the Bombay area and notes on its habits. J. Bombay Nat. Hist. Soc. 66, 386.

Whitaker, R., 1970. Slight reaction from bites of the rear-fanged snakes, Boiga ceylonensis (Gunther) and Dryophis nasutus (Lacepede). J. Bombay Nat. Hist. Soc. 67, 113.

White, J., 1995. Poisonous and venomous animals—the physician's view. In: Meier, J., White, J. (Eds.), CRC Handbook of Clinical Toxicology of Animal Venoms and Poisons. CRC Press, Boca Raton, FL

White, J., 2005. Snake venoms and coagulopathy. Toxicon 45, 951–967.

White, J. 2009. The World Health Organization global antivenom initiative. Venom Week 2009, Alburquerque, New Mexico.

White, J., Dart, R.C., 2008. Snakebite: A Brief Medical Guide. Julian White, Stirling, South Australia.

Williams, F.E., Freedman, M., Kenedy, E., 1954. The bacterial flora of the mouths of Australian venomous snakes in captivity. Med. J. Aust. 2, 190–193.

Williams, D., Gutiérrez, J.M., Harrison, R., Warrell, D.A., White, J., Winkel, K.D., et al. 2010. The Global Snakebite Initiative: an antidote for snake bite. Lancet 375, 89–91.

Wilson, L.D., McCranie, J.R., 2002. Update on the list of reptiles known from Honduras. Herpetol. Rev. 33, 90–94.

Wiwanitkit, V., 2005. Management of acute renal failure due to Russell's viper envenomation: an analysis on the reported Thai cases. Ren. Fail. 27, 801.

Wüster, W., Golay, P., Warrell, D.A., 1998. Synopsis of recent developments in venomous snake systematics. Toxicon 36, 299–307.

Yang, J.Y., Hui, H., Lee, A.C., 2007. Severe coagulopathy associated with white-lipped green pit viper bite. Hong Kong Med. J. 13, 392–395.

Yoshie, S., Ishiyama, M., Ogawa, T., 1982. Fine structure of Duvernoy's gland of the Japanese colubrid snake, Rhabdophis tigrinus. Arch. Histol. Jpn. 45, 375–384.

Yoshie, S., Ogawa, T., Fujita, T., 1988. Histochemical, immunochemical, and ultrastructural characteristics of nerves in the Duvernoy's gland of the Japanese colubrid snake, *Rhabdophis tigrinus*. Arch. Histol. Cytol. 51, 459–466.

Young, R.A., 1992. Effects of Duvernoy's secretions from the eastern hognose snake, *Heterodon platyrhinos*, on smooth muscle and neuromuscular junction. Toxicon 30, 775–779.

Young, B.A., Kardong, K.V., 1996. Dentitional surface features in snakes (Reptilia: Serpentes). Amphibia-Reptilia 17, 261–276.

Zaher, H., 1996. A new genus and species of pseudoboine snake, with a revision of the genus *Clelia* (Serpentes, Xenodontinae). Bull. Mus. Reg. Sci. Nat. Torino 14, 289–337.

Zaher, H., 1999. Hemipenal morphology of the South American xenodontine snakes, with a proposal for a monophyletic Xenodontinae and a reappraisal of colubroid hemipenes. Bull. Am. Mus. Nat. Hist. 240, 1–168.

Zaher, H., Grazziotin, F.G., Cadle, J.E., Murphy, R.W., de Moura-Leite, J.C., Bonatto, S.L., 2009. Molecular phylogeny of advanced snakes (Serpentes, Caenophidia) with an emphasis on South American xenodontines: a revised clasification and descriptions of new taxa. Papéis Avulsos Zool. 49, 115–153.

Zahradnicek, O., Horacek, I., Tucker, A.S., 2008. Viperous fangs: development and evolution of the venom canal. Mech. Develop. 125, 786–796.

Zalisko, E.J., Kardong, K.V., 1992. Histology and histochemistry of the Duvernoy's gland of the brown tree snake, *Boiga irregularis*. Copeia 1992, 791–799.

Zannolli, R., Zazzi, M., Muraca, M.C., Macucci, F., Buoni, S., Nuti, D., 2006. A child with vestibular neuritis. Is adenovirus implicated? Brain Dev. 28, 410–412.

Zotz, R.B., Mebs, D., Hirche, H., Paar, D., 1991. Hemostatic changes due to venom gland extract of the red-necked keel back snake (*Rhabdophis subminiatus*). Toxicon 29, 1501–1508.

Zweifel, R., Norris, K.S., 1955. Contribution to the herpetology of Sonora, Mexico. Am. Midl. Natural. 54 (1), 230–249.

Zwinenberg, A., 1977. *Leptophis ahaetulla*. Aqua. Terr. Z. 30, 64–65.

News Periodicals Cited

Big snake alert defanged. New York Times, October 17, 1990.

Los Angeles bans pet snake after owner is hospitalized. New York Times, September 13, 1981.

Boy killed in dragon attack. The Guardian, June 4, 2007.

Daily Express (Liverpool Edition) July 21, 1967.

Printed in the United States
By Bookmasters